1998
YEAR BOOK OF
DRUG THERAPY®

Statement of Purpose

The YEAR BOOK Service

The YEAR BOOK series was devised in 1901 by practicing health professionals who observed that the literature of medicine and related disciplines had become so voluminous that no one individual could read and place in perspective every potential advance in a major specialty. In the final decade of the 20th century, this recognition is more acutely true than it was in 1901.

More than merely a series of books, YEAR BOOK volumes are the tangible results of a unique service designed to accomplish the following:

- to *survey* a wide range of journals of proven value
- to *select* from those journals papers representing significant advances and statements of important clinical principles
- to provide *abstracts* of those articles that are readable, convenient summaries of their key points
- to provide *commentary* about those articles to place them in perspective

These publications grow out of a unique process that calls on the talents of outstanding authorities in clinical and fundamental disciplines, trained literature specialists, and professional writers, all supported by the resources of Mosby, the world's preeminent publisher for the health professions.

The Literature Base

Mosby and its editors survey more than 1,000 journals published worldwide, covering the full range of the health professions. On an annual basis, the publisher examines usage patterns and polls its expert authorities to add new journals to the literature base and to delete journals that are no longer useful as potential YEAR BOOK sources.

The Literature Survey

The publisher's team of literature specialists, all of whom are trained and experienced health professionals, examines every original, peer-reviewed article in each journal issue. More than 250,000 articles per year are scanned systematically, including title, text, illustrations, tables, and references. Each scan is compared, article by article, to the search strategies that the publisher has developed in consultation with the 270 outside experts who form the pool of YEAR BOOK editors. A given article may be reviewed by any number of editors, from one to a dozen or more, regardless of the discipline for which the paper was originally published. In turn, each editor who receives the article reviews it to determine whether the article should be included in the YEAR BOOK. This decision is based on the article's inherent quality, its probable usefulness to readers of that YEAR BOOK, and the editor's goal to represent a balanced picture of a given field in each volume of the YEAR BOOK. In addition, the editor indicates when to include figures and tables from the article to help the YEAR BOOK reader better understand the information.

Of the quarter million articles scanned each year, only 5% are selected for detailed analysis within the YEAR BOOK series, thereby assuring readers of the high value of every selection.

The Abstract

The publisher's abstracting staff is headed by a seasoned medical professional and includes individuals with training in the life sciences, medicine, and other areas, plus extensive experience in writing for the health professions and related industries. Each selected article is assigned to a specific writer on this abstracting staff. The abstracter, guided in many cases by notations supplied by the expert editor, writes a structured, condensed summary designed so that the reader can rapidly acquire the essential information contained in the article.

The Commentary

The YEAR BOOK editorial boards, sometimes assisted by guest commentators, write comments that place each article in perspective for the reader. This provides the reader with the equivalent of a personal consultation with a leading international authority—an opportunity to better understand the value of the article and to benefit from the authority's thought processes in assessing the article.

Additional Editorial Features

The editorial boards of each YEAR BOOK organize the abstracts and comments to provide a logical and satisfying sequence of information. To enhance the organization, editors also provide introductions to sections or individual chapters, comments linking a number of abstracts, citations to additional literature, and other features.

The published YEAR BOOK contains enhanced bibliographic citations for each selected article, including extended listings of multiple authors and identification of author affiliations. Each YEAR BOOK contains a Table of Contents specific to that year's volume. From year to year, the Table of Contents for a given YEAR BOOK will vary depending on developments within the field.

Every YEAR BOOK contains a list of the journals from which papers have been selected. This list represents a subset of the more than 1,000 journals surveyed by the publisher and occasionally reflects a particularly pertinent article from a journal that is not surveyed on a routine basis.

Finally, each volume contains a comprehensive subject index and an index to authors of each selected paper.

The 1998 Year Book Series

Year Book of Allergy, Asthma, and Clinical Immunology: Drs. Rosenwasser, Boguniewicz, Borish, Nelson, Routes, and Spahn

Year Book of Anesthesiology and Pain Management®: Drs. Tinker, Abram, Chestnut, Roizen, Rothenberg, and Wood

Year Book of Cardiology®: Drs. Schlant, Collins, Gersh, Graham, Kaplan, and Waldo

Year Book of Chiropractic®: Dr. Lawrence

Year Book of Critical Care Medicine®: Drs. Parrillo, Balk, Calvin, Franklin, and Shapiro

Year Book of Dentistry®: Drs. Meskin, Berry, Jeffcoat, Leinfelder, Roser, Summitt, and Zakariasen

Year Book of Dermatologic Surgery®: Drs. Greenway, Papadopoulos, Whitaker, and Barrett

Year Book of Dermatology®: Dr. Thiers

Year Book of Diagnostic Radiology®: Drs. Osborn, Groskin, Dalinka, Maynard, Pentecost, Rebner, Ros, Smirniotopoulos, and Young

Year Book of Drug Therapy®: Drs. Lasagna and Weintraub

Year Book of Emergency Medicine®: Drs. Wagner, Dronen, Davidson, King, Niemann, and Roberts

Year Book of Endocrinology®: Drs. Bagdade, Braverman, Horton, Kannan, Landsberg, Molitch, Morley, Nathan, Odell, Poehlman, Rogol, and Ryan

Year Book of Family Practice®: Drs. Berg, Bowman, Davidson, Dexter, and Scherger

Year Book of Gastroenterology®: Drs. Aliperti and Fleshman

Year Book of Geriatrics and Gerontology®: Drs. Beck, Burton, Ostwald, Rabins, Reuben, Roth, Shapiro, and Whitehouse

Year Book of Hand Surgery®: Drs. Amadio and Hentz

Year Book of Hematology®: Drs. Spivak, Bell, Ness, Quesenberry, Wiernik, and Horowitz

Year Book of Infectious Diseases: Drs. Keusch, Barza, Bennish, Poutsiaka, Skolnik, and Snydman

Year Book of Medicine®: Drs. Klahr, Cline, McCallum, Frishman, Utiger, Malawista, Mandell, and Jett

Year Book of Neonatal and Perinatal Medicine®: Drs. Fanaroff, Maisels, and Stevenson

Year Book of Nephrology, Hypertension, and Mineral Metabolism: Drs. Schwab, Bennett, Emmett, Hostetter, Kumar, and Toto

Year Book of Neurology and Neurosurgery®: Drs. Bradley and Gibbs

Year Book of Nuclear Medicine®: Drs. Gottschalk, Blaufox, Neumann, Strauss, and Zubal

Year Book of Obstetrics, Gynecology, and Women's Health: Drs. Mishell, Herbst, and Kirschbaum

Year Book of Occupational and Environmental Medicine®: Drs. Emmett, Frank, Gochfeld, and Hessl

Year Book of Oncology®: Drs. Ozols, Eisenberg, Glatstein, Loehrer, Tallman, and Wiersma

Year Book of Ophthalmology®: Drs. Wilson, Augsburger, Cohen, Eagle, Grossman, Laibson, Maguire, Nelson, Penne, Rapuano, Sergott, Spaeth, Tipperman, Ms. Gosfield, and Ms. Salmon

Year Book of Orthopedics®: Drs. Morrey, Beauchamp, Currier, Tolo, Trigg, and Swiontkowski

Year Book of Otolaryngology–Head and Neck Surgery®: Drs. Paparella and Holt

Year Book of Pathology and Laboratory Medicine®: Drs. Raab, Cohen, Olson, Sirgi, and Stanley

Year Book of Pediatrics®: Dr. Stockman

Year Book of Plastic, Reconstructive, and Aesthetic Surgery®: Drs. Miller, Bartlett, Garner, McKinney, Ruberg, Salisbury, and Smith

Year Book of Psychiatry and Applied Mental Health®: Drs. Talbott, Ballanger, Frances, Lydiard, Meltzer, Schowalter, and Tasman

Year Book of Pulmonary Disease®: Drs. Jett, Maurer, Ryu, Strollo, and Wenzel

Year Book of Rheumatology®: Drs. Panush, Hadler, LeRoy, Liang, Reichlin, Simon, and Weinblatt

Year Book of Sports Medicine®: Drs. Shephard, Drinkwater, Eichner, Torg, Alexander, and Mr. George

Year Book of Surgery®: Drs. Copeland, Bland, Deitch, Eberlein, Howard, Luce, Seeger, Souba, and Sugarbaker

Year Book of Thoracic and Cardiovascular Surgery®: Drs. Ginsberg, Wechsler, and Williams

Year Book of Urology®: Drs. Andriole and Coplen

Year Book of Vascular Surgery®: Dr. Porter

1998

The Year Book of DRUG THERAPY®

Editors

Louis Lasagna, M.D.

Dean of the Sackler School of Graduate Biomedical Sciences, and Academic Dean, School of Medicine, Tufts University, Boston

Michael Weintraub, M.D.

Director, Office of Drug Evaluation, Food and Drug Administration*

* The opinions and assertions contained herein are the private views of the author and are not to be construed as official or as reflecting the views of the Food and Drug Administration or the Federal Government of the United States.

Mosby

St. Louis Baltimore Boston Carlsbad Naples New York Philadelphia Portland London
Madrid Mexico City Singapore Sydney Tokyo Toronto Wiesbaden

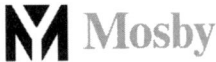

Mosby

Dedicated to Publishing Excellence

A Times Mirror
Company

Publisher: Cheryl A. Smart
Acquisitions Editor: Susan Patterson
Developmental Editor: Kris Horeis, R.N.
Manuscript Editor: Pat Costigan
Project Supervisor, Production: Joy Moore
Production Assistant: Karie House
Manager, Literature Services: Idelle L. Winer
Illustrations and Permissions Coordinator: Phyllis K. Thompson

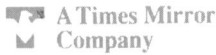

1998 EDITION
Copyright © May 1998 by Mosby, Inc.

Printed in the United States of America
Composition by Reed Technology and Information Services, Inc.
Printing/binding by Maple-Vail

Editorial Office:
Mosby, Inc.
11830 Westline Industrial Drive
St. Louis, MO 63146
Customer Service: customer.support@mosby.com
              www.mosby.com/Mosby/CustomerSupport/index.html

International Standard Serial Number: 0084–3733
International Standard Book Number: 0–8151–5296–5

Table of Contents

Journals Represented

Mosby and its editors survey more than 1,000 journals for its abstract and commentary publications. From these journals, the editors select the articles to be abstracted. Journals represented in this YEAR BOOK are listed below.

Academic Emergency Medicine
Acta Anaesthesiologica Scandinavica
Acta Dermato-Venereologica
Acta Psychiatrica Scandinavica
Age and Ageing
Allergy
American Family Physician
American Journal of Cardiology
American Journal of Epidemiology
American Journal of Gastroenterology
American Journal of Hypertension
American Journal of Medicine
American Journal of Physical Medicine & Rehabilitation
American Journal of Physiology
American Journal of Psychiatry
American Journal of Respiratory and Critical Care Medicine
American Journal of Sports Medicine
American Surgeon
Anaesthesia
Anesthesia and Analgesia
Anesthesiology
Annals of Allergy, Asthma, & Immunology
Annals of Emergency Medicine
Annals of Epidemiology
Annals of Internal Medicine
Annals of Neurology
Annals of Oncology
Annals of Rheumatic Diseases
Annals of the Royal College of Surgeons of England
Archives of Dermatology
Archives of Disease in Childhood
Archives of General Psychiatry
Archives of Ophthalmology
Archives of Pediatrics and Adolescent Medicine
Archives of Physical Medicine and Rehabilitation
Archives of Surgery
Arthritis and Rheumatism
Australian and New Zealand Journal of Obstetrics and Gynaecology
Biological Psychiatry
Blood
British Journal of Anaesthesia
British Journal of Obstetrics and Gynaecology
British Journal of Sports Medicine
British Journal of Urology
British Medical Journal
Canadian Family Physician

Canadian Journal of Anaesthesia
Canadian Journal of Surgery
Canadian Medical Association Journal
Cancer
Cephalalgia
Chest
Circulation
Clinical Cancer Research
Clinical Endocrinology (Oxford)
Clinical Infectious Diseases
Clinical Nephrology
Clinical Pharmacology and Therapeutics
Contraception
Critical Care Medicine
Dermatologic Surgery
Dermatology
Diabetes Care
Diabetic Medicine
Digestive Diseases and Sciences
Epilepsia
European Heart Journal
European Journal of Cancer
European Journal of Dermatology
European Journal of Obstetrics, Gynecology and Reproductive Biology
European Journal of Surgery
European Journal of Vascular and Endovascular Surgery
European Respiratory Journal
Family Practice
Gastroenterology
Gut
Gynecologic Oncology
Headache
Hepatology
Hypertension
Infection Control and Hospital Epidemiology
International Journal of Cancer
International Journal of Dermatology
International Journal of Geriatric Psychiatry
Israel Journal of Medical Sciences
Journal of Acquired Immune Deficiency Syndromes and Human Retrovirology
Journal of Affective Disorders
Journal of Allergy and Clinical Immunology
Journal of Bone and Joint Surgery (American Volume)
Journal of Bone and Joint Surgery (British Volume)
Journal of Clinical Endocrinology and Metabolism
Journal of Clinical Epidemiology
Journal of Clinical Investigation
Journal of Clinical Microbiology
Journal of Clinical Oncology
Journal of Clinical Periodontology
Journal of Clinical Pharmacology
Journal of Clinical Psychiatry

Journal of Clinical Psychopharmacology
Journal of Emergency Medicine
Journal of Family Practice
Journal of General Internal Medicine
Journal of Infectious Diseases
Journal of Internal Medicine
Journal of Neurology
Journal of Neurology, Neurosurgery and Psychiatry
Journal of Pain and Symptom Management
Journal of Pediatric Surgery
Journal of Pediatrics
Journal of Rheumatology
Journal of Sports Sciences
Journal of Thoracic and Cardiovascular Surgery
Journal of Urology
Journal of the American Academy of Dermatology
Journal of the American Board of Family Practice
Journal of the American College of Surgeons
Journal of the American Geriatrics Society
Journal of the American Medical Association
Journal of the Neurological Sciences
Kidney International
Lancet
Laryngoscope
Mayo Clinic Proceedings
Mechanisms of Ageing and Development
Medical Care
Medical Journal of Australia
Medicine
Nephrology, Dialysis, Transplantation
New England Journal of Medicine
New Zealand Medical Journal
ORL (Journal for Oto-Rhino-Laryngology)
Obstetrics and Gynecology
Occupational and Environmental Medicine
Ophthalmology
Orthopedics
Otolaryngology—Head and Neck Surgery
Pain
Pediatric Pathology & Laboratory Medicine
Pediatrics
Pharmacotherapy
Postgraduate Medical Journal
Postgraduate Medicine
Prostate
Psychiatric Services
Psychological Medicine
Respiratory Medicine
Scandinavian Journal of Urology and Nephrology
Schizophrenia Bulletin
Southern Medical Journal
Stroke
Transplantation

Transplantation Proceedings
Urology

STANDARD ABBREVIATIONS

The following terms are abbreviated in this edition: acquired immunodeficiency syndrome (AIDS), cardiopulmonary resuscitation (CPR), central nervous system (CNS), cerebrospinal fluid (CSF), computed tomography (CT), deoxyribonucleic acid (DNA), electrocardiography (ECG), health maintenance organization (HMO), human immunodeficiency virus (HIV), intensive care unit (ICU), intramuscular (IM), intravenous (IV), magnetic resonance (MR) imaging (MRI), and ribonucleic acid (RNA).

NOTE

The YEAR BOOK OF DRUG THERAPY® is a literature survey service providing abstracts of articles published in the professional literature. Every effort is made to assure the accuracy of the information presented in these pages. Neither the editors nor the publisher of the YEAR BOOK OF DRUG THERAPY® can be responsible for errors in the original materials. The editors' comments are their own opinions. Mention of specific products within this publication does not constitute endorsement.

To facilitate the use of the YEAR BOOK OF DRUG THERAPY® as a reference tool, all illustrations and tables included in this publication are now identified as they appear in the original article. This change is meant to help the reader recognize that any illustration or table appearing in the YEAR BOOK OF DRUG THERAPY® may be only one of many in the original article. For this reason, figure and table numbers will often appear to be out of sequence within the YEAR BOOK OF DRUG THERAPY®.

Correction Notice for the **1997 YEAR BOOK OF DRUG THERAPY:**

On page 120, line 3 of the comment, the sentence should read "First, the conversion factor for cholesterol from mg/100 mL to mmol/L is approximately 0.026."

On page 241, the first sentence of the comment should read "This meta-analysis looked at randomized, controlled trials using chemotherapy for non-small cell carcinoma."

On page 351, the first sentence should read "Although exanthemata after systemic corticosteriods are rare, positive patch tests have been reported in 0.2% to 5% of patients, and allergic contact dermatitis occurs after topical use."

We apologize for any inconvenience this may have caused.

Introduction

Periodically, I read something that reminds me that medicine is not practiced the same way in the various countries that exist on this planet of ours.

The New England Journal of Medicine, e.g., published an article last year comparing the use of cardiac procedures in the United States and Canada.[1] The study reported that the rate of revascularization in the United States was five times that in Canada, without convincing evidence that additional benefit accrues to U.S. patients. Several readers took issue with the conclusions.

Then I read a book by Lynn Payer entitled *Medicine & Culture. Varieties of Treatment in the United States, England, West Germany, and France* (Henry Holt and Co., New York, 1996). While these four countries have similar life expectancy rates, medical treatment was shown to differ enormously from country to country. American doctors, e.g., perform more cardiac bypass operations per capita than do English doctors, and many more abortions than their French colleagues.

Then I remembered a 1993 article by the Garattinis[2] and reread it. Let me quote: "When we compared the first 50 pharmaceutical products most sold by value in 1992 in (Italy, France, Germany, and the United Kingdom), we found, to our surprise, that only seven were common to all four lists, although not in the same order...Italy is the only country where a benzodiazepine appears; fluoxetine...appears only in the U.K., and cimetidine...is present only in the U.K. whereas in the other three countries ranitidine is the preferred drug (for peptic ulcer)."

Why these striking differences? The influence of authoritative leaders in the profession? Effective advertising? Cultural pressures in the population or in the medical community? Pricing of medicines? The choice of national health schemes?

Why aren't these differences subject to more academic research? Do these differences translate into health benefit implications for the sick? Is the lack of international harmonization a good thing or a bad thing?

Louis Lasagna, M.D.

References

1. Tu JV, Pashos CL, Naylor CD, et al: Use of cardiac procedures and outcomes in elderly patients with myocardial infarction in the United States and Canada. *N Engl J Med* 336:1500–1505, 1997.
2. Garattini S, Garattini L: Pharmaceutical prescriptions in four European countries. *Lancet* 342:1191–1192, 1993.

1 General Information

Direct-to-Consumer Prescription Drug Advertising
Bradley LR, Zito JM (Univ of Maryland, Baltimore, Md)
Med Care 35:86–92, 1997   1–1

Background.—At its annual meeting in November 1995, the American Public Health Association adopted a resolution on direct-to-consumer advertising of prescription drugs (Rx ads). A brief review of the subject, the rationale for the resolution, and specific follow-up actions for consumers and public health professionals were presented; the entire resolution appears as an appendix to the article.

Description of Rx Ads.—Direct-to-consumer advertising is aimed at the general public and appears in the mass media. Three forms of Rx ads have been identified: (1) health-seeking ads contain information about a disease or condition and advise the consumer to consult a health care provider (no specific drugs or treatments are mentioned); (2) reminder ads contain the name of the drug and limited information; (3) product-specific ads, now the most common, mention the name and use of a specific drug and include safety and efficacy claims.

Regulations.—Except for reminder ads, all ads for prescription drugs must present a brief summary of side effects, warnings, precautions, and contraindications. There must be a fair balance between claims of benefits and disclosure of risk. The first Rx ads aimed at consumers appeared in 1980 and were followed by a 2-year moratorium (1983–1985). Despite a view that Rx ads were not in the public interest, some argued that they served an important educational need. Patients might be more aware of potentially better medications; on the other hand, physicians could be pressured to prescribe newer drugs that might prove risky. In support of Rx ads, some argue that prescription drug prices will drop; others predict that ads will increase the consumer's costs.

Discussion.—It is uncertain whether Rx ads can serve 2 masters: the promotional interest of the manufacturer and the individual's health needs. Advertising seeks to increase consumption rather than to optimize health care. More importantly, there is a danger that conflicts in patient-physician relations may develop. The Food and Drug Administration (FDA) should review prescription advertising and revise regulations; health care professionals should inform the FDA of misleading Rx ads and strengthen their own responsibilities in the selection and monitoring of drug therapy; and consumers should recognize the purpose of Rx ads and seek unbiased drug information sources.

▶ Direct-to-consumer advertising of prescription drugs can take several different forms and, when well done, has the capacity to improve medical care. Improper, misleading, unfair ads are clearly not in the public interest, and the Food and Drug Administration and Federal Trade Commission should lower the boom on those guilty of such practices. Government should not, however, oppose proper direct-to-consumer advertising. (Remember the First Amendment to the Constitution?)

L. Lasagna, M.D.

Over-the-Counter Medication Use in an Older Rural Community: The MoVIES Project
Stoehr GP, Ganguli M, Seaberg EC, et al (Univ of Pittsburgh, Pa)
J Am Geriatr Soc 45:158–165, 1997   1–2

Introduction.—Older people are estimated to use 33% of all prescription drugs in the United States, but the extent of this population's use of over-the-counter (OTC) medications is more difficult to determine. A cross-sectional study of 1,059 older individuals living in a rural community examined the self-reported use of OTC agents and factors associated with their use.

Methods.—Study subjects were drawn from the Monongahela Valley Independent Elders Survey (MoVIES) project, a cohort assembled as part of a population-based dementia registry. The men and women interviewed for prescription and OTC use had a median age of 73; 96.9% were white. They were also asked about recent use of health services and demographic information.

Results.—Four categories of OTC drug use were identified: 0 (13.0%), 1 (32.0%), 2–4 (49.3%), and 5 or more (5.7%). Women were more likely than men to use any OTC drug and reported taking significantly more OTC drugs than men. Age was not associated with extent of OTC drug use, but those with less education used fewer OTC drugs than high school graduates. The most common OTC categories were analgesics, reported by 66.3% of the sample, vitamin and mineral supplements (38.1%), and antacids (27.9%). In all 3 categories, women reported significantly more usage than men. There were no statistically significant associations between OTC use and measures of health service usage, prescription drug insurance, or prescription drug use. Analgesic use decreased significantly and laxative use increased significantly with increasing age.

Conclusion.—Many older community-dwelling individuals use a variety of OTC drugs, especially analgesics and vitamin/mineral supplements. Usage was more common among women and those with a higher level of education. Overall use of OTCs was not related to age and was not associated with health services usage.

▶ The investigators in this study have a really important cohort available to them. This is a group of people that they have been surveying since 1989. The authors have compiled baseline characteristics and drug use information on this group ever since that moment. One thing that has happened, which I'm sure they didn't expect, was the change in the OTC market. More analgesic drugs are available. The availability of H2 blockers may cut into the use of antacids. Thus, the next time they survey these patients, they will find out whether these newer drugs have replaced some of the old ones. Of course, the newer drugs may not totally supplant the older ones, such as happened with ibuprofen, which has been available since 1984 in the OTC market. It seemed not to make great inroads in this rural population. However, anyone who watches TV can tell you that something has happened to OTC drugs in the modern marketplace.

M. Weintraub, M.D.

Pressures on the General Practitioner and Decisions to Prescribe
Weiss MC, Fitzpatrick R, Scott DK, et al (Manchester Research Unit, England; Univ of Oxford, England; John Radcliffe Hosp, Oxford, England)
Fam Pract 13:432–438, 1996   1–3

Purpose.—Several different factors may affect physicians' prescribing rates, including social factors, cost issues, the physician-patient relationship, and patient expectations. Little research has examined the nature and extent of the pressures on general practitioners, particularly given recent changes in the British health care system. The extent of these pressures on general practitioners was evaluated, including their effects on the doctors' prescribing habits.

Methods.—Three hundred eighty-six British general practitioners received a questionnaire covering 4 broad areas associated with prescribing: sense of burden in providing health care, financial constraints and incentives, use of prescriptions to deal with the clinical workload, and perceptions of demanding patients. These concerns were also linked to actual measures of prescribing habits.

Results.—The response rate was 59%. The physicians were very concerned about the pressures they face, but the only issue related to prescribing was concern over the adverse effects of financial pressures on medical decisions. Physicians concerned about financial pressures prescribed more generic drugs, had higher than average practice costs, and had higher overall prescribing rates. Many general practitioners acknowledged prescribing medications to cope with their workload and reported a perceived increase in demanding patients.

Conclusions.—General practitioners' perceptions of financial constraints and incentives appear to affect their prescribing practices, but other areas of concern do not. As the health care environment continues to change, it will be necessary to monitor the effect of the changes on physicians' prescribing behavior.

▶ For some time, Great Britain has experienced low morale and high stress among general practitioners, related in good measure to cost containment pressures. The United States will see the same problems as a consequence of managed care and capitation.

L. Lasagna, M.D.

Prevalence of Potentially Inappropriate Long Term Prescribing in General Practice in the United Kingdom, 1980–95: Systematic Literature Review
Buetow SA, Sibbald B, Cantrill JA, et al (Univ of Manchester, England)
BMJ 313:1371–1374, 1996   1–4

Background.—The government of the United Kingdom is committed to improving the quality of prescribing and reducing the cost and volume of prescription drugs. There are wide variations in prescribing rates and costs in different practices in different geographic regions. Physicians have diverse opinions about the best way to practice medicine and there are no standards for appropriate prescribing for physicians in general practice. Claims that physicians overprescribe drugs of limited clinical value and underprescribe generic drugs and inhaled steroids for asthma lack credibility.

Methods.—A panel of 10 experts was set up to define prescribing appropriateness. This panel defined 19 indicators of appropriate long-term prescribing covering 5 dimensions: indication, choice of drug, drug administration, communication, and review. A review was then conducted of 62 studies identified from electronic databases and reference lists for violations of each indicator.

Results.—The rate of potentially inappropriate prescribing varied by each of the 19 indicators and by chronic condition. The highest rates of potentially inappropriate prescribing were consistently seen in drug dosages outside the therapeutic range. The lowest rates were associated with indicators of inappropriate choice of drug, except for cost minimization. There is less information on communication than on the other dimensions of prescribing.

Discussion.—Inappropriate prescribing in general practice does occur in the United Kingdom, but it is not known to what extent it occurs. There is no evidence of widespread inappropriate prescribing in general practice in the United Kingdom.

▶ This sensible article, while not denying that inappropriate long-term prescribing occurs in the United Kingdom, quite rightly points out that better data are needed to justify (and quantify) sweeping criticisms.

L. Lasagna, M.D.

Paracetamol Prescribing Habits in a Children's Hospital
Anderson B, Anderson M, Hastie B (Auckland Children's Hosp, New Zealand)
N Z Med J 109:376–378, 1996   1–5

Background.—Paracetamol, an analgesic/antipyretic commonly used in children, can cause hepatic and renal damage at dosages exceeding 90 mg/kg/day. No dosing guidelines currently exist for paracetamol use in children younger than 1 month. Paracetamol prescribing habits in 1 university children's hospital were surveyed.

Methods.—An anonymous questionnaire was sent to all medical staff at 1 center eliciting data on paracetamol prescriptions for children in varying age groups. In addition, pharmacists audited the daily prescription charts of inpatients with no hepatic or renal disease for 2 months. Maximum possible daily doses were calculated for each child.

Findings.—Fifty-three of 80 staff members responded to the questionnaire. Lower daily doses tended to be used in the first 2 weeks of life. More practitioners either did not use the drug or did not know safe dosing schedules in children 3 months of age and younger. During the 2-month audit period, 823 prescriptions were written for children 4 months and older, 85 for infants 3 months and younger, and 7 for neonates in the first 2 weeks of life. Twenty-five of 140 prescriptions exceeding 95 mg/kg/day were given to children aged 4 months and older, and 2 of 6 were given to infants 3 months and younger.

Conclusions.—Many staff members were uncertain of current safe dosing regimens for paracetamol, especially in neonates. Previous research suggests that 60–65 mg/kg/day is suitable for infants 1–3 months of age, although this dose was only charted in 16% of the current prescriptions, and pharmacokinetic data suggest the need for a higher dose. In neonates, 30 mg/kg/day produces effective therapeutic levels, but additional studies are needed.

▶ In this study, the authors tried to view what was actually happening in a large children's hospital and see whether they could tease out some intelligent guidelines for the use of acetaminophen or paracetamol in very young children. Unfortunately, it really didn't work out too well. Still, the data remind us of the actual doses used and about the current recommendations.

M. Weintraub, M.D.

The Successful Implementation of Pharmaceutical Practice Guidelines: Analysis of Associated Outcomes and Cost Savings
Lubarsky DA, Glass PSA, Ginsberg B, et al (Duke Univ, Durham, NC)
Anesthesiology 86:1145–1160, 1997   1–6

Background.—Few of the many medical practice guidelines proposed have been implemented and maintained successfully. One attempt to develop and institute practice guidelines to promote more appropriate use of costly anesthetics, to generate and sustain widespread compliance from a large group of physicians, and to reduce costs without adversely affecting clinical outcomes was described.

Methods.—The guidelines were developed by the physicians and their associated care team for the intraoperative use of anesthetic agents. To aid compliance, a drug distribution process was developed. A total of 1,744 patients were studied before and after guideline implementation.

Findings.—Pharmaceutical costs declined from $56 per patient to $32 per patient as a result of adherence to practice guidelines. The patient flow perioperatively was affected only minimally. Time from end of surgery to arrival in the postanesthesia care unit rose from 11 minutes before guideline implementation to 14 minutes after implementation. The admission of inpatients to the postanesthesia care unit needing monitored anesthesia care rose from 6.5% before guideline implementation to 12.9% after implementation. Compliance and cost savings were maintained.

Conclusions.—The current study provides an example of a successful physician-directed program for promoting better utilization of health care resources. Costs were saved with no substantial changes in clinical outcomes.

▶ Seemingly, this program saved the medical center a lot of money without adversely affecting the quality of anesthetic care. To my mind, studies of cost-savings are not helpful unless they do what this research team did— measure quality of care as well as costs.

L. Lasagna, M.D.

Failure to Comply: A Therapeutic Dilemma and the Bane of Clinical Trials
Gibaldi M (Univ of Washington, Seattle)
J Clin Pharmacol 36:674–682, 1996   1–7

Background.—Failure to comply with prescribed drug treatment is a major problem in health care. Poor compliance is a particular problem in children, adolescents, and older adults and has been linked to increased rates of hospitalization and institutionalization. Key issues related to the problem of drug noncompliance were reviewed.

Drug Noncompliance.—Many patients are prescribed effective drug therapy but fail to realize its benefits because of noncompliance. Noncompliance is a major problem in the treatment of tuberculosis, and has led to the apparently successful approach of directly observed therapy. Many factors play a role in noncompliance, including the dosing regimen, family characteristics, patient health beliefs, and the patient-physician relationship. Side effects are one major reason for noncompliance; more complex dosing regimens may be another. Drug costs and reimbursement policies may pose barriers to good compliance.

Adherence has been related to health outcomes, and this is usually explained by selection bias. However, recent studies have ruled out this explanation. There are several different methods of measuring noncompliance, the most common being patient questioning. In clinical trials, misleadingly high compliance rates may lead to incorrect study conclusions. Compliance rates are higher in controlled trials than in actual clinical practice. Patients may be selected for compliance, but this too may bias the results. Discontinuation rates may offer a crude measure of the relative tolerability of various interventions.

Discussion.—The impact of noncompliance on health care is now well recognized. The next step is to find cost-effective approaches to enhancing compliance, both in trials and in clinical practice. Patient education, provider communication, and economic barriers need attention. Also, a consensus is needed on how to handle the problem of compliance in clinical trials.

▶ Milo Gibaldi is one of the most distinguished academic figures in American pharmacy, and he here addresses an extremely important (and seriously neglected) issue—the failure of patients to follow directions. Some noncompliance has been dubbed "intelligent" by my co-editor Mike Weintraub, e.g., when a drug is not working and making you sick. But often, whether it occurs in formal clinical trials or ordinary medical practice, noncompliance is the *cause* of drug failure, not a consequence of it.

Read the whole article. It's excellent.

L. Lasagna, M.D.

Assessing Non-consent Bias With Parallel Randomized and Nonrandomized Clinical Trials
Marcus SM (Jefferson Med College, Philadelphia)
J Clin Epidemiol 50:823–828, 1997   1–8

Background.—A large proportion of patients eligible for randomization in some clinical trials may not consent to be randomized. Nonconsent bias with parallel randomized and nonrandomized clinical trials was discussed.

Discussion.—Nonconsent bias may occur when the randomized subjects differ from the eligible population in characteristics associated with the magnitude of the treatment effect. Some investigators attempt to address this problem by conducting a separate, nonrandomized trial in addition to the randomized trial. This nonrandomized trial is otherwise identical to the randomized trial and consists of patients who wish to choose their treatment. In addition, observed baseline covariate data can be used to adjust for differences between the randomized and eligible populations when estimating the treatment effect for the eligible population. After adjustment, different outcomes for the randomized compared with nonrandomized treated groups and/or the randomized compared with the nonrandomized control groups reflect the presence of hidden nonconsent bias, which results from differences between the trial population and the eligible population with respect to unobserved covariates. Sensitivity analysis can demonstrate how hidden nonconsent bias can account for an imbalance in the treatment groups.

Recommendations for Investigators.—Adding a nonrandomized trial to the randomized trial can provide valuable data for determining whether nonconsent bias exists. Baseline covariate data should be collected because it can be useful in detecting differences between subjects in the randomized trial and those eligible for the trial. Nonconsent bias is less likely to be a threat if the randomized and nonrandomized trial groups are similar at baseline. When there are differences, baseline covariates can be used to adjust for imbalances. When the unadjusted and adjusted treatment effect estimates are similar, nonconsent bias may not be a problem.

▶ Actually, it's amazing to me how many clinical trials turn out to give us a correct answer considering all the things that can go wrong with them. Here's something that many individuals don't even consider, even though the sensitivity of the clinical trial will be diminished by its occurrence.

M. Weintraub, M.D.

The Results of Direct and Indirect Treatment Comparisons in Meta-analysis of Randomized Controlled Trials
Bucher HC, Guyatt GH, Griffith LE, et al (McMaster Univ, Hamilton, Ont, Canada)
J Clin Epidemiol 50:683–691, 1997   1–9

Background.—When trying to decide between 2 different drugs, the physician often has no means of making direct comparisons of their effectiveness. In this situation, indirect comparisons from studies comparing the 2 treatments with a control or placebo may be used. Meta-analysis, or analysis of pooled data from the treatment arms of controlled trials, is increasingly used. However, this approach is no better than comparison of observational study data and carries the possibility of bias. A new approach, comparing the differences between treatment and placebo in 2 sets of clinical trials—one that preserves the randomization of the original studies—was reported.

Methods.—The new approach uses the odds ratio or relative risk as the measure of treatment effect. The approach permits calculation of a summary odds ratio of the indirect comparison between drugs by taking the ratio of the log odds ratio from the studies in question. The resulting estimate is unbiased in large samples, as long as the covariates defining patient subgroups and the magnitude of treatment effect do not interact. This approach was applied to previously reported study data on sulfamethoxazole-trimethoprim vs. dapsone/pyrimethamine as prophylactic agents against *Pneumocystis carinii* in patients with HIV infection.

Results.—The indirect comparison suggested that sulfamethoxazole-trimethoprim was of significantly greater benefit: odds ratio, 0.37; 95% confidence interval, 0.21 to 0.65. In contrast, the findings of directly comparative randomized trials suggested a smaller difference: risk ratio, 0.64; a 95% confidence interval, 0.45 to 0.90.

Conclusion.—If there are no direct comparisons of 2 drugs, the new indirect comparison meta-analysis can evaluate the magnitude of treatment effects across studies. The strength of inferences made by this approach is limited, however, and direct comparisons are preferred. If indirect comparisons are made, they should compare the magnitude of the effect in 2 sets of controlled trials, rather than including only the treatment arms.

▶ Often people call for "head-to-head" comparisons of 1 therapeutic intervention with another. I, myself, have wondered why we do not have more of these head-to-head comparisons. They seem pretty common in Europe where they help to determine the price for an agent. Still—at least in the United States—the pharmaceutical industry is unwilling, in most cases, to test their drug against the industry standard or leader. We are seeing more comparisons but, perhaps, not enough. Therefore, the abstracted article seems to be quite important and may be important enough to be read in its entirety. The model that the authors used is based on a meta-analysis, but it is also based on the treatment effects and their magnitude in randomized trials of the intervention compared with either control groups or placebo. Perhaps this will decrease the necessity for comparisons on a head-to-head basis. If I were running an HMO, I would view this technique as worth a try.

M. Weintraub, M.D.

Moving Promising Research Findings to the Clinic: Methodological Issues in the Design and Conduct of Clinical Trials of Retinoids
Arnold A (McMaster Univ, Hamilton, Canada)
Int J Cancer 70:467–469, 1997   1–10

Background.—Retinoids have been successful in the treatment of acute promyelocytic leukemia and in decreasing secondary primary head and neck cancers. Some unexpected negative clinical results have also been reported. The methodologic issues that arise when promising laboratory or epidemiologic retinoid findings are tested in a clinical setting were discussed.

Discussion.—As the potential for retinoid use extends from chemoprevention to the treatment of advanced disease, the clinical challenge is to obtain drug levels in human beings that approximate active doses in experimental systems. Tolerance depends on the exact clinical situation, the likelihood of a positive outcome, and the duration of retinoid use. Strategies for reducing or overcoming retinoid toxicity are the use of co-interventions such as lipid-lowering drugs and emollients to decrease skin toxicity, the inclusion of drug holidays, and pharmacologic monitoring to titrate toxic retinoid levels. These stratgies need further study.

Extrapolating data from epidemiologic studies and in vivo or in vitro studies can be problematic. Epidemiologic research generates hypotheses and confirms findings from case reports but does not prove the efficacy of retinoids. Risks are also associated with attempts to reproduce laboratory findings in the clinic.

The performance of chemoprevention trials can yield much useful information. Examining methodologic issues, such as compliance, drug levels, and assessment of the accuracy of the study end point, may provide possible explanations for negative study results, which can be used in the design of subsequent research. Understanding the reasons for differences among responses to retinoids is also important.

Conclusions.—Introducing retinoids into clinical practice has been frustrating, especially for chemoprevention. Carefully controlled studies are needed. Older paradigms about clinical trial design and drug development strategies need to be challenged if more progress is to be made.

▶ Although this abstracted paper is mostly about cancer chemotherapy and retinoids in the treatment of cancer, the lessons learned are terrific. They include using epidemiologic or case reports as a starting place, moving from studies done in "little glass dishes" to studies done in whole animals and in people, getting something out of nothing (negative studies), learning from important clinical differences, and arranging the drug development plan. All these things are critical parts of the way we study medications. This short article is very worthwhile to read in its unabstracted form. All you have to do is substitute words. Every time they talk about oncology, you can substitute another field in which you are interested.

M. Weintraub, M.D.

Is Good Clinical Research Practice for Clinical Trials Good Clinical Practice?
Yastrubetskaya O, Chiu E, O'Connell S (Univ of Melbourne, Kew, Australia)
Int J Geriatr Psychiatry 12:227–231, 1997   1–11

Introduction.—Randomized controlled trials are key to modern research in medical therapy. Specific guidelines have been developed to control the recruitment of patients into ethical research studies. The circumstances of a phase III trial should reflect the normal conditions of use as closely as possible for the therapeutic safety and value of a new drug to be established. Currently, it is common to use near-perfect patient selection criteria that reduce sample heterogeneity. Data drawn from a homogeneous sample have greater statistical power, but efficacy analyses of a larger, heterogeneous sample can identify more practical questions regarding choice of therapy.

A Phase III Trial.—The authors participated in a phase III study of a new antidepressive drug in elderly patients. Of 188 patients screened, 171 patients had a Hamilton Depression Rating Scale score of more than 18 and met inclusion criteria, but only 8 could be recruited after applying exclusion criteria (Fig 1). These 8 patients were not seen as representative

RECRUITMENT FOR TRIAL

Referred between 30/10/92 and 28/02/94

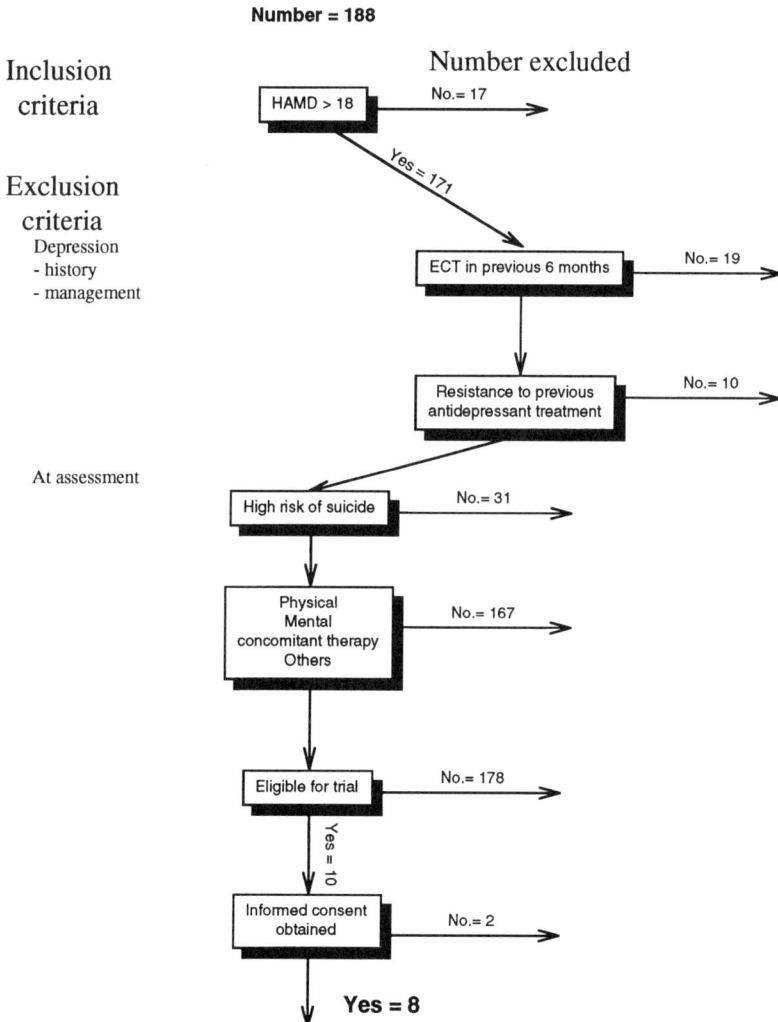

Number = 188

Inclusion criteria

Exclusion criteria
Depression
- history
- management

At assessment

Number excluded

HAMD > 18 — No.= 17

Yes = 171

ECT in previous 6 months — No.= 19

Resistance to previous antidepressant treatment — No.= 10

High risk of suicide — No.= 31

Physical Mental concomitant therapy Others — No.= 167

Eligible for trial — No.= 178

Yes = 10

Informed consent obtained — No.= 2

Yes = 8

FIGURE 1.—Selection of depressed patients for trial. (Courtesy of Yastrubetskaya O, Chiu E, O'Connell S: Is good clinical research practice for clinical trials good clinical practice? J Geriatr Psychiatry 12:227–231, copyright 1997. Reprinted by permission of John Wiley & Sons Ltd. Reproduced with permission.)

of the total sample. The referring doctors believed that the new drug had something to offer and were disappointed that such stringent criteria excludes so many patients from participating in the study and possibly benefiting from the drug.

Discussion.—If the new antidepressive drug is marketed in the future, clinicians will not be provided with information regarding its efficacy in elderly patients with depressive symptoms who have significant comorbidity or concomitant therapy or a history of affective or nonaffective psychiatric disorders, or who are generally frail. The conclusions drawn by studies with stringent exclusion criteria do not reflect the clinical environment in which the product will be used. The relevance of currently accepted clinical research guidelines to actual clinical practice needs to be examined further.

▶ This important paper reminds us that although rigid inclusion criteria often help to keep the "noise" down and increase the likelihood of demonstrating a difference between treatments, the very process of choosing patients for a trial leads to a "hothouse" situation in which the results simply cannot be generalized to patients with characteristics that would have excluded them from the trial.

L. Lasagna, M.D.

Surrogate End Points in Clinical Trials: Are We Being Misled?
Fleming TR, DeMets DL (Univ of Washington, Seattle; Univ of Wisconsin, Madison)
Ann Intern Med 125:605–613, 1996   1–12

Introduction.—The primary end point of a phase 3 trial should be a clinically relevant event, such as death, loss of vision, symptomatic events of AIDS, the need for ventilatory support, or other events precipitating a reduction in quality of life. This level of trial often is long and expensive. There is recent interest in the use of surrogate end points, such as increased CD4 cell counts or decreased viral load measures for trials of therapy for HIV infection or AIDS; suppression of ventricular arrhythmias or reductions in cholesterol levels or blood pressure in cardiology trials; and tumor regression in cancer therapy trials. The basic requirements that surrogates must meet to be used as the replacement outcome were described.

Surrogate End Point Requirements.—It is not true that if an outcome is a correlate, it can be used as a valid surrogate end point (i.e., a replacement for the true clinical outcome). A surrogate must be a correlate of the true clinical outcome and must capture completely the net effect of treatment on the clinical outcome. Several factors may explain the failure of surrogate end points. Although it is a correlate of disease progression, a surrogate end point may not involve the same pathophysiologic processes that result in the clinical outcomes. An intervention may affect only the pathway mediated through the surrogate end point or pathways independent

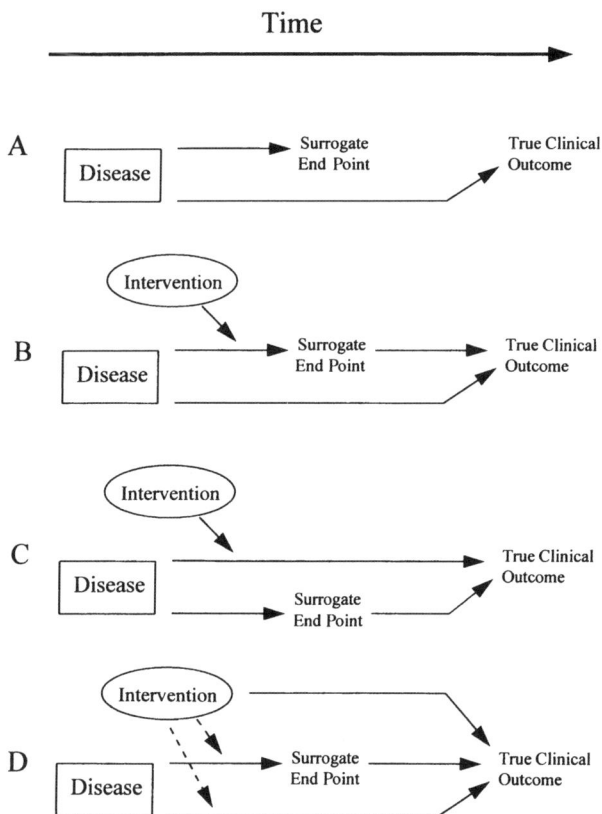

FIGURE 1.—Reasons for failure of surrogate end points. **A**, the surrogate is not the causal pathway of the disease process. **B**, of several causal pathways of disease, the intervention affects only the pathway mediated through the surrogate. **C**, the surrogate is not in the pathway of the intervention's effect or is insensitive to its effect. **D**, the intervention has mechanisms of action independent of the disease process. *Dotted lines* indicate mechanisms of action that might exist. (Courtesy of Fleming TR, DeMets DL: Surrogate end points in clinical trials: Are we being misled? *Ann Intern Med* 125:605–613, 1996.)

of the surrogate end point. An intervention may affect the true clinical outcome by unintended mechanisms of action independent of the disease process. Finally, the effects of the intervention mediated through the intended mechanisms may be offset substantially by unintended, unanticipated, or unrecognized mechanisms (Fig 1).

Conclusion.—Surrogate end points perform best when used in screening for promising new therapies through evaluation of biologic activity in preliminary phase 2 trials. Surrogate end points in definitive phase 3 trials may provide valuable insight into an intervention's mechanism of action, but the primary goal is to collect direct evidence regarding the intervention's effect on safety measures and true clinical outcomes.

▶ Surrogate end points are important not only in giving clues as to whether a drug at least deserves further study but also in predicting benefits that are worthwhile per se. As such, surrogate end points have long enjoyed utility (e.g., blood sugar levels, blood pressure readings, serum cholesterol determinations). However, it is important that we not be misled into believing that a surrogate is the same as a clinical outcome. For example, CD4 lymphocyte counts seem to correlate with the severity of AIDS, but it is not necessarily true that a drug that moves CD4 counts in the right direction will cut down on AIDS-related illness or prolong life. Some end points are desirable in any case, such as a decrease in opportunistic infections in patients with AIDS. Such a decrease may or may not prolong the life of a patient with AIDS (because there are so many ways in which to die of that dreaded disease), but it is certainly a welcome achievement.

L. Lasagna, M.D.

The Elderly and Their Medication: Understanding and Compliance in a Family Practice
Blenkiron P (York, England)
Postgrad Med J 72:671–676, 1996   1–13

Background.—Up to 75% of elderly patients make errors in medication compliance, a quarter of which are potentially serious. Elderly patients were directly questioned in the current study to determine the extent and nature of prescribing to those aged 75 and older in one rural dispensing practice.

Methods and Findings.—Eighty patients aged 75 and older were interviewed to assess their level of knowledge, degree of compliance, and problems with their medications. Fifty-nine patients had regularly prescribed medications. These patients took a total of 206 drugs. The purpose of 72% of the medications was correctly stated. The dosage regimen was accurately recalled for 75%. The correct name was given for 64% of the drugs. The patients reported that they never missed a dose for 77% of the drugs prescribed. However, there was a poor correlation between such self-ratings and the level of compliance on computer records of repeat prescriptions, though the latter showed that compliance was accurate for 80% of the medications taken. Removing the tops of medicine containers was a significant problem for the patients, including half of those taking analgesics or nonsteroidal anti-inflammatory agents.

Conclusions.—Regular explanations of medications by the family physician may further improve comprehension and compliance among elderly patients. The widespread use of child-resistant containers often creates problems for the elderly.

▶ Child-resistant medicine containers are all too often adult-resistant as well. They make no sense for elderly (or even young) adults who don't live with children.

L. Lasagna, M.D.

Recombinant Protein and Therapeutic Monoclonal Antibody Drug Development in the United States From 1980 to 1994

Gosse ME, DiMasi JA, Nelson TF (Tufts Ctr for the Study of Drug Development, Boston)

Clin Pharmacol Ther 60:608–618, 1996   1–14

Background.—Biopharmaceuticals produced through the use of recombinant DNA technology are now an integral part of drug development in the United States. Recombinant protein and therapeutic monoclonal antibody drug development from 1980 to 1994 were discussed.

Methods.—Data regarding recombinant proteins and therapeutic monoclonal antibody products tested in U.S. clinical studies were analyzed to better determine the successes and failures of biopharmaceutical agents. Data were acquired from company surveys and public access sources.

Data Synthesis.—The early investigational new drug (IND) applications were generally successful, with 9 of the first 23 IND filings marketed in the United States. Even if the 2 recombinant versions are removed from the analysis, 38 percent were clinically effective and were approved by the FDA. Subsequent products were not as successful, with a fivefold to eightfold reduction in the percentage approval for the products filed after 1984. Data also suggest that the products made by this industry are most likely to be tested in a phase II protocol. During the 15-year period, the recombinant proteins entered phase II at a rate of 80%. Product failures appeared to shift from phase II between 1985 and 1989 to phase III in the early 1990s. The overall clinical success of the recombinant proteins tested in patients between 1980 and 1989 was comparable to that of the new recombinant entities tested clinically during that time.

Conclusion.—This analysis underscores the growth of the biotechnology industry. It also provides a foundation for the study of the effects of present and future regulatory and legislative efforts to facilitate the biopharmaceutical development process.

▶ The early successes of the new biotechnology industry led to an unrealistic euphoria regarding future successes. Venture capitalists need to realize that a quick and predictable return on their investment in biotechnology is unlikely. One can predict that many of the 1,500 or so U.S. biotechnology companies will either fail or be absorbed by one of the few successful biotechnology firms or by a traditional pharmaceutical company with deep pockets and an income stream from marketed products.

L. Lasagna, M.D.

Whither Triazolam?

Johnson RE, McFarland BH, Woodson GT (Kaiser Permanente Northwest Division, Portland, Ore)
Med Care 35:303–310, 1997   1–15

Background.—Triazolam, a sedative/hypnotic agent used for short-term management of insomnia, was banned in a number of countries because of reported behavioral side effects. Safety concerns were also widely publicized in the United States from 1987 on. Despite such findings, triazolam remained the most frequently prescribed benzodiazepine hypnotic in the Kaiser Permanente Northwest Division (KPNW) through 1991. In April 1992, the Regional Formulary and Therapeutics Committee of the KPNW decided to delete triazolam from the drug formulary. The effect of that decision on the prescribing and use of triazolam was discussed.

Methods.—The KPNW is an HMO with more than 410,000 enrollees; more than 80% have prepaid drug benefits. Data on all prescriptions dispensed were obtained from an automated outpatient prescription database. The number of triazolam users, their sex and ages, total annual exposure, estimated daily doses, and total days of annual exposure were compared before (1989–1991) and after (1992–1993) the drug's deletion from the formulary.

Results.—Triazolam was the most frequently dispensed short-acting benzodiazepine in the HMO in 1989, accounting for 18.8% of all benzodiazepine dispensings in that year. The drug had fallen to 1.3% of the total by 1993, however, and the total number of users decreased 91% from the year before its deletion through the second year after its deletion. Most long-term users were aged 65 years or older.

Conclusion.—Deletion of triazolam from this HMO's formulary committee led to a marked decrease in the number of new and continuing users of the drug. Many patients were switched from triazolam to other benzodiazepines or to antidepressants. Even in an HMO setting with an open, advisory-type formulary, decisions about a drug's inclusion in the formulary can have a considerable impact on prescribing behavior.

▶ One of the features of this paper is the fact that the formulary was, in fact, an open, advisory-type one. That is, all medications were available; prescribers could choose any drug whether it was on the formulary or not; and any patient with a prepaid drug benefit could be reimbursed for prescription fees if that patient obtained a nonformulary drug from an outside pharmacy. Even the very modest restrictions on physician prescribers had quite a dramatic effect on prescribing of triazolam. The percentage went from approximately 19% of the population receiving triazolam to 2%, whereas lorazapam and temazepam increased. In fact, temazepam (around 10%) and lorazapam (around 15%), together superseded, by a significant amount, the percentage of triazolam previously prescribed. Even if one subtracts the temazepam use at the time triazolam was removed from the formulary (8%), the sum of the 2 added up to just about the same percentage as triazolam.

Triazolam prescribing was decreasing, admittedly at a slow rate, in the years before it was removed.

In a paper my colleagues and I published,[1] we showed that benzodiazepine use was declining before the institution of New York State requirements for use of a triplicate prescription with benzodiazepine. One thing that the abstracted paper did not look at was the use of other than benzodiazepine sleeping pills, for example, meprobamate and chlorohydrate, which increased dramatically according to the study that we did.

M. Weintraub, M.D.

Reference

1. Weintraub M, Singh S, Byrne L, et al: Consequences of the 1989 New York State triplicate prescribing regulations for benzodiazepines. *JAMA* 266:2392–2397, 1991.

A Technique for Population Pharmacodynamic Analysis of Concentration–Binary Response Data

Bailey JM, Gregg KM (Emory Univ, Atlanta, Ga; Stanford Univ, Calif)
Anesthesiology 86:825–835, 1997   1–16

Background.—Pharmacodynamic research often involves the binary assessment of the response to a defined stimulus in many patients. The concentration-effect relation is typically given in terms of C_{50}, the drug concentration associated with a 50% probability of drug effect, and parameter γ, which determines the shape of the concentration-probability curve. The accurate estimation of this parameter, which described the entire curve, is as important as that of C_{50}, a single point on the curve. Usually, interpatient variability is not considered in the analysis of pharmacodynamic data. Accounting for such variability may improve the accuracy of γ estimations and allow for the estimation of C_{50} variability.

Methods and Findings.—A probit-based model characterized by C_{50} and γ was assumed for the individual concentration-response relation. This assumption was validated by comparing probit regression with the more commonly used logistic regression of data from individual patients. The model was extended to population data analysis, assuming that C_{50} has a log-normal distribution. Three parameters were used in the population data analysis: (C_{50}), the mean value of C_{50} in the population; ω, the standard deviation of the distribution of the logarithm of C_{50}; and γ. Simulated data were generated for a range of γ and ω values, assuming that C_{50} and γ had a log-normal distribution. Population analysis with the extended probit model accurately estimated (C_{50}), γ, and ω for a range of values.

Conclusions.—A method for population analysis of binary pharmacologic data was presented. This probit-based method of pharmacodynamic analysis of pooled population data facilitates accurate estimation of the concentration-response curve.

▶ The anesthesiologists have been among the most consistent users of the binary response, probably because so many of their pharmacodynamic data can provide a "yes or no" answer. I am hopeful that investigators in other areas of medicine, and especially in clinical pharmacology, will also use the binary response whenever possible. For example, if one chooses a clinically meaningful end point and assesses whether the patient achieved that end point, be it for a blood pressure of 140/90 mm Hg or "no-vomiting" after cancer chemotherapy, the quality of the data will be much improved. Physicians will be able to deal with their patients in a way that both of them understand. They'll be able to say, "You have this chance of achieving this response." In any case, we've got to worry more about any defects in this binary response for clinical judgements and, hopefully, use it correctly.

M. Weintraub, M.D.

Folate Intake in Young Women and Their Knowledge of Preconceptional Folate Supplemenation to Prevent Neural Tube Defects
Wild J, Schorah CJ, Maude K, et al (Univ of Leeds, England)
Eur J Obstet Gynecol Reprod Biol 70:185–189, 1996   1–17

Background.—In the United Kingdom, the Department of Health's Expert Advisory group has recommended that women should take supplementary folic acid, 0.4 mg, daily before conception and in the early months of pregnancy. However, recent research has shown that most women are unaware of these recommendations at the beginning of pregnancy. Young women's knowledge of periconceptional folate for preventing neural tube defect (NTD) and their folate intake were investigated.

Methods and Findings.—One hundred fifty adolescents, aged 16 to 19 years, and 150 undergraduate women were interviewed. A food frequency questionnaire was administered to determine folate intake. Fourteen percent of the adolescents and 41% of the undergraduates knew that folate intake should be increased before conception. Estimated median folate intakes were 235 and 248.5 µg/day in the adolescents and undergraduates, respectively. In both groups, more than one fourth had folate intakes of less than the reference nutrient intake of 200 µg/day, below which the prevalence of NTD increases markedly. Thus these women would be at increased risk of having a child with NTD if an unplanned pregnancy were to occur.

Conclusions.—Even highly educated young women have little knowledge of the importance of periconceptional folic acid. Strategies are needed to increase such knowledge and increase folate intake among young women.

▶ These data, of course, were very worrisome, particularly in the 16–19 year-olds. Only 14% of them knew that their folate level had to be increased if they became pregnant. Of course, I'll bet that the data are no better in the United States because we have such a heterogeneous population and because the importance of folate hasn't reached mass communication. There have been meetings in Washington and a short flurry of articles in newspapers. But there really hasn't been a lot on television, which is the major place that most of the people that we're trying to reach get their news. In Britain, they started a campaign with posters and pamphlets and pictures in 1996. I hope they'll have a chance to redo this kind of study and help the United States inform the same population groups.

M. Weintraub, M.D.

Study of Eight Cases of Cancer in 426 Rheumatoid Arthritis Patients Treated With Methotrexate
Bologna C, Picot M-C, Jorgensen C, et al (CHU Laperyronie, Montpellier, France)
Ann Rheum Dis 56:97–102, 97   1–18

Objective.—Although weekly low-dose methotrexate is a common treatment for rheumatoid arthritis, there have been no large, long-term studies of the oncogenicity of the drug. In a retrospective study, 426 patients with rheumatoid arthritis were treated long-term with methotrexate.

Methods.—Medical and surgical history, current treatment, and the time and reason for methotrexate withdrawal were obtained for 426 patients with rheumatoid arthritis who received methotrexate once weekly for at least 12 months between January 1, 1985, and March 31, 1994, and who were followed up for an average of 4.65 years. The number of hospitalizations and incidence of cancers were recorded and compared with data from 420 controls with rheumatoid arthritis and with a regional population. The data were analyzed statistically.

Results.—There were 8 cancers in the methotrexate group (1.88%) and 6 cancers in the control group (1.43%). Life-table analysis showed that the control group had a significantly higher incidence of cancer, with age established by multivariate analysis as the only significant risk factor. The incidence of cancer in a regional population of 812,344 was 0.79%. Using the indirect standardization method after adjusting for age, there was no significant incidence of cancer in either populations with rheumatoid arthritis.

Conclusion.—Weekly long-term methotrexate therapy for patients with rheumatoid arthritis did not appear to cause an increased incidence of cancer in this study. Longer-term prospective studies are recommended.

▶ The oncogenic potential of methotrexate has long been debated. This study is somewhat reassuring on this matter.

L. Lasagna, M.D.

2 Drug Action

Vitamins and Analgesics in the Prevention of Collagen Ageing

Malik NS, Meek KM (Open Univ, Oxford, England)
Age Ageing 25:279–284, 1996
2–1

Background.—Collagen modifications play a key role in the aging of connective tissues. Protein glycation is a nonenzymic reaction involving sugar. It may be involved in the development of various physical changes of aging as well as in diabetic retinopathy, neuropathy, renal failure, and atherosclerosis. In studies using human corneal and scleral tissue, glycation leads to increases in collagen intermolecular spacing, comparable to the increases noted in studies of collagen aging in these tissues. Certain compounds were studied for their ability to inhibit protein glycation in vitro.

Methods.—Studies were performed in cultured corneal and scleral tissue. The inhibitors investigated included aspirin, vitamin C, and vitamin E. Their ability to inhibit protein glycation was studied by x-ray diffraction. Measurements of collagen-associated fluorescence were performed as well.

Results.—All compounds studied, including aspirin and aspirin-like compounds and vitamins C and E, inhibited the sugar-induced expansion of the corneal collagen network. Expansion of the corneal collagen network at 24 days was 49% under control conditions vs. 2% to 11% with inhibitors. All inhibitors also reduced fructose-induced fluorescence of corneal collagen.

Conclusions.—Aspirin, certain vitamins, and other common compounds appear to prevent sugar-induced molecular changes in corneal and scleral collagen. These compounds might thus be useful in the prevention of collagen aging and age-related complications.

▶ Rat tail tendon is often employed in vitro to study the aging of collagen. These authors use human corneal and scleral tissue, which has been shown to undergo changes after incubation with glucose that are similar to the changes seen in aging. Their work suggests a possible role for aspirin-like compounds and certain vitamins (C and E) in preventing some of the undesirable effects of aging.

L. Lasagna, M.D.

Pharmacokinetics of Morphine and Its Glucuronides After Intravenous Infusion of Morphine and Morphine-6–Glucuronide in Healthy Volunteers
Lötsch J, Stockmann A, Kobal G, et al (Univ of Erlangen-Nürnberg, Germany)
Clin Pharmacol Ther 60:316–325, 1996   2–2

Introduction.—Morphine is metabolized to morphine-3–glucuronide (M-3-G) and morphine-6-glucuronide (M-6-G). Evidence suggests that M-6-G is a potent analgesic with an improved therapeutic index. However, consistent pharmacokinetic data are available on this agent, which makes it difficult to suggest a dosing regimen for pharmacodynamic studies. The steady-state pharmacokinetics of morphine, M-6-G, and M-3-G after IV dosing with morphine or M-6-G were investigated.

Methods and Findings.—Initial studies in 4 volunteers were performed to calculate a dosing regimen. The regimens were the following: for morphine, IV loading dose of 0.24 mg/kg of body weight for 5 minutes, followed by IV infusion of 0.069 mg·kg$^-$·hr^{-1} for 4 hours; and for M-6-G, loading dose of 0.011 mg/kg for 5 minutes followed by infusion of 0.006 mg·kg$^-$·hr^{-1} for 4 hours. In another 4 volunteers, these doses produced plasma concentrations close to predefined target levels: 35.0 ng/mL for morphine and 45.5 ng/mL for M-6-G. The latter was well tolerated and did not lead to the euphoria or nausea that occurred with morphine.

Conclusions.—The dosing regimen used in this study can achieve the same steady-state plasma M-6-G concentration whether morphine or M-6-G itself is given. It can be used in future pharmacodynamic studies comparing the analgesic effects of morphine and M-6-G. The study includes data on the kinetics of M-6-G, calculated as a function of time with a linear systems approach to estimate the rate and fraction of morphine's glucuronidation to M-6-G.

▶ Two glucuronides represent the major end points of morphine's metabolism in the human body. The 6-glucuronide seems to be equivalent, or perhaps even superior, to the parent opioid and appears to produce fewer side effects. The present study provides a basis for picking dosage regimens that can now be compared in clinical analgesic trials.

L. Lasagna, M.D.

Meperidine-induced Generalized Seizures With Normal Renal Function
Marinella MA (Univ of Michigan, Ann Arbor)
South Med J 90:556–558, 1997   2–3

Background.—Meperidine is an opioid analgesic commonly prescribed in a variety of clinical settings. Though the parent compound has a CNS depressant effect, its sole active metabolite, normeperidine, is a CNS excitatory agent with the ability to cause seizures, especially in patients with renal failure. Meperidine rarely causes seizures in patients with normal renal function, but it can cause seizures when used in large doses at frequent dosing intervals. A patient with normal renal function in whom meperidine caused a tonic-clonic seizure is described.

> *Case Report.*—Man, 40, with chronic abdominal pain from alcohol-related chronic pancreatitis, was hospitalized for an increase in abdominal pain and vomiting. He had been taking methadone daily for more than 1 year. Dextrose-containing IV fluids, pain control, and antiemetic treatment were begun. Meperidine at 75 mg IM every 2 to 3 hours was administered, along with prochlorperazine at 10 mg IV every 6 hours as needed. The route of meperidine administration was switched to IV at the patient's request. A total of 750 mg meperidine (300 mg by the IV route) was delivered in 17 hours. A generalized tonic-clonic seizure lasting about 1 minute occurred about 30 minutes after a dose of meperidine. A thorough neurologic examination revealed no abnormality in focal findings. No postictal myoclonus or tremor occurred. Meperidine was discontinued, and the patient had no further seizure activity.

Conclusions.—Meperidine carries a definite risk for CNS toxicity, especially in patients with impaired renal function. This case report illustrates that even patients with normal renal function are at risk for adverse CNS events. Generalized seizure activity can occur in patients given the drug at frequent intervals or in addition to phenothiazines.

▶ CNS toxicity, including nervousness, hyperreflexia, tremors, myoclonus, and (rarely) generalized seizures can occur after administration of meperidine, presumably from the impact of its metabolite, normeperidine. These troubles have usually been seen in patients with renal failure (and thus higher levels of normeperidine). This article suggests that CNS toxicity can occur after meperidine administration in patients with normal renal function if the analgesic is given at frequent intervals or in addition to phenothiazines.

L. Lasagna, M.D.

Decrease of Plasma and Urinary Oxidative Metabolites of Acetaminophen After Consumption of Watercress by Human Volunteers
Chen L, Mohr SN, Yang CS (Rutgers Univ, Piscataway, NJ; Univ of Medicine and Dentistry of New Jersey, New Brunswick)
Clin Pharmacol Ther 60:651–660, 1996   2–4

Background.—Experimental research has shown that phenethyl isothiocyanate (PEITC), a component derived from watercress, inhibits 4-(methylnitrosamino)-1-(3-pyridyl)-1-butanone–induced lung carcinogenesis and N-nitrosobenzylmethylamine–induced esophageal tumors in animals. The effect of watercress consumption on xenobiotic metabolism in humans was investigated by studying the pharmacokinetics of acetaminophen and its metabolites after ingestion in the presence or absence of watercress.

Methods and Findings.—A 1-g oral dose of acetaminophen was given 10 hours after 50 g of watercress homogenates was ingested. When compared with acetaminophen only, watercress ingestion significantly decreased the area under the plasma cysteine acetaminophen (Cys-acetaminophen) concentration-time curve and the peak plasma Cys-acetaminophen concentration by 28% and 21%, respectively. The Cys-acetaminophen formation rate constant and Cys-acetaminophen formation fraction were reduced by 55% and 52%, respectively. Total urinary excretion of Cys-acetaminophen in 24 hours was also decreased, consistent with the results obtained from the plasma. Mercapturate acetaminophen, a Cys-acetaminophen metabolite, was also reduced in the plasma and urine samples. However, watercress ingestion did not significantly change the plasma pharmacokinetic processes and urinary excretion of acetaminophen, acetaminophen glucuronide, and acetaminophen sulfate.

Conclusions.—Watercress consumption causes a reduction in the levels of oxidative metabolites of acetaminophen. This is probably a result of the inhibition of oxidative metabolism of this drug.

▶ This impact of a watercress-derived ingredient on oxidative metabolism raises the possibility of using phenethyl isothiocyanate or watercress itself to lower the risk from certain drugs (such as hepatotoxicity from acetaminophen).

L. Lasagna, M.D.

Interaction Between Cyclosporin A and Nonsteroidal Antiinflammatory Drugs
Tugwell P, Ludwin D, Gent M, et al (Univ of Ottawa, Canada; McMaster Univ, Hamilton, Canada; Univ of Sydney, Darwin, Australia)
J Rheumatol 24:1122–1125, 1997   2–5

Introduction.—Most patients with rheumatoid arthritis (RA) who take cyclosporin A (CyA) also require nonsteroidal anti-inflammatory drugs (NSAIDs) for relief of joint pain and stiffness. Because both CyA and NSAIDs can affect renal function, there is concern that their combination might result in a clinically important difference in calculated creatinine clearance. This was examined in a study of 35 patients.

Methods.—The patients with RA received CyA when aspirin and other NSAIDs and at least 1 slow-acting antirheumatic drug failed to improve symptoms or had toxic effects. They were started at 2.5 mg/kg CyA/day, with the dosage increased carefully to 5 mg/kg/day or less if serum creatinine rose by ≥30% above baseline. After stabilization of the CyA dose (mean 171.43 mg/day), patients were randomized to 4-week periods of acetaminophen, indomethacin, ketoprofen, and sulindac. Data from the multiple crossover design were evaluated for joint count and pain level and for increases in calculated creatinine clearance.

Results.—Thirty-two patients completed the acetaminophen and at least 1 of the NSAID treatment periods. On average, the calculated creatinine clearance was increased by 2.79 mL/min (3.5%) for acetaminophen versus all 3 NSAIDs (6% for indomethacin, 2.3% for ketoprofen, and 2.6% for sulindac). This was well below the 25% increase regarded as clinically important, and in no patient did the calculated creatinine clearance increase or decrease by more than 15% after any treatment period. Acetaminophen was slightly less effective than the 3 NSAIDs in relieving joint pain and stiffness.

Conclusion.—Although sulindac is reported to have a lesser renal effect than other NSAIDs, none of the agents studied here produced a clinically important difference in the calculated creatinine clearance. Patients with RA should be able to continue with the NSAIDs of their or their physician's choice.

▶ In this case, the investigators were trying to find out whether different nonsteroidal antiinflammatory medications (NSAIDs) would differ in raising creatinine and blood pressure in cyclosporin-treated patients. The good news is that the 3 drugs studied, indomethacin, ketoprofen, and sulindac, did not differ among themselves or decrease renal function. The bad news is that sulindac was the same as the other 2 medications. It had been hoped that sulindac would be different from the other NSAIDs, and it wasn't.

M. Weintraub, M.D.

δ-Aminolevulinic Acid Dehydratase Genotype Modifies Four Hour Urinary Lead Excretion After Oral Administration of Dimercaptosuccinic Acid

Schwartz BS, Lee B-K, Stewart W, et al (Johns Hopkins, Baltimore; Soonchunhyang Univ, Chonan, Republic of Korea; Harvard School of Public Health, Boston)
Occup Environ Med 54:241–246, 1997   2–6

Background.—The binding of lead by δ-aminolevulinic acid dehydratase (ALAD) may vary by ALAD genotype. Whether ALAD genotype modifies urinary lead excretion (dimercaptosuccinic acid [DMSA] chelatable lead) after the oral administration of DMSA was determined.

Methods.—Fifty-seven male lead battery manufacturing workers in South Korea were selected randomly from 2 ALAD genotype strata from among 290 current workers. The 38 men with ALAD1–1 were frequency matched with 19 men with ALAD1–2 for duration of employment in the lead industry. The subjects were given 5 mg/kg oral DMSA, and urine was obtained for a 4-hour period.

Findings.—Concentrations of blood lead ranged from 11 to 53 μg/dl, with a mean of 25.4 μg/dl. After DMSA was taken, the workers excreted a mean 85.4 μg lead during the 4-hour urine collection. Workers with ALAD1–2 excreted a mean of 24 μg less than those with ALAD1–1, controlling for blood lead levels, exposure duration, current tobacco use, and body weight. The relation between plasma δ-aminolevulinic acid (ALA) and DMSA chelatable lead was modified by ALAD genotype. Men with ALAD1–2 excreted more lead after DMSA, with increasing plasma ALA, than did the men with ALAD1–1.

Conclusions.—DMSA chelatable lead may partially reflect the stores of bioavailable lead. The current findings indicated that men with ALAD1–2 have lower stores than those with ALAD1–1 and support the notion that ALAD genotype modifies the toxicokinetics of lead, possibly by differential binding of current lead stores or by differences in long-term retention and deposition of lead.

▶ Obviously, the genetic polymorphisms of many proteins are critically important to understanding drug effects such as metabolism and perhaps even pharmacodynamic outcomes. They are also important in the understanding of the relation between the chemical or toxin and the toxicity in people. Who would have thought you'd have to have a genetic polymorphism test to work in, for example, a factory making lead batteries.

M. Weintraub, M.D.

Potentiation of Mivacurium by Rocuronium Is Age- and Time-dependent: A Study in Children, Adolescents, and Young and Elderly Adults
Goudsouzian N, Martyn JA (Harvard Med School, Boston)
J Clin Pharmacol 37:649–655, 1997   2–7

Background.—The coadministration of rocuronium, a steroidal muscle relaxant, and mivacurium, a benzylisoquinolinium relaxant, results in potentiation. The effects of time and age on this interaction were investigated.

Methods.—Fifteen children, 15 adolescents, 15 young adults, and 15 elderly individuals were studied. The ulnar nerve–evoked force of contraction of the adductor pollicis (twitch response) was monitored. Paralysis was induced by administering 600 μg/kg of rocuronium. During recovery, mivacurium infusion was begun and maintained for at least 90 minutes to retain the twitch response at 1% to 9% of baseline tension.

Findings.—Rocuronium, 600 μg/kg, induced a greater than 95% paralysis in 57 of the 60 patients within 2.2 minutes. The recovery period to 5% of baseline twitch height was longest in the eldery and briefest in the adolescents (at 30.1 and 16.5 minutes, respectively). The amount of mivacurium infusion needed to maintain 95% paralysis was greatest in the children, increasing progressively with time. The infusion rates in young and elderly adults remained lower than in children and did not change with time. The incidence of satisfactory spontaneous recovery within 20 minutes was highest in the children, followed by the adolescents and young adults, and was lowest in the elderly individuals. The residual neuromuscular effect of rocuronium on the subsequent mivacurium infusion was most marked in the elderly, followed by the young adults, adolescents, and children.

Conclusions.—These findings suggest that mivacurium should not be administered after neuromuscular blockade with rocuronium to achieve relaxation for a short duration. The administration of the short-acting relaxant mivacurium results in paralysis of a longer duration than expected given its pharmacologic properties when used alone. This effect is more pronounced in adults, especially in the elderly. The potentiating effect may last for 2 hours or more after the initial dosage.

▶ The use of a nondepolarizing relaxant with a muscle relaxant of another type (benzylisoquinolinium in this case) shows potentiation of their neuromuscular effects. This study was done in groups of children, adolescents, young adults, and elderly patients so that careful monitoring of any differences among them would be possible. As is frequently the case, the children needed much less time to recover and the elderly needed more time to recover. I think this may be, in this case, related to the differences in pharmacokinetics between children and elderly patients in the elimination of rocuronium. However, the recovery of receptors—the authors suggest as a mechanism only 30% have to recover to show muscle twitching—may also play a role. We don't really know why potentiation occurred, just that it did, and it was more profound in the older patients.

M. Weintraub, M.D.

Progesterone-induced Changes in Sleep in Male Subjects
Friess E, Tagaya H, Trachsel L, et al (Max Planck Inst, Munich)
Am J Physiol 272:E885–E891, 1997   2–8

Background.—Progesterone administration is known to induce fatigue or reduce vigilance during wakefulness. Previous studies suggest that this effect is mediated by neuroactive metabolites that interact with the γ-aminobutyric acid$_A$ (GABA$_A$) receptor complex. Agonistic ligands of this complex shorten sleep onset latency, suppress the amount of rapid eye movement (REM) sleep, and increase non-REM sleep. A double-blind study was designed to investigate the effects of progesterone administration on the sleep electroencephalogram (EEG).

Methods.—Only men participated in the study so that interference from variations in endogenous progesterone secretion could be avoided. The 9 healthy volunteers had a mean age of 24.7 years. None had sleep disturbances or a family or personal history of psychiatric or neurological disorder. Two experimental sessions were conducted in a sleep laboratory. Polysomnographic recordings, including sleep stage-specific spectral analysis, were obtained at the same time as plasma concentrations of progesterone and its GABA-active metabolites were measured. In a crossover design, a single oral dose of 300 mg micronized progesterone or placebo was administered at 9:30 PM.

Results.—Administration of progesterone resulted in a clear elevation of progesterone concentration and of the reduced metabolites allopregnanolone and pregnanolone. Changes in non-REM sleep also occurred during the progesterone condition, with the amount of non-REM sleep showing a significant increase. The EEG spectral power during non-REM sleep decreased significantly in the slow wave frequency range (0.4 to 4.3 Hz), whereas there was a tendency toward elevated spectral power in the higher frequency range (less than 15 Hz).

Conclusion.—The progesterone-induced changes in sleep architecture and sleep-EEG power spectra are similar to those induced by agonistic modulators of the $GABA_A$ receptor complex. Such changes appear to be mediated in part by conversion of progesterone into its GABA-active metabolites allopregnanolone and pregnanolone.

▶ Who would have guessed that progesterone would be metabolized to $GABA_A$? Although crossover studies are, in general, less able to answer questions because of their carryover effects, this study was probably OK to run as a crossover. Although one may ask: "why study another chemical for its effect on sleep?" I think that the world needs a sleeping pill which can be given for long periods of time or can be used in patients who are resistant to the effects of other sleeping pills. Perhaps someone will be able to identify a portion of the progesterone molecule, or another aspect of this medication, which does not have the hormonal effects but still has the sleep-inducing properties.

M. Weintraub, M.D.

Bromfenac Disposition in Patients With Impaired Kidney Function
Ermer JC, Boni JP, Cevallos WH, et al (Wyeth-Ayerst Research, Princeton)
Clin Pharmacol Ther 61:312–318, 1997   2–9

Introduction.—Bromfenac, a new nonsteroidal anti-inflammatory drug with rapid clearance and a short half-life, has been used for pain relief after oral surgery and orthopedic surgery. The pharmacokinetic behavior of bromfenac in normal subjects, renally compromised patients, and patients with end-stage renal disease was compared to determine the need for dosage adjustment in chronic renal disease.

Methods.—Forty adults were enrolled in the study, 18 with normal kidney function, 12 with decreased kidney function, and 10 who were dialysis-dependent. After an overnight fast, participants were given a single 50 mg oral dose of bromfenac with 240 mL water. Venous blood samples were collected at various time points in the 24 hours after the 8 AM dose. Urine output was also collected from the normal and impaired groups. Members of the dialysis group took part in an intradialysis evaluation of bromfenac on the following day.

Results.—Mean peak concentrations of bromfenac ranged from 3.3 to 3.9 µg/ml in the 3 study groups; mean areas under the concentration versus time curve ranged from 5.1 to 6.9 µg·hr/ml. The mean unbound fraction in the dialysis group (0.29%) was nearly twice that in the impaired (0.16%) and normal (0.17%) groups. There were no differences in clearance, volume of distribution, or their free fraction-corrected counterparts in the 3 groups. Although half-life of the drug nearly doubled in the impaired and dialysis groups, it was shorter than the anticipated 8-hour dose interval. Concentrations of bromfenac in arterial and venous plasma during hemodialysis were not significantly different. The amount of bromfenac in urine accounted for less than 2% of the administered dose. Eleven adverse events were reported, but none led to withdrawal from the study.

Discussion.—Bromfenac is eliminated by hepatic metabolism, and renal dysfunction can lead to changes in the pharmacokinetics of compounds that are predominantly hepatically metabolized. The findings of this study do not indicate a need for dosage adjustment in patients with kidney impairment, but routine clinical monitoring is appropriate.

▶ Bromfenac is a recently released new analgesic medication for short-term (less than 10 days) administration. Many drugs are now coming to market with a renal study done in patients with decreased renal function and, in fact, in patients receiving chronic dialysis. This is to help doctors dose the drug for renal insufficiency and also to meet FDA requirements. These studies are somewhat harder to do than general pharmacokinetic studies, but they're worth doing.

M. Weintraub, M.D.

Ranitidine Improves Lymphocyte Function After Severe Head Injury: Results of a Randomized, Double-blind Study

Rixen D, Livingston DH, Loder P, et al (New Jersey Med School, Newark)
Crit Care Med 24:1787–1792, 1996   2–10

Background.—Ranitidine, which can reduce gastric acid secretion, is often prescribed for the prophylaxis or treatment of gastric/duodenal ulcer disease and for the prevention of gastrointestinal stress bleeding in the critically ill. This drug's potential immunomodulatory effect is important because critically ill patients are often immunosuppressed, and the immunomodulatory effect of H_2-receptor blockade in such patients is not known. The immunodulatory effect of ranitidine in severely head-injured patients admitted to the ICU was investigated in a randomized, prospective, double-blind study.

Methods.—Twenty patients with a Glasgow Coma Scale score of less than 10 were included. Nine patients received a continuous infusion of ranitidine, 6.25 mg/hr, and 11 received placebo for 5 days or less.

INTERLEUKIN-1
(Ref.1)

MAST CELLS   BASOPHILS

ANTIBODY SYNTHESIS (IgG) ↓
(Ref.2)

B-CELLS

HELPER T-CELLS ⟶ INTERLEUKIN-2 ↓
↓ (Ref.3)
INTERFERON GAMMA ↓

HISTAMINE

SUPPRESSOR T-CELLS
↓ (Ref.4)
HISTAMINE SUPPRESSOR FACTOR (HSF)

MONOCYTES ⟶ INTERLEUKIN-1 ↓ (Ref.5)

TUMOR NECROSIS FACTOR ALPHA ↓ (Ref.6)

PROSTAGLANDINS ↑ (Ref.7)

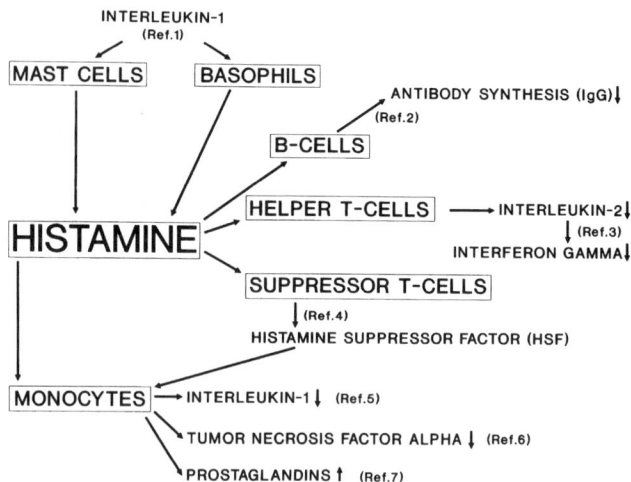

FIGURE 1.—Role of histamine in immunodepression. This bioamine is released from mast cells and basophils on contact with inflammatory stimuli. Histamine influences B lymphocytes, T lymphocytes, and monocytes, resulting in an overall immunodepression, with a downregulation of proinflammatory lymphokines (interleukin-2, interferon-γ) and monokines (interleukin-1, tumor necrosis factor-α) and an upregulation of immunosuppressive prostaglandins. (Courtesy of Rixen D, Livingston DH, Loder P, et al: Ranitidine improves lymphocyte function after severe head injury: Results of a randomized, double-blind study. *Crit Care Med* 24(II):1787–1792, 1996.)

Findings.—Ranitidine treatment increased CD4+ lymphocytes significantly, from 33% to 49%, and significantly reduced CD8+ lymphocytes, from 41% to 27%. Placebo had no effect on these values. The mitogen-stimulated interferon-γ production rose from 121 to 269 pg/mL in ranitidine recipients but was unchanged in placebo recipients. The 2 groups did not differ significantly in interleukin-2 production or circulating B-cell concentrations (Fig 1).

Conclusions.—These data are consistent with the notion that ranitidine has an immunostimulatory effect. A more thorough understanding of the benefits and risks of H₂-receptor antagonists in the treatment of critically ill and immunocompromised patients is needed.

▶ As shown in Figure 1, histamine has a complex role in the regulation of B and T cells in the regulation of immunodepression. It would seem logical then that ranitidine could cause an immunostimulatory effect by blocking histamine if the effect was histamine₂ mediated. Sometimes, in settings like this, one can find a reason for the effect of a medication on some sort of transmitter that is related to many things. Certainly, it's been true of many receptors and factors. Unfortunately, the human organism is so complex that it really will take several years to work out all the modulation of the immune system that ranitidine seems to be causing. It may, in fact, be true that ranitidine causes all the effects: however, it's also possible that it's an epiphenomenon.

M. Weintraub, M.D.

3 Adverse Reactions, Poisoning, and Drug Abuse

Factors Related to Errors in Medication Prescribing
Lesar TS, Briceland L, Stein DS (Albany Med Ctr, NY; Albany College of Pharmacy, NY; Albany Med College, NY)
JAMA 277:312–317, 1997   3–1

Introduction.—Errors in the prescribing and management of drug therapy are major causes of adverse drug events in hospitalized patients. A survey of prescribing errors in a tertiary care teaching hospital was designed to characterize specific factors associated with the errors.

Methods.—From July 1994 through June 1995, every third prescribing error detected and averted by pharmacists at the study institution was analyzed for potential adverse outcome and likely contributing factors. A physician and 2 pharmacists retrospectively evaluated the errors in order to reach a consensus on error type and significance.

Results.—During the 1-year study period, 2,103 errors of potential clinical importance were identified. The overall rate of errors was 3.99 per 1,000 medication orders. Of the 696 errors considered capable of causing adverse patient effects, 41.8% involved overdoses. Other error types were underdoses (16.5%) and prescribing drugs to which the patient was allergic (12.9%). The medications most often involved in prescribing errors were antimicrobials (39.7%) and cardiovascular agents (17.5%). Forty-three errors (6.2%) were rated as potentially fatal or severe, and a large proportion (83.7%) of these errors were related to the presence of patient allergy history. Errors related to knowledge and the application of knowledge regarding drug therapy accounted for 30% of incidents; knowledge and use of knowledge involving patient factors were implicated in 29.2%.

Conclusion.—Most prescribing errors involve a lack of knowledge of drug therapy or of patient characteristics. Recommended strategies to improve accuracy and reduce the risk to patients include standardization of processes, simplification of the system, computerization of the prescribing process, better prescriber education, and greater use of the expertise of pharmacists.

The Costs of Adverse Drug Events in Hospitalized Patients

Bates DW, Spell N, Cullen DJ, et al (Harvard Med School, Boston)
JAMA 277:307–311, 1997   3–2

Introduction.—Drugs are a leading cause of adverse events during hospitalization, and many adverse drug events (ADEs) are preventable. A previous study found that the average ADE increased hospital costs by almost $2,000, not including malpractice costs or the costs of injuries to patients. A prospective study was undertaken to better define ADE-associated costs.

Methods.—The study cohort included 4,108 admissions to medical and surgical units in 2 tertiary-care hospitals over a 6-month period. Cases were patients with an ADE; a control for each case was the patient on the same unit with the most similar pre-event length of stay. Incidents were identified by nurses, pharmacists, and chart review by nurse investigators. Two physician reviewers confirmed that an event was an ADE and classified it as preventable or not preventable.

Results.—Of the 247 identified ADEs, 57 were excluded as multiple episodes and length-of-stay outliers. Sixty of the remaining 190 ADEs were preventable. Approximately half of preventable ADEs were caused by 4 classes of drugs: analgesics (29%), sedatives (10%), antibiotics (9%), and antipsychotics (7%). Cardiovascular (21%), central nervous system (19%), and respiratory (9%) complications were most common among preventable ADEs. Multivariate analyses found the additional length of stay associated with all ADEs was 2.2 days; the increase in cost was $3,244. For preventable ADEs, hospitalization was increased by 4.6 days and costs by $5,857. In a 700–bed teaching hospital, annual costs are estimated to be $5.6 million for all ADEs and $2.8 million for preventable ADEs.

Conclusion.—Adverse drug events, particularly those that are preventable, add significantly to the cost of a patient's hospitalization. Malpractice costs and the costs of injuries to patients would further increase costs. In addition, admissions related to ADEs experienced by outpatients are projected to cost $76.6 billion nationwide on an annual basis.

▶ Many of the factors related to errors in prescribing medication will be corrected by the wider use of computers in ordering medications and calculating their doses (Abstract 3–1). This is important because of the dramatic costs related to adverse drug events and is detailed in the second study (Abstract 3–2). This study used a very good way to select the control group, choosing a patient with approximately the same duration of hospitalization before the adverse event occurred. Thus, the investigators could calculate the lengthening of hospitalization due to the adverse event. The detection of adverse events in the study patients was also excellent. They were detected by nurses, pharmacists, and chart review. I'm always a little mistrustful of the numbers on amount of money saved or, more particularly, spent on treating patients with adverse effects. Nonetheless, the figures quoted in this paper are conservative and reasonable. What we have to do is find out if we can prevent adverse drug reactions.

M. Weintraub, M.D.

Can Adverse Drug Reactions Be Detected Earlier? A Comparison of Reports by Patients and Professionals

Egberts TCG, Smulders M, de Koning FHP, et al (Utrecht Univ, The Netherlands; Netherlands Pharmacovigilance Found, Tilburg, The Netherlands)
BMJ 313:530–531, 1996   3–3

Background.—When a new drug is marketed, it is common for previously unknown adverse reactions to surface. Because these adverse reactions should be reported as soon as possible, some have suggested that patients report adverse events. Results of a study of patient vs. health care professional reporting times for adverse reactions to a newly introduced antidepressant drug are presented.

Methods.—A telephone information service sponsored by the Dutch Ministry of Health and the Royal Dutch Association for the Advancement of Pharmacy was set up to take calls about adverse drug reactions from patients.

Results.—Between 1992 and 1994, 120 of 23,625 calls reported adverse reactions to paroxetine, an antidepressant drug, whereas 89 of 7,665 adverse reactions reported by health care professionals to the Netherlands Pharmacovigilance Foundation were related to paroxetine. The average time lag for patient reporting was 229 days less than that for health care professional reporting. Nine new adverse reactions were identified by both reporting systems.

Conclusion.—Patient reporting of adverse reactions identifies new reactions sooner than does health care reporting; however, patient reporting tends to be less complete and may lead to false alarms. A combination of patient and health care professional reporting is probably the best system.

▶ The premise of this article, that patients can call in adverse reactions through a pharmacy quicker than do physicians, is a helpful one. The example is also good. However, patients should see their physician and report the adverse reaction. Patients and physicians should both think about reporting the reaction to the drug company and directly to the government. The Med Watch system here in the United States allows just that. It is run by the Food and Drug Administration and the phone number is (800) 332–1088. Physicians, patients, and pharmacists can report by telephone or by fax, with the assurance that someone will review the reports.

M. Weintraub, M.D.

Adverse Drug Events in Hospitalized Patients: Excess Length of Stay, Extra Costs, and Attributable Mortality
Classen DC, Pestotnik SL, Evans RS, et al (LDS Hosp, Salt Lake City, Utah)
JAMA 277:301–306, 1997   3–4

Introduction.—Adverse drug events (ADEs) account for a major proportion of drug-related morbidity and mortality, and may be responsible for as many as 140,000 deaths in the United States each year. Approximately 30% of hospitalized patients have an adverse event attributable to drugs during their stay. There are no specific data regarding the effects of ADEs on mortality, length of hospital stay, or resource utilization. The impact of ADEs during hospitalization on length of stay, costs, and mortality was analyzed.

Methods.—The case-control study included 1,580 patients with ADEs occurring during their stay at a tertiary care hospital. They were matched to 20,197 control subjects for primary discharge diagnosis related group, age, sex, acuity, and year of admission. The 2 groups were compared for mortality and length of stay, both crude and attributable to ADEs. Hospital costs were compared as well.

Results.—The rate of ADEs during the 4-year period studied was 2.43 per 100 hospital admissions. The crude mortality rate was 3.5% for the patients with ADEs vs. 1.05% for the controls. The mean length of stay was 7.69 days for cases vs. 4.46 days for controls, with an extra 1.74 days attributable to ADEs. The mean hospital costs were $10,010 vs. $5,355, with an extra cost of $2,013 attributable to ADEs. On linear regression analysis, an ADE increased the length of stay by 1.91 days and hospital costs by $2,262. In a logistic regression analysis, patients with an ADE had a 1.88 times higher risk of death.

Conclusions.—Adverse drug events carry a significant impact for hospitalized patients. These events are associated with increased lengths of stay, higher hospital costs, and a nearly doubled risk of death. Adverse drug events have major potential costs to the hospital as well as to the nation as a whole. The authors advocate a system-wide approach to improving the processes of drug use, including monitoring for ADEs.

▶ There is no doubt about the somatic, psychic, and economic costs of ADEs. But the emphasis, in my view, should not be on collective hand-wringing, but rather on how to prevent the preventable. It is the latter I resent, not the ADEs that could neither have been predicted nor forestalled.

L. Lasagna, M.D.

Adverse Nondrug Reactions: An Update

Meyer FP, Tröger U, Röhl F-W (Otto-von-Guericke Univ, Magdeburg, Germany)

Clin Pharmacol Ther 60:347–352, 1996   3–5

Introduction.—Thirty years ago, Reidenberg and Lowenthal reported on psychopharmacologic problems in healthy medical student volunteers in Philadelphia. Seventy-four percent reported they had experienced symptoms in the preceding 72 hours that were typically described as side effects of drugs. This investigation was repeated in a different cultural area (Central Europe) to determine whether the findings from 30 years ago are still relevant today.

Methods.—One hundred thirty medical students completed the "Questionnaire for Side Effects of Drugs," the same tool used in 1968 by Reidenberg and Lowenthal. Respondents were asked whether any symptoms listed in the questionnaire had occurred in the previous 72 hours. Personality traits, motivation, and emotional state were evaluated using the Freiburg Personality Inventory, the Motivational Q-Sort, and the State-Trait Anxiety Inventory, respectively. None of the volunteers were taking any drugs at the time of evaluation.

Results.—The most frequent complaints of healthy volunteers not taking any medications were fatigue (65%), nasal congestion (30%), and headache (25%). Only 11% of respondents reported they had no symptoms. Three percent reported more than 6 symptoms. Volunteers who had less than 3 complaints were less nervous, had higher motivation, were more stable emotionally, and were less anxious than respondents who had 3 or more symptoms.

Conclusions.—The incidence of fatigue and of headache were markedly higher in the present group, compared to the Philadelphia group of 30 years ago. There was a weak positive correlation between having more than 3 symptoms and being more nervous, having lower motivation, having less emotional stability, and having more anxiety.

▶ In 1968, Reidenberg and Lowenthal[1] reported that, of 239 healthy medical students and hospital staff, only 16% had not experienced any symptoms in the previous 3 days that could be considered side effects of drugs. This recent study confirms the 1968 findings and reminds us of the value of placebo controls in distinguishing between true drug side effects and spontaneous adverse events unrelated to the drug under study.

L. Lasagna, M.D.

Reference

1. Reidenberg MM, Lowenthal DT: Adverse nondrug reactions. *N Engl J Med* 279:678–679, 1968.

Safety Issues in Herbal Medicine: Implications for the Health Professions

Drew AK, Myers SP (Newcastle Mater Misericordiae Hosp, Australia; Southern Cross Univ, Lismore, Australia)

Med J Aust 166:538–541, 1997

3–6

Introduction.—The increased use of herbal medicine in developed countries raises concerns about the safety of these preparations and the possibility of adverse drug reactions (ADRs). An Australian study proposes a classification of ADRs of herbal medicines and recommends that physicians question patients on their use of "complementary and alternative medicine" (CAM).

Use and Regulation of Herbal Medicines.—A 1993 survey in South Australia found that 48.5% of respondents had used at least 1 form of CAM preparation in the previous year; 20% had visited at least 1 alternative practitioner. Products for human medicinal use are listed or registered in Australia by the Register of Therapeutic Goods. Listed products contain substances of low public health concern and cannot claim to "treat" conditions. Registered products contain agents that are restricted or raise health concerns and require documentation of clinical trial work. In practice, most CAM preparations are not exposed to the same premarketing evaluation process as prescription and scheduled proprietary medicines. Many "natural" products have been associated with ADRs, but it is difficult to find information about effects of a specific preparation in the medical literature.

Proposed Classification of Adverse Effects.—The ADRs of herbal medications may be intrinsic (caused by the herb itself) or extrinsic (caused by failure of good manufacturing process). Type A intrinsic reactions are predictable and dose-dependent, whereas type B intrinsic reactions are unpredictable and idiosyncratic. Causes of extrinsic adverse effects include misidentification of ingredients, product variation, contamination, and inappropriate labeling or advertising.

Conclusion.—It is essential that ADRs be reported for CAM products. Physicians should routinely question patients about CAM use and include CAM products in ADR reports. Because of batch-to-batch variations, a CAM used long term without ill effects may subsequently be the cause of an ADR. There should also be some way for consumers and alternative practitioners to report adverse effects of CAM preparations.

▶ Although this study is from Australia, the same considerations exist here in the United States. Physicians have to learn to take better patient histories, including use of complementary or alternative medicine as well as the use of prescription drugs and over-the-counter medications. Also, as we have seen, the herbal medications may be contaminated with prescription drugs. The doses of medication may differ from batch to batch and also cause major adverse effects. For the alternative medications, the authors recommend a special data base to promote adverse drug reaction reporting. This will be difficult but worth the effort, if we can only figure out how to do it.

M. Weintraub, M.D.

Adulteration by Synthetic Therapeutic Substances of Traditional Chinese Medicines in Taiwan

Huang WF, Wen K-C, Hsiao M-L (Inst of Health and Welfare Policy; Natl Yang-Ming Univ; Natl Labs of Foods and Drugs, Taipei, Taiwan; et al)
J Clin Pharmacol 37:344–350, 1997   3–7

Background.—The adulteration of traditional Chinese medicines by synthetic therapeutic substances is a public health concern in Taiwan. In 1992, a large-scale effort was begun to screen traditional Chinese medicines suspected of adulteration.

Methods.—Eight major general hospitals in Taiwan collected a total of 2,609 samples through physicians' referrals during patient visits. Hospital pharmacists analyzed the samples using standard procedures compared with references by thin-layer chromatography.

Findings.—A mean 23.7% of the samples were found to be adulterated. Four samples with a rheumatoid or anti-inflammatory indication contained 6 different kinds of adulterants. Fifty-three percent of the adulterated medicines contained at least 2 adulterants.

Conclusions.—Taiwanese health authorities should continue to monitor and provide screening services to detect adulteration in traditional Chinese medicines. Public education on the health hazards of affected medicines is also warranted.

Herbal Products in Canada: How Safe Are They?

Kozyrskyj A (Univ of Manitoba, Winnipeg, Canada)
Can Fam Physician 43:697–702, 1997   3–8

Background.—A resurgence of interest in herbal medicine has occurred in North America in the past 10 years, attributed to the current trend toward naturalness. A recent survey showed that 1 in 5 Canadians has used some form of alternative treatment. The safety of herbal products was discussed.

Methods and Findings.—The Canadian Food and Drug Act and findings of an Expert Advisory Committee on Herbs and Botanical Preparations provided an overview of herbal product regulation in Canada. In addition, case reports of herbal toxicity were identified. In Canada, herbal products that are not registered as drugs are sold as foods. These products are exempt from the drug review process that assesses safety and efficacy. Thus, the public is at risk of undesired effects from herbal products adulterated with other substances and of missing effective conventional treatment. Consumers are also exposed to a great deal of information that portrays herbal products as harmless.

Conclusions.—Most of the herbal products assessed were ineffective or unsafe or had not been studied to determine efficacy. Physicians need to be aware that herbal treatments can be harmful. In Canada, some progress has been made by registering herbal products as drugs.

Association of Nonsteroidal Antiinflammatory Drugs With Outcome in Upper and Lower Gastrointestinal Bleeding
Wilcox CM, Clark WS (Emory Univ, Atlanta, Ga; Grady Mem Hosp, Atlanta, Ga)
Dig Dis Sci 42:985–989, 1997   3–9

Objective.—Nonsteroidal antiinflammatory drugs (NSAIDs) are strongly associated with lower gastrointestinal bleeding (LGIB). Because there are few studies documenting the outcome of such bleeding, incidences of upper gastrointestinal bleeding (UGIB) or LGIB and their relationship to prescription and over-the-counter NSAID use were evaluated prospectively.

Methods.—Between August 1, 1990, and September 30, 1994, NSAID use among consecutive patients with UGIB (n=785) or LGIB (n=161) in a large hospital was determined. Endoscopy, transfusions, hospitalization, surgery, and death were recorded.

Results.—The use of NSAIDs was associated with 60% of UGIB and 52% of LGIB. The most common causes of UGIB were gastric ulcer (24%), duodenal ulcer (24%), esophageal varices (8%), and Mallory-Weiss tear (6%). The most common causes of LGIB were diverticulosis (55%), colonic ulcer (9.3%), colon cancer (6%), and vascular ectasia (5%). NSAID users with UGIB were significantly older and female, but they had significantly fewer rebleeding episodes, shorter hospitalization stays, and lower mortality. When age and sex were controlled for, these latter 3 variables remained significant. NSAID users and nonusers with LGIB differed only by sex; significantly more NSAID users were male.

Conclusion.—NSAID users with gastrointestinal bleeding did not have a worse prognosis than nonusers. NSAID users with UGIB had significantly fewer rebleeding episodes, shorter hospitalization stays, and lower mortality when compared with nonusers.

▶ The data in this epidemiologic study may have occurred just by chance, but they are worth looking at and evaluating in future studies. The patients with UGIB were, again, the usual excess of female and older persons. However, the people who had used NSAIDS had a shorter hospital stay, less rebleeding, and less hospital mortality. The population was quite different, however, as it was predominantly black and inner-city. As might be predicted, the course of LGIB was not affected by having taken NSAIDS. Still, it's a puzzlement as to why the data turned out this way. The observations fly in the face of other epidemiologic data. Perhaps the investigators at Grady Hospital should resurvey their population.

M. Weintraub, M.D.

Evidence of Aspirin Use in Both Upper and Lower Gastrointestinal Perforation

Lanas A, Serrano P, Bajador E, et al (Hosp Clinico, Zaragoza, Spain; Hosp Miguel Servet, Zaragoza, Spain)
Gastroenterology 112:683–689, 1997   3–10

Background.—Neither the risk factors for gastrointestinal perforation nor the association between gastrointestinal perforation and nonsteroidal anti-inflammatory drugs (NSAIDs) are well known. Results of various studies of the relationship between use of NSAIDs and ulcer perforation have been inconsistent. The use of this type of drug may be related to upper and lower gastrointestinal bleeding, but a relationship to lower gastrointestinal perforation is not clear.

Methods.—In an attempt to find a relationship, 76 consecutive patients with gastrointestinal perforation and 152 control subjects were studied. Blood samples were tested for platelet cyclooxygenase activity and *Helicobacter pylori*. A clinical history and information about drug use were obtained in an interview.

Results.—Of the 76 patients, 78.9% had upper gastrointestinal perforation and 21% had lower gastrointestinal perforation. There was evidence of use of NSAIDs in 71% of patients and 26.9% of control subjects. Serology tests showed evidence of aspirin use in 12.7% more patients than those who reported using aspirin. In 66.6% of cases, the NSAID used was aspirin, and in 59.25% of cases, the NSAID used was nonprescription. Independent risk factors were smoking, alcohol, and a history of arthritis or peptic ulcer, but not a positive serology test for *H. pylori*.

Discussion.—In these patients, a strong association between the use of NSAIDs and upper and lower gastrointestinal perforation was found. The role of aspirin in gastrointestinal perforation may be underestimated.

▶ Aspirin and the newer NSAIDs are now acknowledged by all to increase the risk of gastrointestinal bleeding. The risk of gastrointestinal perforation from these drugs has been less well studied, but it looks as though in both the upper and the lower gastrointestinal tract, bleeding sites, perforations, or both can develop.

L. Lasagna, M.D.

Acetaminophen-related Acute Renal Failure Without Fulminant Liver Failure
Eguia L, Materson BJ (Univ of Miami, Fla)
Pharmacotherapy 17:363–370, 1997   3–11

Background.—Acetaminophen toxicity can cause acute renal failure, typically occurring in the setting of fulminant hepatic failure. The associated mortality rate is high and hepatorenal syndrome or acute tubular necrosis from hypotension in the terminal stage of illness is common. Acute renal failure from acetaminophen toxicity can also occur without fulminant liver failure, hepatic encephalopathy, hypotension, or evidence of liver disease.

Methods.—The medical records of patients with acetaminophen toxicity, but no fulminant hepatic failure or hypotension were reviewed. One patient was treated by the authors and 34 patients were identified from the literature. Clinical and laboratory features of acetaminophen nephrotoxicity were examined.

Results.—Of 31 patients, 23 had oliguria. Peak serum creatinine levels were similar in patients treated and not treated with N-acetylcysteine. Acute renal failure occurred 2 to 5 days after overdose. Peak serum creatinine levels occurred 3 to 16 days after overdose. Hemodialysis was required in 13 patients, 12 of whom were oliguric. In all patients, renal failure was spontaneously reversible.

Discussion.—Acute renal failure from acetaminophen toxicity can occur without fulminant hepatic failure, although this is uncommon. Acetaminophen-induced acute hepatic failure can also occur without renal toxicity. Acute acetaminophen toxicity must be considered in the differential diagnosis of hepatic and renal disease.

▶ Acetaminophen is generally regarded as a hepatotoxin but innocent with regard to renal toxicity. This article reminds us that the literature testifies to the rare, but real, nephrotoxicity seen with this excellent analgesic. I especially liked the admission by the authors that their electronic record search failed to identify their own index case!

L. Lasagna, M.D.

Late Increase in Acetaminophen Concentration After Overdose of Tylenol Extended Relief
Bizovi KE, Aks SE, Paloucek F, et al (Univ of Illinois, Chicago; Mercy Hosp and Med Ctr, Chicago; Northwestern Mem Hosp, Chicago)
Ann Emerg Med 28:549–551, 1996   3–12

Objective.—There are few data on the management of patients who take an overdose of extended-release acetaminophen (Tylenol Extended Relief). A patient with a late rise in acetaminophen concentration after taking this preparation was seen.

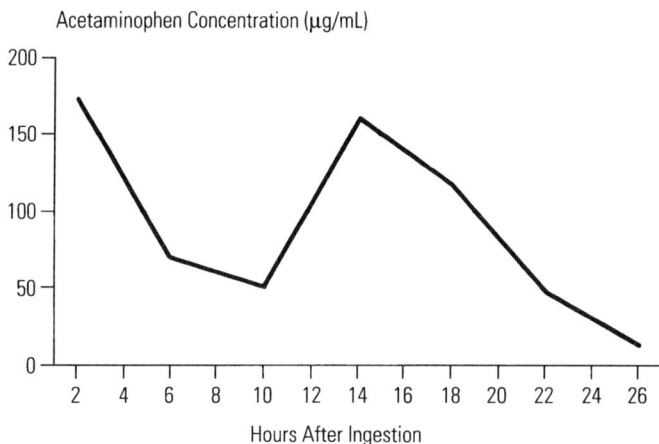

Acetaminophen Concentration (µg/mL)

Hours After Ingestion

FIGURE.—Acetaminophen levels after ingestion. The drug was undetectable 30, 34, 38, and 42 hours after ingestion. (Courtesy of Bizovi KE, Aks SE, Paloucek F, et al: Late increase in acetaminophen concentration after overdose of Tylenol Extended Relief. *Ann Emerg Med* 28[5]:549–551, 1996.)

Case.—Woman, 25, was seen 1.5 hours after a suicide attempt. She had taken up to 67 extended-release acetaminophen tablets plus 8 ounces of Nyquil. Her total acetaminophen dose was estimated at 43.55 g for the tablets plus another 4.5 g from the Nyquil. Her serum acetaminophen concentration reached hepatotoxic levels at 14 hours after ingestion and thereafter, according to the Rumack-Matthew nomogram (Figure). The patient recovered after treatment with activated charcoal and *N*-acetylcysteine.

Discussion.—This patient had a late increase in serum acetaminophen concentration after taking an overdose of extended-release acetaminophen. It is difficult to draw conclusions because of her concomitant ingestion of drugs known to slow gastrointestinal tract motility. However, this case questions the use of the Rumack-Matthew nomogram in patients who have overdosed on extended-release acetaminophen. Prolonged monitoring of drug concentrations is indicated in patients overdosing on Tylenol Extended Relief plus drugs that slow gastrointestinal tract motility.

► Overdose with ordinary acetaminophen is well understood and can be rationally treated. Extended-release acetaminophen (Tylenol Extended Relief) has not been the subject of extensive scrutiny in the overdose situation.

The present case is admittedly complicated, because the patient took not only a lot of Tylenol but a big dose of liquid Nyquil to commit suicide. In addition, she was taking paroxetine, synthroid, thioridazine, clonidine, omeprazole, and Bactrim. Whew!

The available data on extended-release acetaminophen in the *absence* of co-ingestants would not lead me to expect a delayed second peak level in the blood. The findings in this case are probably explainable by a combination of factors—rapid absorption of the acetaminophen in the liquid Nyquil and much delayed absorption of the Tylenol as a consequence of the intake of dextromethorphan and doxylamine in the Nyquil.

The better part of valor, however, is to *not* just measure serum acetaminophen 4 hours after ingestion of Tylenol Extended Release and again 4–6 hours later, but to run a few extra blood samples later on.

L. Lasagna, M.D.

Perioperative Acute Renal Failure Associated With Preoperative Intake of Ibuprofen
Sivarajan M, Wasse L (Univ of Washington, Seattle; Veterans Affairs Puget Sound Health Care System, Seattle)
Anesthesiology 86:1390–1392, 1997   3–13

Purpose.—Nonsteroidal anti-inflammatory drugs (NSAIDs) inhibit the synthesis of prostaglandin, which is required for renal blood flow, especially when circulating blood volume is reduced. This has led to the recommendation that NSAIDs be withheld before surgery, to avoid renal dysfunction. However, there have been no reports of such renal dysfunction resulting from NSAID administration, leading some to suggest that the perioperative restrictions on its use be loosened. A case of perioperative acute renal failure in a patient who took ibuprofen before surgery was reported.

> *Case.*—Man, 38, with a long history of back pain, was admitted for lumbar diskectomy. He had a history of alcohol abuse and drug-seeking behavior, and was taking prescribed acetaminophen/codeine and meperidine up to the day before surgery. Preoperative physical examination, hemogram, and urinalysis were normal. The patient's urine output fell dramatically during the operation, and persisted overnight. Laboratory tests suggested renal failure, with no evidence of urinary tract obstruction on renal ultrasound. The patient admitted taking ibuprofen, 600 mg 4 times a day up to the night before surgery, despite having been instructed to stop taking it the week before. The diagnosis of acute tubular necrosis was made. Renal function improved with conservative treatment using IV potassium-free solutions. The patient was fully recovered at 6-week follow-up.

Discussion.—A case of perioperative acute tubular necrosis in a patient who took ibuprofen before back surgery was reported. Ibuprofen is a possible cause of renal injury in this case, although other possibilities must be considered in this unreliable patient. The prognosis of NSAID-related acute tubular necrosis is good, if recognized early.

▶ While preoperative and postoperative analgesics benefit patients undergoing minor outpatient procedures, it is important to remember that drug-induced benefit of any kind is likely to be associated with some risk.

This young patient's acute renal failure was deemed attributable to NSAID-induced acute tubular necrosis. If recognized early, the drug culprit stopped, and K⁺-free parenteral solutions administered, prompt recovery can be expected in such cases.

L. Lasagna, M.D.

Comparative Effects of Nabumetone, Sulindac, and Ibuprofen on Renal Function
Cook ME, Wallin JD, Thakur VD, et al (LSU Med School, New Orleans; Tulane Univ, New Orleans, La; SmithKline Beecham, Philadelphia)
J Rheumatol 24:1137–1144, 1997   3–14

Background.—Various renal syndromes have been linked to nonsteroidal anti-inflammatory drugs (NSAIDs), whether through inhibition of prostaglandin synthesis or idiosyncratic reactions. Among these conditions is reversible, hemodynamically mediated, acute renal failure, with the evidence suggesting that different NSAIDs vary in their potential to cause this effect. The renal effects of 3 different NSAIDS—ibuprofen, sulindac, and nabumetone—were compared.

Methods.—Seventeen patients aged 56 years or older who had hypertension, treated with hydrochlorothiazide and fosinopril, and osteoarthritis requiring NSAID treatment were studied. They received nabumetone, sulindac, and ibuprofen in random order to compare the renal effects of these drugs. Each drug was given for 1 month, with 2-week control periods in between. The effects on renal function were assessed by measuring inulin and para-amunophippurate clearances and urinary prostaglandins.

Results.—There were no statistically significant differences between the 3 NSAIDs. However, 4 patients had a clinically significant decrease in renal function during ibuprofen treatment. During sulindac treatment, 1 of these same patients had another reduction in renal function. There were no such occurrences during nabumetone treatment. In the overall sample, estimated glomerular hydrostatic pressure and afferent and efferent arteriolar resistances were unchanged during the 3 treatments. However, in the patients who had decreased renal function while taking ibuprofen, glomerular hydrostatic pressure decreased by 15% while afferent arteriolar resistance increased by 85%. Along with these changes, the patients with ibuprofen-related decreases in renal function showed marked reductions in vasodilatory prostaglandins.

Conclusions.—Various NSAIDs differ in their effects on renal function in patients at risk. These effects are linked to specific alterations in suppression of the cyclo-oxygenase system cascade, and to changes in hemodynamic control of glomerular filtration. A risk of decreased renal function with ibuprofen was demonstrated in hypertensive patients treated with diuretics and angiotensin-converting enzyme inhibitors; more research is needed to assess patients with other at-risk conditions.

▶ The NSAIDs can cause a variety of renal syndromes, for which the elderly seem in general more at risk, as are individuals with decreased effective arterial blood volume. While this group of drugs have some things in common, differences also exist. This article supports the contention that these differences may at times be clinically important.

L. Lasagna, M.D.

Outcome of Acetaminophen Overdose in Pediatric Patients and Factors Contributing to Hepatotoxicity
Rivera-Penera T, Gugig R, Davis J, et al (Univ of California, Los Angeles; Valley Children's Hosp, Fresno, Calif; Cedars-Sinai Med Ctr, Los Angeles; et al)
J Pediatr 130:300–304, 1997   3–15

Objective.—Acetaminophen is a widely used drug that causes liver toxicity in overdose. Research has shown that adolescents are unaware of the dangers of this drug. This study evaluates the outcomes of pediatric acetaminophen overdose, including factors contributing to hepatotoxicity.

Methods.—The retrospective study included 73 children and adolescents with acetaminophen overdose and no previous history of liver disease. Thirty-eight percent of patients had abnormal liver test results. All of these patients had severe hepatotoxicity, and 6 required a liver transplant. The remaining patients were managed medically, with most receiving and responding to treatment with N-acetylcysteine (NAC). Two-thirds of the patients with normal liver function tests had toxic serum acetaminophen levels and were given NAC. None of this group had liver failure develop. The patients with abnormal liver tests tended to be younger and had longer delays in getting to the hospital. The patients with normal liver test results had earlier symptoms, often after taking a single, massive overdose. When severe hepatotoxicity developed in a young child, it was always related to multiple overdoses mistakenly given by the parents.

Conclusions.—Liver toxicity caused by acetaminophen overdose is a serious problem. In young children, mistaken overdose by parents is the major cause; in adolescents, it may result from "suicide gestures." The public and physicians alike need to be made aware of the dangers of acetaminophen overdose.

▶ Acetaminophen is safe and effective for most patients. But overdose can produce severe hepatic damage and may necessitate liver transplantation. Parental misguidance and suicide gestures were major causes of overdose in these patients.

L. Lasagna, M.D.

Refining the Level for Anticipated Hepatotoxicity in Acetaminophen Poisoning

Brandwene EL, Williams SR, Tunget-Johnson C, et al (Univ of California, San Diego; San Diego Regional Poison Ctr, Calif)
J Emerg Med 14:691–695, 1996   3–16

Introduction.—The treatment of an acetaminophen (APAP) overdose is frequently based on the position of the 4-hour APAP concentration on the Rumack-Matthew nomogram. The level at which clinically relevant hepatotoxicity occurs has not been determined. Data from the San Diego Regional Poison Control Center were reviewed to determine the level of clinically relevant hepatotoxicity in all acute adult formulation APAP exposures reported from 1986 to 1993.

Methods.—A chart review of all adult formulation APAP exposures during a 7-year period was conducted retrospectively. All patients with 4-hour serum APAP levels of 150–200 µg/mL, or the extrapolated equivalent on the treatment nomogram, were identified. Patients with significant risk of hepatotoxicity who were treated with N-acetylcysteine (NAC) when the overdose level fell within possible toxicity range were excluded.

Results.—A total of 3,329 patients with adult formulation APAP exposures were reported. Most ingestions were not significant and treatment was not indicated. Of 28 patients identified as falling into the possible toxicity range on the nomogram, 5 patients were excluded and treated with a full course of NAC because of risk factors; 6 were treated with a maximum of 2 doses of NAC; and 17 patients received no NAC. There were no fatalities, and there was no clinical or laboratory evidence of hepatotoxicity in patients either treated or not treated with NAC. All patients were symptom-free on telephone follow-up at 24 and 48 hours postingestion.

Conclusions.—A review of 7 years of data from a poison center revealed that there was no evidence of hepatotoxicity with adult formulation APAP poisoning in patients with no risk factors and APAP levels in the "possible risk" range. These patients may not need NAC therapy.

▶ This is another counterintuitive review of 7 years of data from the San Diego Regional Poison Center. The authors found no evidence of hepatotoxicity in patients whose acetaminophen levels fell in the toxic range and who did not have either decreased glutathione stores or increased mixed-function oxidase activity. Their conclusion is that those patients may not need NAC treatment. The reason this is so counterintuitive is that individuals would tend to be more sensitized than less sensitized to acetaminophen toxicity. However, doctors in the United Kingdom use a blood level range from 100 to 200 µg/mL, and that really doesn't provide my confidence great support and comfort. A large prospective study needs to be done with careful monitoring of everything, including risk factors.

M. Weintraub, M.D.

Treatment of Toad Venom Poisoning With Digoxin-specific Fab Fragments

Brubacher JR, Ravikumar PR, Bania T, et al (New York City Dept of Health; Bellevue Hosp Ctr, New York)
Chest 110:1282–1288, 1996   3–17

Introduction.—Many toads will secrete a protective venom that is similar in structure to digoxin from their parotid glands when threatened. In China, dried toad venom, otherwise known as Chan Su, is used as traditional medication. There have been reports of human poisonings from toad venom in Taiwan and the United States. The treatment of a series of patients with severe toxic reactions after the ingestion of a topical aphrodisiac similar to Chan Su that was marketed in New York City was described.

Methods.—Six patients, who were previously healthy young men, ingested the product marketed as a topical aphrodisiac. They all developed vomiting and bradycardia, and a clinical course that was similar to digoxin toxicity. Digoxin immunoassay showed that they all had positive apparent digoxin levels. Despite resuscitative attempts, the first 4 patients died of cardiac dysrhythmia. Digoxin Fab fragments (Digibind) were used successfully to treat the other 2 patients.

Results.—An analysis of the product showed that when dissolved, it was strongly positive for digoxin. It was sold in New York City as "Rock Hard" or "Love Stone." Bufotenine, a hallucinogen found in a South American plant and in toad venom, was identified. If the topical aphrodisiac were made from toad venom, it could cause the desired "aphrodisiac" effect by delaying ejaculation by decreasing penile sensation because toad venom is a potent local anesthetic.

Conclusions.—This was the first use of digoxin Fab fragments to treat patients poisoned by toad venom; previous treatments have included gastric decontamination and supportive care. The decision to administer digoxin-specific antibody fragments must be made on clinical grounds, given the lack of accurate prognostic markers. The empiric administration of large doses of digoxin Fab fragments (10 vials) is recommended for all patients with suspected cardioactive steroid overdose who have hyperkalemia or any abnormalities in cardiac rhythm. This recommendation is justified by the high fatality rate of these patients and apparent efficacy of digoxin Fab fragments.

▶ Although dried toad venom is a traditional remedy in China and other Asian countries, it is also potentially a cause of serious toxicity. These cases certainly resembled digitalis toxicity, they were positive for apparent serum digoxin levels by immunoassay, and 2 were treated successfully by these smart scientists with digoxin-specific Fab fragments. We are told that these alleged aphrodisiacs are no longer being exported to the United States. I hope that is true, but in case it is not, remember the successful application of Fab fragments to counteract cardioactive non-digoxin steroids such as are found in red squid, oleander, and toad venom.

L. Lasagna, M.D.

Minocycline-induced Scleral Pigmentation
Fraunfelder FT, Randall JA (Oregon Health Sciences Univ, Portland)
Ophthalmology 104:936–938, 1997   3–18

Objective.—Minocycline rarely causes important adverse effects, although cases of skin pigmentation have been reported. Four previously reviewed cases and 3 new cases of scleral pigmentation were discussed.

Discussion.—Scleral color bands of 3 to 5 mm in width associated with oral minocycline have been described as blue-gray and also as dark metallic blue, black, or brownish. Color may be deeper in light-exposed areas. The discoloration may take 4 years or more to fade or may be permanent, and discoloration may be reason to discontinue the medication. The cause of the pigmentation is unknown, but iron-containing products are suspected.

Conclusion.—Minocycline can cause blue sclerae that can last for 4 or more years or can become permanent.

▶ Minocycline can cause pigmentation in skin, teeth, nails, mucosa, thyroid, and bones. Scleral involvement is rare; these reports on 3 cases join 4 published previously and 2 cases reported to the National Registry of Drug-Induced Ocular Side Effects. There are apparently 27 medical explanations for blue sclerae.

L. Lasagna, M.D.

Serious Adverse Reactions Induced by Minocycline: Report of 13 Patients and Review of the Literature
Knowles SR, Shapiro L, Shear NH (Univ of Toronto)
Arch Dermatol 132.934–939, 1996   3–19

Objective.—Serious and rare adverse reactions have been associated with the antiacne drug minocycline. Reports of patients with hypersensitivity syndrome reaction (HSR), serum sickness–like reaction (SSLR), and drug-induced lupus (DIL) and a review of the literature on adverse reactions associated with minocycline are presented.

Methods.—The records of 160 patients admitted to the Adverse Drug Reaction Clinic at Sunnybrook Health Science Centre, Toronto, with any of the 3 aforementioned adverse reactions possibly induced by minocycline were reviewed. The records review identified 6 patients with HSR, 6 with SSLR, and 1 with DIL. The literature review found 11 reports of HSR, 1 of SSLR, and 24 of DIL.

Case 1.—Girl, 16 years, had fever and headache 3 weeks after starting minocycline therapy. Although minocycline therapy was discontinued and erythromycin therapy was begun, a rash on her face spread, lymphadenopathy developed, and she had a fever of 40°C and abnormal liver function test results.

Case 2.—Woman, 22, experienced urticarial eruptions 9 days after beginning minocycline therapy. Despite treatment with epinephrine and diphenhydramine, fever, conjunctivitis, arthralgia, and lymphadenopathy developed. The patient was treated successfully with parenteral steroids, antihistamine, and oral prednisone.

Case 3.—Woman, 43, had polyarthritis after 10 days of taking minocycline. She discontinued the medication and her symptoms resolved. When she resumed the medication, her arthritis returned. She was found to have synovitis and elevated erythrocyte sedimentation rate, alanine aminotransferase level, aspartate aminotransferase level, and antinuclear antibodies. Her symptoms resolved when she stopped taking the drug.

Conclusion.—Fever, rash, and internal organ involvement can herald possibly life-threatening adverse reactions in patients taking the antiacne drug minocycline. Recognizing these side effects early is critically important.

▶ The most interesting thing about this article is where it comes from. It was written by individuals who work in the Adverse Drug Reactions Clinic, as well as in other parts of a Canadian hospital. I am not aware of too many adverse reaction clinics in the United States. With the merger mania in hospitals and therefore, the inclusion of more patients, although in separate buildings, we may need similar clinics. Also, with the new-drug quick approvals by the Food and Drug Administration, an adverse drug reaction clinic will be helpful in guiding physicians practicing at an institution.

P.S. Minocycline has been studied as a potential treatment for rheumatoid arthritis. Therefore, patient 3 is of particular interest.

M. Weintraub, M.D.

Sulfadiazine-associated Nephrotoxicity in Patients With the Acquired Immunodeficiency Syndrome
Becker K, Jablonowski H, Häussinger D (Heinrich Heine Univ, Düsseldorf, Germany)
Medicine 75:185–194, 1996   3–20

Objective.—*Toxoplasma gondii* infection is a common CNS infection in patients with AIDS. Sulfadiazine in combination with pyrimidine as therapy can result in formation of the crystalline precipitate acetylsulfadiazine, which can in turn can cause irritation and possibly extensive renal damage. Results of a review of the literature that identified 35 HIV-positive patients with this adverse reaction and a synopsis of the epidemiologic, pathophysiologic, and clinical features and current recommendations and treatment were presented.

Methods.—When the literature between 1984 and 1995 was reviewed for sulfadiazine-associated renal impairment, the incidence among HIV-negative patients varied from 1% to 4% and among HIV-positive patients was 1.9% to 7.5%.

Results.—In 24 of 35 patients, renal function was normal before the initiation of sulfadiazine therapy. Fluid imbalance was common as a result of decreased fluid intake because of nausea, dysphagia, general lethargy, vomiting, diarrhea, fever, or sweating. Symptoms include pain on urination, blood in the urine, difficulty urinating, hydronephrosis, stones, and albumin in the urine. The condition is rarely fatal, and crystal formation depends on serum and urine concentrations of the drug. Microscopic "sheaves" or "shocks of wheat" crystals in the urine are characteristic of the problem. Spectral analysis of stones is also diagnostic. Urinary pH is frequently in the 5–6 range. Therapeutic options consist of reducing the dosage or discontinuing treatment with the drug and vigorous parenteral rehydration and alkalinization of the urine. Short-term hemodialysis or treatment with furosemide, spasmolytics, and antibiotics was necessary for some patients. Treatment and discontinuation of sulfadiazine therapy usually resolve the symptoms quickly and normalize renal function. If antitoxoplasmic therapy is continued, alternative medications such as pyrimethamine alone or a combination of clindamycin and pyrimethamine can be used.

Conclusion.—In HIV-positive patients there is a higher prevalence of sulfadiazine-associated nephrotoxicity than in HIV-negative patients. Early recognition of symptoms, and discontinuing treatment with the drug, and possibly replacing it with alternative medications will usually resolve the symptoms.

▶ Sulfadiazine is used prophylactically to prevent *T. gondii* infection. The authors have collected 34 cases of adverse reactions and added 1 of their own to the world's literature. AIDS can cause the presence of both *T. gondii* and its adverse effects or change the expected incidence of adverse effects. In the case of sulfadiazine-induced renal dysfunction, there aren't many specific predictive factors, with the possible exception of hypoalbuminemia. Apparently, low albumin increases the free serum level. The authors provide several points about avoiding renal toxicity and its therapy. They include, stopping the sulfadiazine, forced diuresis, alkalinization of the urine with a pH goal of more than 7.15, and less commonly, the need for ureteral stents or a renal pelvic fistula for the installation of sodium bicarbonate as well as drainage or a need for hemodialysis.

M. Weintraub, M.D.

Comparison of Adverse Events Associated With Use of Mefloquine and Combination of Chloroquine and Proguanil as Antimalarial Prophylaxis: Postal and Telephone Survey of Travellers

Barrett PJ, Emmins PD, Clarke PD, et al (Medical Advisory Service for Travellers Abroad, London; London School of Hygiene and Tropical Medicine) *BMJ* 313:525–528, 1996   3–21

Objective.—A retrospective study was conducted to determine the frequency of adverse events from the antimalarial drugs mefloquine and chloroquine plus proguanil taken prophylactically in areas where malaria resistant to chloroquine is widespread.

Methods.—A questionnaire requesting information regarding adverse events was sent to travelers to malarious areas who had been advised to use either mefloquine or chloroquine plus proguanil.

Results.—Adverse events were reported by 41% of the mefloquine users and 40.6% of the chloroquine plus proguanil users. Significantly more chloroquine plus proguanil users reported gastrointestinal problems and mouth ulcers. More mefloquine users reported grade 3 gastrointestinal adverse events than did chloroquine plus proguanil users. Significantly more mefloquine users reported neuropsychiatric effects at all grades except grade 4. An equal number of chloroquine plus proguanil and mefloquine users reported changing or stopping treatment with the drug. Two mefloquine and 1 chloroquine plus proguanil users were admitted to hospitals for adverse events related to the drug. Twelve chloroquine plus proguanil and 31 mefloquine users reported grade 3 or 4 neuropsychiatric effects, with 9 mefloquine and 1 chloroquine plus proguanil users reporting disabling effects. These differences were significant. Overall, 1.1% of the mefloquine users and 0.3% of the chloroquine plus proguanil users had serious to disabling neuropsychiatric adverse events.

Conclusion.—Prophylactic use of mefloquine resulted in a significantly higher rate of neuropsychiatric adverse events of grade 3 or 4 than did chloroquine plus proguanil.

▶ In addition to giving us a great deal of information about neuropsychiatric adverse effects, particularly with mefloquine, this study and article helped us understand how one can categorize severity of the effects. In general, I think we should be more interested in how the adverse effects have an impact on patients' lives. I was therefore very interested in the categories "bad enough to interfere with daily activities" or "bad enough to make you seek medical advice." In some ways, these are as important as the serious adverse effects. They may portend the more serious reactions, but they are also important because in and of themselves they are life disrupting.

M. Weintraub, M.D.

Cancer Risk in Users of Calcium Channel Blockers

Olsen JH, Sorensen HT, Friis S, et al (Danish Cancer Society, Copenhagen; Univ of Aarhus, Denmark; Internatl Epidemiology Inst, Rockville, Md; et al)

Hypertension 29:1091–1094, 1997   3–22

Background.—Recent evidence suggests that drug users are at increased risk for cancer, especially of the colon. The regular use of Ca^{2+} channel blockers has been hypothesized to increase the risk of cancer, which may occur through inhibition of apoptosis or the reduction of intracellular Ca^{2+} in certain tissues. This cancer risk was further explored.

Methods.—A total of 17,911 residents of 1 Danish county receiving at least 1 Ca^{2+} channel-blocker prescription from 1991 through 1993 were included in the study. Cancer occurrences and rates were calculated using Danish Cancer Registry data and compared with county-specific incidence rates for various categories of cancer.

Findings.—Among Ca^{2+} channel-blocker users, 412 cancers occurred, compared with 414 expected. The age- and sex-standardized incidence ratio was 1.00. No excess risk was apparent in the subgroup of likely long-term users or users of specific drugs. The standardized incidence ratio of colon cancer was 0.8 (based on 34 cases).

Conclusions.—Although these findings are reassuring, the lack of association between Ca^{2+} use and cancer risk may reflect the relatively short follow-up period after registration in the prescription database. Further research is warranted.

▶ Calcium channel blockers have come under attack of late, having been accused of all sorts of harm, including an increased risk of cancer. Unfortunately, these dramatic accusations get a lot of attention in the media, whereas reports discrediting the accusations receive little attention. Instead of "no news is good news," the motto of too many reporters is "no good news is news."

This report shows no hint of an increased risk of cancer in these Danish consumers of calcium channel blockers.

L. Lasagna, M.D.

Headache Induced by a Nitric Oxide Donor (Nitroglycerin) Responds to Sumatriptan: A Human Model for Development of Migraine Drugs

Iversen HK, Olesen J (Univ of Copenhagen)

Cephalalgia 16:412–418, 1996   3–23

Objective.—Reproducible vascular headaches induced in healthy volunteers by nitroglycerine (NTG) would be useful as a migraine headache model if they responded to migraine treatments. Results of a double-blind, randomized, placebo-controlled crossover study substantiating the relevance of the NTG model in migraine drug development are presented.

Changes in headache, sumatriptan

Changes in headache, placebo

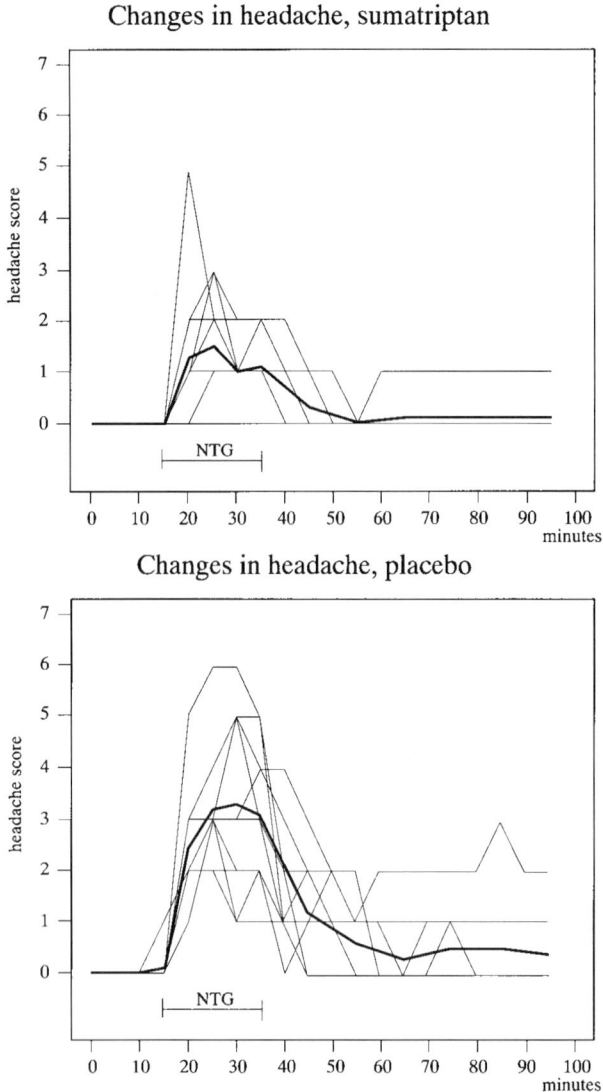

FIGURE 1.—Headache during NTG infusions after pretreatment with sumatriptan, 6 mg subcutane-ously, *left*, and placebo, *right*. Individual responses are shown and the bold line represents a mean of 10 subjects ($n = 10$). Sumatriptan significantly decreased te NTG-induced headache. (Reprinted by permis-sion of Scandanavian University Press from Iversen, HK, Olesen J: Headache induced by a nitric oxide donor [nitroglycerin] responds to sumatriptan: A human model for development of migraine drugs. *Cephalalgia* 16:412–418, 1996.)

Methods.—Ten healthy volunteers, aged 26 to 37 years, who experi-enced headache after 0.5 mg sublingual NTG, were given 6 mg sumatrip-tan subcutaneously or placebo followed 20 minutes later by 0.12 γ/kg/min infusion of either NTG or placebo. The luminal diameter of the radial and temporal arteries was measured using ultrasound 10 and 15 minutes after subcutaneous injection, every 5 minutes during NTG infusion, and every 10 minutes for the next hour. Patients scored their headaches on a 10-point scale and recorded side effects.

Results.—Nitroglycerine induced headache in 10 volunteers after placebo and in 8 after sumatriptan treatment. Sumatriptan treatment significantly decreased severity of headache and significantly delayed onset of headache, compared with placebo, from 2.5 to 5 minutes (Fig 1). The sumatriptan group had headache relief in 7.5 minutes, whereas the placebo group had relief from headache in 22.5 minutes. Diameters of the temporal and radial arteries increased significantly after NTG infusion. Compared with baseline values, sumatriptan, but not placebo, significantly decreased both diameters by 75% and 86%, respectively, but did not change the magnitude of the initial dilatation response. Sumatriptan significantly increased diastolic but not systolic blood pressure compared with placebo. Sumatriptan did not affect skin temperature.

Conclusion.—Although sumatriptan's mechanism of action is unclear, the drug significantly decreases the severity and time of onset of migraine. The NTG-induced vascular headache has sufficient similarities with migraine to make it a useful model for studying migraine in humans.

▶ The problem with models is that they tend to find the same kinds of medications as used in developing the paradigm. However, this is really a new model, and it certainly picked up sumatriptan, which is a relatively new medication for the treatment of migraine headache. As shown in the graph, the medication was effective in blocking the headache and also in blocking the dilation of the temporal artery and the radial artery as well. As an intermediate step between animal models of vascular constriction and sick patients, this model might be very helpful in normal volunteers.

M. Weintraub, M.D.

Sex Difference in Risk of Torsade de Pointes With *d,l*-Sotalol

Lehmann MH, Hardy S, Archibald D, et al (Sinai Hosp, Detroit; Bristol-Myers Squibb Co, Princeton, NJ)
Circulation 94:2534–2541, 1996   3–24

Background.—Women appear to be more prone to torsade de pointes (TdP) development with *d,l*-sotalol than men. This hypothesis was tested in a defined cohort of patients exposed to this QT-prolonging antiarrhythmic agent.

Methods and Findings.—Data on 3,135 adults in 22 clinical trials were analyzed. All had received oral *d,l*-sotalol and were followed up for a median of 164 days. Torsade de pointes developed in 44 men (1.9%) and 33 women (4.1%). In a logistic regression analysis, being female, initially having an arrhythmia of sustained ventricular tachycardia or fibrillation, having a history of congestive heart failure, and receiving a *d,l*-sotalol dose exceeding 320 mg/day were the strongest predictors of TdP. Also, a serum creatine level exceeding 1.4 mg/dL in women and exceeding 1.6 mg/dL in men weakly predicted the development of TdP. When these risk factors were adjusted for, women were found to have a threefold greater odds of developing TdP than men. The sex difference in TdP risk was independent of age and not explained by differential dose-related bradycardic responses in women as opposed to men.

Conclusions.—The risk of TdP development during *d,l*-sotalol administration was increased in women. In general, greater caution in using QT-prolonging drugs in women is advised.

▶ The problem with a report such as this one is that the way it's constructed, the way the data were gathered, really are hypothesis-generating techniques. This means that what should happen is that the next studies, if possible, should investigate this factor because this is *post hoc* rummaging through the data to see what can be found. Really, the only thing that can be learned from a study like this is that perhaps women should be dosed more in conjunction with their weight and shouldn't be overdosed with sotalol, or any other medication of any type.

M. Weintraub, M.D.

Tyramine Content of Previously Restricted Foods in Monoamine Oxidase Inhibitor Diets
Walker SE, Shulman KI, Tailor SAN, et al (Univ of Toronto)
J Clin Psychopharmacol 16:383–388, 1996   3–25

Objectives.—To determine the tyramine content of various foods and beverages that have been restricted from the diets of individuals taking monamine oxidase inhibitors, but whose tyramine content is unclear or unknown, and to evaluate the effect of freshness on the tyramine content of some foods.

Background.—Monoamine oxidase inhibitors are important in the treatment of refractory depressive illnesses, anxiety, and eating disorders. They have been associated with hypertensive crisis resulting from an interaction with foods containing tyramine. The list of restricted foods linked to hypertensive crisis has grown to more than 70 items. The danger of over-inclusive diets is that if a patient ingests a prohibited food and has no negative reaction, he or she may become careless and indulge in other restricted foods that may be more dangerous. The restricted foods and beverages have now been classified as containing high or low amounts of tyramine. The authors have received requests for information on specific foods for which there is little or no reliable information.

Methods.—The tyramine content of various foods and beverages was tested by liquid chromatography; 51 samples were tested, including samples of the inside and skin or peel of sausages and bananas.

Results.—Foods with dangerously high levels of tyramine include chicken liver aged 9 days, air-dried sausage, soy sauce, and sauerkraut. No tyramine was found in Italian Chianti wine. Part-skim mozzarella cheese had extremely low amounts of tyramine. Although only one beer was analyzed and found to have small amounts of tyramine, alarmingly high amounts of tyramine were found in 4 tap beers in a previous report. This indicates that storage and hose contamination may encourage the production of tyramine. The pulp of bananas, even overripe bananas, had acceptable levels of tyramine. Raspberries contained low concentrations of tyramine.

Discussion.—The hypertensive response is variable and depends on many factors. Therefore, patients may be able to ingest 6 mg or more of tyramine and not have a response, but the danger of an increase in blood pressure is always present and may occur the next time a restricted food or beverage is ingested. The amount of ingested tyramine should remain below 6 mg. Most of the reported fatal and nonfatal hypertensive reactions associated with monamine oxidase inhibitors have involved the ingestion of cheese. Although all aged cheese has traditionally been restricted, not all cheeses need be prohibited. Tap beer should be avoided. Foods that have been improperly stored or are spoiled may contain higher amounts of tyramine. Only foods with dangerously high levels of tyramine should continue to be restricted. All other foods are safe or safe in moderation. Patients should be given a diet that clearly identifies these two groups of foods. These findings should be combined with findings from similar studies to develop accurate and comprehensive lists of foods that must be absolutely restricted for these individuals.

▶ Hurray! Chianti wine gets another clean bill of health for patients who are taking monoamine oxidase inhibitors. It has no tyramine in it. Actually, patients will have a much easier time following this diet than they will following a traditional monoamine oxidase inhibition diet. Really, it appears that many things that were once worries have been cleaned up and become acceptable. Some items are still taboo, however, and these include soy sauce and aged chicken livers. The symptoms sometimes do not correlate with hypertension. We have to be very careful attributing everything to a hypertensive crisis with monoamine oxidase inhibitors and diet is one factor. There are still many things that happen to patients which are not caused by tyramine.

M. Weintraub, M.D.

Systemic Toxicity From Ocular Homatropine

Reilly KM, Chan L, Mehta NJ, et al (Albany Med Ctr, New York)
Acad Emerg Med 3:868–871, 1996   3–26

Objective.—A case of systemic toxicity associated with ocular application of homatropine was presented.

Case Report.—Woman, 55, with agitation, paranoid ideation, and pressured speech had elevated vital sign readings, flushed and dry skin and mucous membranes, and pupils reactive to light. She had tachycardia, a distended abdomen, and diminished bowel sounds. Two weeks earlier she had begun treatment with 5% homatropine drops and 1% prednisolone acetate drops for uveitis. The patient was treated with lorazepam and hydration. During the next 48 hours, her symptoms improved. The patient admitted to using more than the prescribed dose.

Discussion.—Drop runoff should be wiped from the eye, the solution should be chilled to help patients feel the drop so that only 1 drop is instilled, the eyes should be closed for 5 minutes, the lowest dose and longest treatment interval should be used, the nasolacrimal duct should be closed by pressure to limit absorption by this route, possible interactions with other drugs should be checked, and the patient should be cautioned that no extra benefit will accrue from increasing the dosage.

Conclusion.—Ocular administration of anticholinergic agents can cause severe side effects. These agents are commonly used in geriatric patients.

▶ Too often we think that ocular drugs do not really have systemic toxicity. However, this article disabuses us of that idea. There are several important predictors of toxicity, for example, passage of the drug directly to the target organ for toxicity when it is administered through the conjunctiva and absorbed through the tear ducts. Another is a calculation of the amount in the suspension solution. Toward the end of the bottle, the fluid in which the drug is dissolved will have decreased from evaporation. More importantly, suspensions of the drug can also have increased concentrations at the end of the bottle because the drug has settled out, particularly if it had not been shaken properly. And then there is a whole host of less important factors, including inflammation, genetic predispositions that can increase response to medications, patient age, technique of application, and many others. The authors provide a list of 9 ways to avoid toxicity. They believe that excessive medication should be wiped from the eye, patients should administer 1 drop at a time, the eyedrop bottle should be chilled to restrict the flow and to tell the patient when a drop has been applied, the eyelid should be closed for 5 minutes, the label should be checked, the lowest dose and longest effective interval should be chosen, patients should apply fingertip pressure to block the lacrimal duct, the patient should learn about interactions with other medications, ointments are less well absorbed into the systemic circulation, and patients should be instructed on the use of their eye medication and warned that only the proper dose and duration of dosing should be used.

M. Weintraub, M.D.

Propylthiouracil-induced Fulminant Hepatitis: Case Report and Review of the Literature
Deidiker R, deMello DE (St Louis Univ, Mo; Cardinal Glennon Children's Hosp, St Louis, Mo)
Pediatr Pathol Lab Med 16:845–852, 1996   3–27

Introduction.—Propylthiouracil (PTU), a drug often used in the treatment of hyperthyroidism, has a number of side effects. Although PTU-related hepatitis is usually transient and mild, the patient reported here experienced severe hepatotoxicity.

> *Case Report.*—Girl, 13, was seen for complaints of agitation, heat intolerance, insomnia, increased appetite, and changes in school performance. Her health and development had otherwise been normal, and she had no history of thyroid or liver disease. Laboratory studies led to a diagnosis of hyperthyroidism. Treatment with PTU (250 mg/day) and propranolol (20 mg 3 times a day) was started. Four months later, when the patient began to experience jaundice, fatigue, fever, and diarrhea, PTU was discontinued. The patient was admitted for work-up after hyperbilirubinemia and profound elevation of liver enzymes were detected. Her condition worsened and orthotopic liver transplantation was performed on hospital day 7. The patient's clinical course declined rapidly, and she died despite extensive therapeutic measures. Death was attributed to cerebral and cerebellar herniation secondary to metabolic encephalopathy.

Discussion.—Seven of 17 previously reported cases of PTU-associated hepatitis were in children, and this case represents only the second PTU-related fatality in a child. Diagnosis of PTU-induced fulminant hepatitis in this case was based on the timing of the symptoms, the form of hepatic injury, and the absence of other identifiable risk factors.

▶ Propylthiouracil is a common treatment for hyperthyroidism but can produce a variety of side effects including rash, fever, blood disorders, vasculitis, and kidney disease. Hepatitis has been repeatedly observed but is usually transient and mild. This case adds a sixth PTU-related death to those previously described in the literature.

L. Lasagna, M.D.

Polymyositis Associated With Simvastatin
Giordano N, Senesi M, Mattii G, et al (Univ of Siena, Italy)
Lancet 349:1600–1601, 1997   3–28

Objective.—Some lipid-lowering drugs have been associated with reversible muscular disease. A case of polymyositis linked to simvastatin is discussed.

Case.—A man, 42, with myocardial infarction and hypercholesterolemia had severe proximal muscle weakness, myalgia, arthralgia, and increased serum creatine kinase (CK) 3 months after beginning simvastatin (20 mg). His cholesterol, CK, aldolase, and lactic-acid dehydrogenase were elevated. Blood, hormone, and immune factors were normal. Radiographs were normal, but an electromyogram was myogenic and neurogenic with spontaneous activity. A deltoid muscle specimen showed muscle-fiber necrosis, fragmentation, and inflammatory cell infiltration. He was diagnosed with polymyositis. Most cells were activated T-cells and macrophages. Simvastatin was discontinued. The patient received NSAIDs for 5 days followed by 6-methylprednisone (4 mg weekly) when laboratory abnormalities failed to resolve. Remission was rapid (within days) and myopathy did not recur when steroids were discontinued 4 months later.

Conclusion.—Myopathy linked to simvastatin is not spontaneously reversible primarily because it is mediated by a cellular immunologic mechanism. Complement activation could also be an important component of the pathogenic process.

▶ Fortunately, the incidence of muscle damage is quite low and very rarely gets to be this serious compared with the beneficial effects of the "statin" drugs. Nonetheless, we have to be on the lookout for a polymyositis syndrome.

M. Weintraub, M.D.

Late-afternoon Ethanol Intake Affects Nocturnal Sleep and the Sleep EEG in Middle-aged Men
Landolt H-P, Roth C, Dijk D-J, et al (Univ of Zürich, Switzerland)
J Clin Psychopharmacol 16:428–436, 1996   3–29

Background.—Recent studies have shown some unexpected effects of alcohol, suggesting that it affects some unknown processes involved in the homeostatic regulation of human sleep. These studies have been conducted mainly in young men, whereas sleep quality is subjectively impaired in middle age. Many people drink alcohol in the early evening hours, with no further intake before bedtime. The effects of this alcohol intake pattern on sleep quality was investigated in healthy middle-aged men.

Methods.—The study included 10 middle-aged male volunteers (mean age 62 years). All received a moderate dose of ethanol, 0.55 g/kg of body weight, at 17:00 hours, 5 hours before their scheduled bedtime. The effects of this ethanol dose on performance, nighttime sleep, and sleep electroencephalography (EEG) were compared with effects seen with a control condition in which the men received mineral water.

Findings.—When they went to sleep, all participants had a breath ethanol concentration of zero. The men reported more superficial sleep after receipt of alcohol than after receipt of mineral water. This was supported by the finding of reduced sleep efficiency, total sleep time, stage 1 sleep, and rapid eye movement sleep. Wakefulness during the second half of sleep increased 2-fold. Significant EEG changes were noted in rapid-eye movement (REM), non-REM, and slow-wave sleep.

Conclusions.—Moderate drinking of alcohol in the late afternoon may alter the sleep pattern in middle-aged men after the ethanol has been almost eliminated. Sleep consolidation was disrupted, sleep-stage distribution changed, and sleep EEG findings were altered. Ethanol may have a delayed effect, similar to that documented for benzodiazepines.

▶ Drinking alcoholic beverages at evening "happy hours" clearly disrupts normal sleep at a time when the drug is no longer detectable in the breath. These delayed effects (possibly a "rebound") have also been previously documented for benzodiazepines.

L. Lasagna, M.D.

Gym and Tonic: A Profile of 100 Male Steroid Users
Evans NA (Cardiff Royal Infirmary, Wales)
Br J Sports Med 31:54–58, 1997   3–30

Purpose.—Many athletes continue to use anabolic/androgenic steroids despite the risk of adverse effects. These steroid users are often seen by medical practitioners. There are few data regarding the type of unsupervised steroid regimens being used by athletes. An anonymous questionnaire was used to gather information on unsupervised anabolic steroid regimens.

Methods.—Questionnaire responses were received from 100 athletes from 4 different weight-training gymnasiums. The athletes were asked about the steroid drugs and dosages they were currently using, as well as about side effects, withdrawal symptoms, and physical signs.

Findings.—Two thirds of the respondents were recreational athletes, and one third were competitive bodybuilders. Sixty-four percent had been using steroids for 1–5 years. The weekly dose of anabolic steroid ranged from 250 to 3,200 mg/week, with 50% of respondents using less than 500 mg/week. Twelve percent of respondents took a dose of more than 1,000 mg/week. The respondents used various drugs in combination, including injectable and oral drugs, in 4- to 12-week cycles. Other drugs, in addition to steroids, were used by 86% of respondents for reasons such as additional anabolic effects, minimization of steroid-related side effects, and withdrawal symptoms. The main reported side effects of steroid use were acne, striae, and gynecomastia.

Conclusion.—When using unsupervised steroids, athletes may take several different kinds in very high doses, often self-administered in cyclical fashion. Most of these athletes misuse other drugs as well. Practitioners should be alert to the common physical signs of steroid use, including muscular hypertrophy, acne, striae, and gynecomastia.

▶ I picked this article only in part because I love the title. It reminds us of the spectrum of untoward events that follows chronic use of large doses of steroids by athletes.

L. Lasagna, M.D.

A High Prevalence of Abnormal Personality Traits in Chronic Users of Anabolic-Androgenic Steroids

Cooper CJ, Noakes TD, Dunne T, et al (Univ of Cape Town, South Africa; Sports Science Inst of South Africa, Newlands)
Br J Sports Med 30:246–250, 1996   3–31

Background.—The use of anabolic-androgenic steroids is no longer restricted to highly trained athletes who engage in competition. Today, recreational and noncompetitive athletes and school children are the primary users of anabolic-androgenic steroids. The psychological and behavioral effects of these agents are not well understood. Because of ethical considerations, the effects of large nontherapeutic doses of steroids must be studied in a free-living population. A series of studies have linked the use of anabolic-androgenic steroids to significant psychiatric effects, including personality disorders.

Methods.—The first author became a member of a group of body builders who used anabolic-androgenic steroids but did not use steroids himself. A subgroup of body builders who had been using steroids for 18 months or less was identified. Control subjects who claimed they had never used steroids were also recruited. All subjects were interviewed using an interview schedule based on the *Diagnostic and Statistical Manual of Mental Disorders,* ed III, revised, criteria for personality trait disorders. Friends and family provided additional information about the subjects.

Results.—Subjects who used anabolic-androgenic steroids were heavier than control subjects and also exhibited abnormal personality traits. The personality traits of steroid users before they began steroid use were evaluated retrospectively and compared with the personality traits of nonusers; no significant differences were found. Significant differences were found in the personality traits of steroid users before and after the onset of steroid use.

Discussion.—These findings suggest that anabolic-androgenic steroids significantly increase the incidence and severity of symptoms of personality disorders. There is a growing body of evidence of the dangers of using anabolic-androgenic steroids. This study is limited by its inability to directly assess the premorbid personality traits of these subjects.

▶ The illicit use of anabolic-androgenic steroids continues to mushroom, now affecting not only "power" athletes and body builders but all sorts of athletes, school children included. This was a tough study to plan, and the authors deserve a lot of credit for their imaginative protocol. My guess is that people who abuse these steroids are "funny" before *and* after taking them.

L. Lasagna, M.D.

Oxidants, Antioxidant Nutrients and the Athlete
Packer L (Univ of California, Berkeley)
J Sports Sci 15:353–363, 1997   3–32

Background.—Although physical exercise has many beneficial effects, evidence suggests that free radical production increases during exercise, resulting in oxidative damage in the muscles, liver, blood, and possibly other tissues. Oxidants and antioxidant nutrients during exercise were discussed.

Discussion.—The oxidative stress that occurs during strenuous activity may have a number of sources. These include mitochondrial superoxide production, ischemia–reperfusion mechanisms, and autooxidation of catecholamines. Antioxidant defenses include vitamin E and C and thiol antioxidants, which are interlinked in an antioxidant network. Severe or prolonged exercise can overwhelm antioxidant defenses as well as antioxidant enzymes. Evidence for the occurrence of oxidative stress and damage during exercise comes from direct measures of free radicals, measures of lipid and DNA damage, and measures of antioxidant redox status, especially glutathione. Little evidence of improved performance with antioxidant supplementation exists. However, a large body of research suggests that bolstering antioxidant defenses may alleviate the damage caused by exercise. Thus, the benefits of antioxidant treatment may be long-term rather than short-term.

▶ Most medications taken by athletes are intended to improve competitive performance and might be categorized as "melioristic pharmacology." This paper is a pleasant change. It poses the possibility of decreasing long-term, exercise-induced damage caused by the oxidative stress of strenuous physical activity.

It's helpful to be reminded that although regular physical exercise can provide all sorts of benefits, such as improved cardiovascular function, greater muscle strength and endurance, and decreased osteoporosis, it also can produce harm.

L. Lasagna, M.D.

Serious Cardiovascular Side Effects of Large Doses of Anabolic Steroids in Weight Lifters
Nieminen MS, Rämö P, Viitasalo M, et al (Helsinki Univ; Central Military Hosp, Helsinki)
Eur Heart J 17:1576–1583, 1996   3–33

Introduction.—Anabolic steroids have been shown to increase ventricular wall thickness, end-diastolic volume, and left ventricular mass and significantly prolong isovolumetric relaxation time in weight lifters. Anabolic steroids are considered atherogenic and have been linked to arterial occlusion in several reports. The pathologic cardiovascular manifestations in 4 young men who used high doses of anabolic steroids for several years in combination with weight training were reviewed.

Methods.—Patients were referred for evaluation because of long history of massive anabolic steroid use (patient 1); ventricular fibrillation during exercise (patient 2); clinically manifest heart failure (patient 3); and arterial thrombus in the lower left leg (patient 4). Ages ranged from 27 to 33 years. All patients underwent history, physical examination, and cardiovascular evaluation.

Results.—All 4 patients had cardiac hypertrophy. Two patients who underwent endomyocardial biopsy had diffuse myocardial fibrosis. Patients 3 and 4 had signs of heart failure, patient 2 had impairment of coronary flow, and patient 3 had impairment of perfusion. A large lobular intraventricular thrombus was observed in both the left and right ventricles of patient 4 during echocardiography. Two patients had improved left ventricular function after cessation of anabolic steroids. Despite warnings, both patients restarted use of anabolic steroids.

Conclusion.—Two of the 4 weight lifters using anabolic steroids had potentially lethal side effects—malignant ventricular arrhythmia in 1 and massive intracardiac thrombosis in the other. All 4 men had cardiac hypertrophy. Physicians and athletes should be warned about the serious risks involved in continuous use of large doses of anabolic steroids.

▶ Massive doses of anabolic steroids may help a weightlifter to win a competition, but the cardiovascular risks are very, very real.

L. Lasagna, M.D.

4 AIDS

Should We Embrace New Drugs With Open Arms? Experience From a Community-based, Open-arm, Randomized Clinical Trial of Combination Antiretroviral Therapy in Advanced HIV Disease
Montaner JSG, Hogg R, Srour LF, et al (British Columbia Centre for Excellence in HIV/AIDS; Univ of British Columbia, Canada)
J Acquir Immune Defic Syndr Hum Retrovirol 13:422–426, 1996   4–1

Background.—The rapid spread of lethal HIV infection in the 1980s made accelerated drug development a priority. An "open arms" design for new drug studies was proposed, in which an additional arm was added for participants to freely choose between the treatments being compared in the randomized part of the start. Concerns have been raised about this strategy. Some authorities believe that the existence of an open arm would slow enrollment and eventually ethically compromise the randomized arm of the trial. The current prospective study investigated the effects of an open arm in a randomized study of combination antiretroviral therapy in patients with advanced HIV disease.

Methods.—Zidovudine (ZDV) plus didanosine (ddI) was compared with ZDV plus zalcitabine (ddC). HIV-infected patients were eligible for the study if they were ddI and ddC naive, had CD4 counts of 50–350mm^3, and were residents of British Columbia. Participants were allowed to choose between open-label ZDV/ddI, ZDV/ddC, or randomization to open-label ZDV/ddI or ZDV/ddC. The study drugs were free of charge and were not available by any other means in the province.

Findings.—Enrollment was begun in November 1992, and closed in March 1994, when the target size of 120 evaluable participants in the randomized arm was met. A total of 138 patients enrolled in the randomized arm, and 444 enrolled in the open arm. In the latter group, 72% were initially given ZDV/ddI, and 28% were given ZDV/ddC. The enrollment rate in the open arm was strikingly higher than it was in the randomized arm, with 168 patients enrolling during the first 2 months in the former and 138 patients enrolling during 17 months in the latter. The 2 groups did not differ significantly.

Conclusions.—The coexistence of an open arm makes study recruitment challenging. If randomized clinical studies are to be carried out with coexistent open arms, an increased commitment by all interested parties will be needed.

▶ Patients and doctors concerned with AIDS treatment understandably like the option of an open arm while a randomized trial is in progress because the open arm leaves no doubt about what the patient will get, whereas the randomized trial only promises the patient one or the other treatment arm. As might be expected, recruitment into the randomized trial is likely to suffer in this situation.

L. Lasagna, M.D.

Combination Treatment With Zidovudine, Didanosine, and Nevirapine in Infants With Human Immunodeficiency Virus Type 1 Infection
Luzuriaga K, Bryson Y, Krogstad P, et al (Univ of Massachusetts, Worcester; Univ of California at Los Angeles; Univ of Connecticut, Farmington; et al)
N Engl J Med 336:1343–1349, 1997   4–2

Introduction.—There is a need for some type of treatment for infants and children with maternally acquired HIV-1 infection. Therapy with a single inhibitor of reverse transcriptase has proved to be of limited efficacy. Studies in adults suggest that the best approach to preventing HIV-1 disease after infection is to control viral replication as early as possible. A 3-drug regimen of zidovudine, didanosine, and nevirapine was studied for safety and efficacy in infants with maternally acquired HIV-1 infection.

Methods.—In a phase 1–2 study, this drug combination was used in 8 HIV-1 infected infants aged 2 to 16 months. All drugs were given orally. The children underwent serial measurements of plasma HIV-1 RNA, quantitative plasma cultures, and quantitative cultures of peripheral blood mononuclear cells. Potential toxic effects were assessed as well.

Results.—There were no significant adverse events. All of the patients had rapid declines in plasma HIV-1 RNA with treatment. Seven of the 8 patients achieved a reduction of at least 96% — i.e., a 1.5 log reduction in the number of copies per milliliter — within 2 to 4 weeks. Two infants who started the 3-drug combination by 2.5 months of age had sustained control over HIV-1 replication during the 6-month study period. Of the other 6 infants, 5 had 0.5 to 1.5 log reductions in plasma RNA levels.

Conclusions.—Preliminary study shows good results with a combination of zidovudine, didanosine, and nevirapine in infants with maternally acquired HIV-1 infection. The treatment is well tolerated and has lasting efficacy in the control of HIV-1 replication. To reduce the chances of antiretroviral resistance and enhance the opportunity for long-term control of HIV-1 replication, infants with maternally acquired infection should be treated as early as possible, preferably within the first 2 to 4 weeks.

▶ Infants and children seem to handle HIV infection even more poorly than adults. This 3-drug combination regimen looks like a step in the right direction and should probably be instituted as early as possible after documentation of maternally acquired infection.

L. Lasagna, M.D.

Long-term Efficacy and Safety of Dronabinol for Acquired Immunodeficiency Syndrome-associated Anorexia
Beal JE, Olson R, Lefkowitz L, et al (St John's Hosp, Tulsa, Okla; Oaklawn Physician's Group, Dallas; Vanderbilt Univ, Nashville, Tenn; et al)
J Pain Symptom Manage 14:7–14, 1997   4–3

Objective.—Anorexia and wasting commonly occur during last-stage AIDS mainly as a result of inadequate caloric intake. After a randomized, double-blind, placebo-controlled study of dronabinol in AIDS patients showed trends toward increased body weight with mild to moderate CNS side effects, a follow-up, multicenter, open-label, long-term study was conducted to re-evaluate the safety and efficacy of up to 12 months of dronabinol therapy in late-stage AIDS patients from the previous trial.

Methods.—Between July 1991 and January 1993, 94 patients, average age 37.2, 48 who had previously received placebo, with a mean weight loss of 9.2 kg, received oral dronabinol 2.5 mg twice daily (90%) or 2.5 mg once daily. Appetite was measured on a 100-mm visual analogue scale for hunger (VASH) in which 100 represented extremely hungry and 0 represented not hungry at all.

Results.—Although 93 patients were evaluable for efficacy, only 22 patients completed the study. Of the 71 who terminated early, 36 did so before 3 months. There were 24 noncompliant patients. Increase in appetite from baseline ranged from 48.6% to 76.1% for previous dronabinol patients and from 27.3% to 69.9% for previous placebo patients. Dronabinol increased appetite approximately by a factor of 2 from baseline. Previous placebo patients increased their appetite scores from baseline by 48.5% at month 1, 66.9% at month 2, 69.9% at month 3, and 58.7% at month 4. Adverse events affected 41 patients, with 2 experiencing severe adverse events, primarily anxiety, confusion, somnolence, depersonalization, dizziness, euphoria, and thinking abnormality. In 19 patients discontinued early, treatment-related adverse events included CNS effects, asthenia, palpitations, tachycardia, and alcohol intolerance.

Conclusion.—Dronabinol is safe and effective for long-term use as a treatment for anorexia associated with weight loss in AIDS patients.

▶ This was a long-term follow-up of a short-term (too short) 6-week study of dronabinol in AIDS patients. However, patients who had received placebo in the initial group did continue to lose weight even when they were placed on dronabinol in an open-label follow-up. The investigators in this study looked for differences between the treatment groups and found only an increased variability. There have been trials of at least 6 other agents in AIDS wasting, none really effective. It appears from this study that dronabinol will have maintained efficacy, although one would have to be wary of the initial negative response on placebo being maintained. This may be another one of those mind/body connections where there was a learned response to placebo that could not be overcome by exposure to the active therapy.

M. Weintraub, M.D.

Recombinant Human Growth Hormone in Patients With HIV-associated Wasting: A Randomized, Placebo-controlled Trial
Schambelan M, and the Serostim Study Group (San Francisco Gen Hosp; Veterans Affairs Med Ctr, San Francisco; Cedars-Sinai Med Ctr, Los Angeles; et al)
Ann Intern Med 125:873–882, 1996   4–4

Introduction.—Body wasting is a frequent AIDS-defining condition. It is linked with impaired function and decreased quality of life and is an independent predictor of death. A study found that 1 week of treatment with growth hormone leads to weight gain and nitrogen retention in patients with HIV-associated body wasting. However, the long-term effects of this treatment are unknown. The long-term effects of growth hormone treatment on body weight, body composition, functional performance, and quality of life were assessed.

Methods.—The randomized, double-blind, placebo-controlled trial included 178 patients with HIV-associated body wasting. All had unintentional weight loss of 10% or more or weight less than 90% of the lower limit of ideal. The patients were randomly assigned to receive treatment with 0.1 mg of recombinant human growth hormone per kilogram per day, or placebo. The dose in the growth hormone group was 6 mg/day. Clinical and laboratory outcome measures included weight, body fat, lean body mass, bone mineral content, total body water, extracellular water, work output, and quality of life.

Results.—Weight increased significantly in the growth hormone group, by a mean of 1.6 kg. Lean body mass increased by 3.0 kg; body fat decreased by 1.7 kg. None of these measures was significantly changed in the placebo group. The differences between groups were significant at 12 weeks. Treadmill output increased by a greater amount in the growth hormone group. There were no differences in quality of life, days of disability, or use of medical resources. Treatment was well tolerated, with no increase in clinical events, AIDS progression, CD4+ or CD8+ cell count, or viral burden.

Conclusions.—Treatment with recombinant human growth factor appears to be beneficial for patients with HIV-associated body wasting. It increases body mass, lean body mass, and treadmill work output while reducing fat body mass. The treatment is well tolerated; the cost is still to be determined.

▶ Body wasting is an all-too-common complication of AIDS. It impairs performance, decreases the quality of life, and contributes to a fatal outcome. Nutritional supplementation and attempts at appetite stimulation do not consistently restore lean tissue. It is nice to learn that growth hormone is a safe way to help such patients regain weight and improve their physical performance.

L. Lasagna, M.D.

Recombinant Human Growth Hormone, Insulin-like Growth Factor 1, and Combination Therapy in AIDS-associated Wasting: A Randomized, Double-blind, Placebo-controlled Trial
Waters D, Danska J, Hardy K, et al (Univ of New Mexico, Albuquerque; Univ of Texas, Dallas)
Ann Intern Med 125:865–872, 1996   4–5

Background.—Wasting is a serious complication of AIDS. Recombinant human insulin-like growth factor 1 (rhIGF-1) and recombinant human growth hormone (rhGH) have positive effects on lean body mass. Therefore, patients with AIDS-associated wasting were administered rhIGF-1, rhGH, or both to increase lean body mass and improve health status.

Methods.—A randomized, double-blind, placebo-controlled clinical trial was conducted in 60 patients with AIDS-associated wasting. The patients were divided into 4 groups of 15 patients each. Group 1 received 1.4 mg of rhGH once daily plus placebo twice daily. Group 2 received 5 mg of rhIGF-1 twice daily and placebo once daily. Group 3 received 5 mg of rhIGF-1 twice daily plus 1.4 mg of rhGH once daily. Group 4 received placebo 3 times daily. Body weight, body composition, muscle strength, protein catabolism, quality of life, and immune status were evaluated at baseline, and at 6 and at 12 weeks.

Results.—At 6 weeks, lean body mass had increased and total fat mass had decreased in groups 1, 2, and 3. Group 3 had the most increase in lean body mass. The increase was maintained in group 3 at 12 weeks, but not in the other groups. Only the patients in group 1 had improvement in muscular strength of the knees and upper body and improvement in quality of life. Immunologic function was not improved in any of these groups over the time course of the study.

Conclusions.—Administration of rhGH alone or in combination with rhIGF-1 increased the lean body mass of patients with AIDS-associated wasting. However, this increase in body mass did not consistently lead to improvements in muscle strength, immunologic recovery, or quality of life. Therefore, therapy involving these hormones at the doses used in this study cannot be recommended for patients with AIDS-associated wasting.

▶ The wasting associated with AIDS is a dreaded complication of this viral infection, and its pathogenesis is probably multifactorial. Because lean body mass seems to be increased by both rhGH and rhIGF-1, it would seem logical to try both together in such patients. The combination *did* look better in this trial, but there were so many dropouts that conclusions (and enthusiasm) had to be muted. The most frequent side effects were edema, arthralgia, and myalgia.

L. Lasagna, M.D.

Malariotherapy for HIV Patients

Heimlich HJ, Chen XP, Xiao BQ, et al (Heimlich Inst, Cincinnati, Ohio; Municipal Health and Anti-Epidemic Station of Guangzhou, Guandong, China)
Mech Ageing Dev 93:79–85, 1997   4–6

Background.—Techniques that enhance immune response in patients with HIV infection include exogenous cytokine infusion, therapeutic vaccination with inactivated HIV, and malariotherapy to stimulate cytokine production. The current study determined whether patients with HIV treated with malariotherapy benefit from immunologic change without iatrogenic complications.

Methods.—Asymptomatic patients who were HIV positive were inoculated with *P. vivax*, a curable form of malaria. The malaria infection was permitted to run a predetermined course according to standard malariotherapy protocols and then cured with chloroquine. Initially, 2 men, aged 23 and 40 years, volunteered for the study, neither of whom had been treated previously for HIV. After these patients were followed up for 18 months, 6 additional men were enrolled in the study.

Findings.—In the initial 2 patients, CD4 counts increased significantly over measures obtained before malariotherapy. The CD4 counts in these men remained at normal levels for 2 years with no further treatment of any type. Both patients remained clinically well during follow-up. The other 6 patients also remained clinically well after malariotherapy during their 6-month follow-up.

Conclusions.—Malariotherapy results in increased CD4 counts in patients who are HIV positive. These increases persist for at least 2 years after the malaria is cured.

▶ This paper is quite controversial, but it is interesting. Dr. Heimlich and his colleagues have very cleverly moved from the effects of malaria therapy in patients with neurosyphilis to the scourge of modern times, HIV. However, in parts of Africa, malarial attacks are universal. Perhaps the immunity achieved before HIV infection prevents the development of high temperatures. It may be time for a well-controlled clinical trial to be carried out so that we can tell whether this form of treatment will be valuable for more patients.

M. Weintraub, M.D.

Thalidomide for the Treatment of Oral Aphthous Ulcers in Patients With Human Immunodeficiency Virus Infection

Jacobson JM, for the National Institute of Allergy and Infectious Diseases AIDS Clinical Trials Group (Bronx Veterans Affairs Med Ctr, NY; et al)
N Engl J Med 336:1487–1493, 1997   4–7

Background.—Apthous ulceration in the mouth and oropharynx can be extensive and debilitating in patients with advanced HIV infection. Preliminary studies suggest that thalidomide may facilitate oral aphthous ulcer healing.

Methods.—Fifty-seven patients completed a double-blind, randomized, placebo-controlled study of thalidomide treatment for oral aphthous ulcers. Thalidomide, 200 mg, or placebo was taken orally for 4 weeks.

Findings.—Fifty-five percent of the patients in the thalidomide group and only 7% in the placebo group showed complete healing of ulcers after 4 weeks. Active treatment decreased pain and improved ability to eat. Adverse effects included somnolence and rash, in 7 patients each. Six of the 29 thalidomide recipients quit treatment because of toxicity. Levels of HIV RNA were increased in the active treatment group, and there were unexpected increases in the plasma levels of TNF-α and soluble TNF-α receptors.

Conclusions.—Though severe aphthous ulcers are not common in HIV-infected persons, they can be devastating when they do occur. Thalidomide is an effective treatment for this condition.

▶ In almost every volume of the YEAR BOOK OF DRUG THERAPY, Dr. Lasagna and I include 1 or more articles about treatment for aphthous ulcers. Unfortunately, none of the treatments seems to work very well, although the paper we are reviewing seems to be positive. Of course, almost no aphthous ulcers are as large and aggressive and even life-changing as in HIV infection. In this study, thalidomide was effective in helping the patients heal their ulcers. The incidence of sedation was relatively high, although it did not reach statistical significance. This study did not have the power to determine adverse effects. Rash and sensory neuropathy also occurred. The sensory neuropathy affected just a few more in the thalidomide group, because of the short duration of therapy and the fact that patients who have AIDS and take other medications may already have sensory neuropathy. The most troublesome aspect about this study was the increased numbers of copies of HIV RNA, but the results were within the statistical significance of the test. In addition, the patients were not taking modern antiretroviral therapy. Still, thalidomide may be useful as a palliative treatment for aphthous ulcers in end-stage AIDS patients.

M. Weintraub, M.D.

Adverse Reactions to Thalidomide in Patients Infected With Human Immunodeficiency Virus

Haslett P, Tramontana J, Burroughs M, et al (Rockefeller Univ, New York)
Clin Infect Dis 24:1223–1227, 1997   4–8

Background.—Certain complications of HIV infection respond to treatment with thalidomide. Although thalidomide is considered well tolerated, there have been reports of unusual toxicity in patients with HIV infection. The authors' experience suggests that thalidomide has more frequent and severe toxic effects in patients with HIV infection.

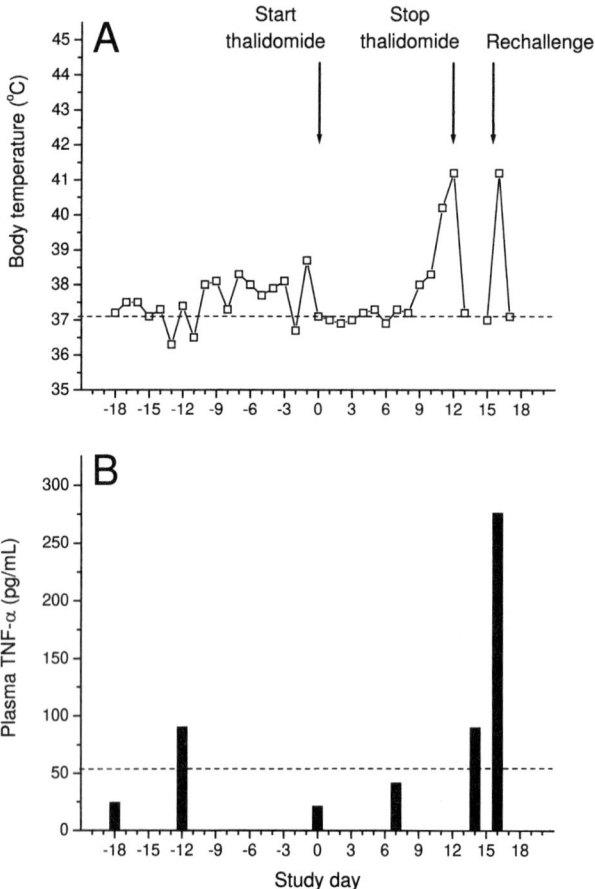

FIGURE 2.—Daily maximum body temperature (**A**) and plasma TNF-α levels (**B**) in an HIV-infected patient treated with thalidomide who developed a drug-induced fever and had an accelerated sepsis-like reaction upon rechallenge. The plasma TNF-α level was measured by ELISA. The *horizontal dotted line* in **A** indicates the normal body temperature (37°C), and that in **B** the lower limit of accuracy of the TNF-α assay (50 pg/mL). (Courtesy of Haslett P, Tramontana J, Burroughs M, et al: Adverse reactions to thalidomide in patients infected with human immunodeficiency virus. *Clin Infect Dis* 24:1223–1227, 1997. Published by The University of Chicago. Copyright 1997 by The University of Chicago. All rights reserved.)

Patients.—The experience included 56 HIV-infected patients treated with thalidomide in 3 prospective studies. Thalidomide treatment was given for 2 or 3 weeks. Forty-three percent of patients discontinued treatment because of adverse reactions, most commonly cutaneous or febrile reactions or both. The mean interval to reactions was 10 days. Median CD4 T lymphocyte count was 53/mm³ in reactors vs. 242 cells/mm³ in nonreactors. Hypersensitivity was noted in 4 patients who were rechallenged with thalidomide (Fig 2); 1 of these patients had hypotension. Almost all patients experienced sedation, which was moderate to severe in only 13%. Nine percent had moderate to severe constipation. Four percent had severe neuropathic symptoms and mood changes.

Discussion.—Thalidomide appears to have increased toxicity in patients with HIV infection. This risk must be considered with the increasing use of thalidomide to treat complications of HIV infection. The range of possible toxic effects should be appreciated so as to promote early recognition.

▶ Thalidomide's ability to produce phocomelia in fetuses whose mothers took the drug early in pregnancy was responsible for the passage of the 1962 Kefauver-Harris Amendments to the food and drug laws. But the drug lives on because it can help patients with a variety of uncommon but serious ailments.

The latest development is the drug's promise in managing several complications of HIV infection such as severe aphthous ulceration of the oral mucosa, the wasting syndrome, and an itchy nodular eruption called prurigo nodularis.

Although thalidomide is generally well tolerated, the drug seems more likely to produce adverse events in HIV patients, especially (but not exclusively) cutaneous and febrile reactions.

L. Lasagna, M.D.

5 Asthma

Compliance With Inhaled Medication and Self-treatment Guidelines Following a Self-management Programme in Adult Asthmatics
van der Palen J, Klein JJ, Rovers MM (Univ of Nijmegen, The Netherlands)
Eur Respir J 10:652–657, 1997   5–1

Background.—Patient compliance with any drug regimen can be vexing, and it is extremely important that patients comply with self-management programs for asthma. Two key factors in patient self-management are that patients use the inhaled medications at the correct doses and times, and that they adhere to the written guidelines for modifying therapy when necessary. These 2 factors were evaluated in a self-management program of adults with asthma.

Methods.—Twenty-four patients with stable asthma and regular corticosteroid use were enrolled. Baseline data, including compliance with inhaled steroids and peak expiratory flow, were recorded for 2 weeks, to arrive at a "personal best" peak expiratory flow measurement. Thereafter, all patients participated in 4 group sessions that instructed them about the proper use of the inhaler and provided them personal written instructions as to when they should adjust their therapy. Specifically, patients were to measure their peak expiratory flow on the same day each week. If the measurement was between 60% and 80% of their personal best value on 2 consecutive days, they were to double their dose of inhaled steroids. If the measurement was less than 60% of their personal best value, they were to begin oral prednisolone.

Findings.—Mean compliance improved from 81% during the 2-week run-in period to 93% in the follow-up period. Individual patient compliance ranged from 21% to 200%. Ten patients experienced a peak expiratory flow between 60% and 80% of their personal best, and thus should have doubled their inhaler use; however, compliance actually decreased by 28% in this group (individual compliance 46% to 94%). In 5 patients whose peak expiratory flow rate dropped below 60% of their personal best, only 4 started taking oral prednisolone (self-reports).

Conclusions.—Despite 4 sessions of instruction, patient compliance with doubling the dose of inhaler averaged only 65%. Three patients doubled their dose, and 3 did not change their dose, but 4 increased their dose somewhat without ever actually doubling it. This indicates that patients may hesitate to double the dose if they think "just a little increase is enough." Thus, patient education about the safety of doubling the dose of inhaled steroids may result in improved compliance.

▶ This study shows what many people have often noted, that patients really are very conservative with their medications, even when being conservative is probably being wrong. Even teaching patients that they need to double their medication or start an oral course of steroids may not be enough to get them to do it. Although we always say that patients say, "If one is good, 2 is really good, and 4 may be fantastic," we really have very little evidence that patients act in such a way.

M. Weintraub, M.D.

Hospitalization of Adults for Asthma and Inhaled Corticosteroid Use in an Island Population
Cacciottolo JM, Balzan MV, Buhagiar A (Univ of Malta; St Luke's Hosp, Malta)
Respir Med 91:411–416, 1997   5–2

Background.—Despite improvements in asthma treatment, hospital admission rates for asthma among adults at a population level are increasing. Hospitalization rates and corticosteroid use among Maltese adults were reported.

Methods.—The prevalence rate of hospital admission among individuals aged 15–59 years between 1989 and 1993 was determined retrospectively. The concurrent annual total dispensal of inhaled corticosteroids for the whole population was also calculated.

Findings.—The age-specific hospital admission rates for asthma declined from 96.2 per 100,000 in 1989 to 38.1 per 100,000 in 1993. Prevalence rates of admission from asthma dropped from 67.6 to 30.6 per 100,000 between 1989 and 1993. Inhaled beclomethasone dipropionate (BDP) dispensal rose from 0.99 defined daily dose (DDD) per 1,000 in 1989 to 3.28 DDD per 1,000 in 1993. A logistic regression analysis demonstrated that increasing inhaled BDP dispensal by 1 DDD per 1,000 reduced the odds of an admission from asthma to 0.71 times their previous value. The odds of an individual being admitted for asthma declined to 0.75 times their previous value.

Conclusions.—Between 1989 and 1993, hospital admission rates for asthma among Maltese adults progressively declined. This trend was well correlated with the increasing use of inhaled corticosteroids at a community level. However, the increase in the use of anti-inflammatory treatment also probably reflects improved general and widespread care for asthma.

Systemic Corticosteroid Rapidly Reverses Bronchodilator Subsensitivity Induced by Formoterol in Asthmatic Patients

Tan KS, Grove A, McLean A, et al (Univ of Dundee, Scotland; Astra Draco, Lund, Sweden; Univ Hosp of Nottingham, England)
Am J Respir Crit Care Med 156:28–35, 1997   5–3

Background.—Downregulation and desensitization of airway β_2-adrenoceptors (β_2-AR) appear to develop after continuous exposure to long-acting β_2-agonists such as formoterol and salmeterol. The facilitatory effects of the acute administration of systemic corticosteroid on bronchodilator subsensitivity, as may occur in acute asthma, were investigated.

Methods.—Twelve patients with moderately severe asthma and a mean forced expiratory volume in 1 second (FEV_1) of 66% predicted were included in the study. All were receiving inhaled corticosteroids. By random assignment, the patients received inhaled placebo or inhaled formoterol (FM), 24 µg, twice a day for 4 weeks in a double-blind crossover design. The patients were genotyped for β_2-AR polymorphism at loci 16 and 27. Dose-response curves (DRCs) and duration-time profiles for FM, 12–108 µg, were generated 1 hour after placebo administration and after injection at 3 weeks, and 1 hour after the administration of oral prednisolone, 50 mg, and IV hydrocortisone, 200 mg, at 4 weeks.

Findings.—Compared with placebo, the DRC showed a significant rightward shift after FM for ΔFEV_1 and ΔFEF_{25-75}. Steroid significantly reversed these shifts. Lymphocyte β_2-AR density showed significant upregulation 3 hours after steroid. Subsensitivity occurred with FM for heart-rate response, which was reversed by steroid. This corticosteroid-induced reversal appeared to be generally independent of β_2-AR polymorphism at loci 16 and 27.

Conclusions.—Bronchodilator subsensitivity occurs after regular inhaled FM in asthmatic patients. Systemic corticosteroid rapidly reverses this. In acute asthma, therefore, systemic corticosteroid should be given as soon as possible to restore normal airway β_2-AR sensitivity, especially in patients receiving regular long-acting β_2-agonists.

▶ On the island of Malta, the use of steroids increased dramatically from 1989 to 1993. At the same time, the age-specific hospital admissions and the rates of admission from asthma decreased. In the setting of improved asthma care, over a short period, these changes are impressive, decreasing the odds of an admission to a significant degree. That may, in part, be due to the information transmitted in the second paper (Abstract 5–3) which found, in acute asthma, systemic corticosteroids were helpful in restoring bronchodilator subsensitivity.

M. Weintraub, M.D.

Comparison of Regularly Scheduled With As-Needed Use of Albuterol in Mild Asthma

Drazen JM, for the National Heart, Lung, and Blood Institute's Asthma Clinical Research Network (Harvard Med School, Boston; Univ of California, San Francisco; Milton S Hershey Med Ctr, Pa; et al)

N Engl J Med 335:841–847, 1996   5–4

Introduction.—In the past, the standard recommendation was that in-haled-agonists should be used on a regular basis for optimal asthma control. More recent studies have suggested that regularly scheduled use of these medications may actually worsen asthma control. Previous studies have not had been adequate to resolve the debate over the safety and efficacy of β-agonist medications. The effects of regularly scheduled vs. as-needed albuterol were compared in a randomized, double-blind trial.

Methods.—The study included 255 patients with mild, clinically stable asthma, with an FEV_1 of no more than 70% of predicted, among other characteristics. Those assigned to regular albuterol were to take 2 inhala-tions 4 tmes daily plus albuterol as needed; those assigned to as-needed albuterol received placebo on the same regular schedule plus albuterol as needed. The patients followed their assigned treatment for 16 weeks.

Results.—Peak morning expiratory air flow was not significantly differ-ent before and after treatment for either group: about 415 L/min in the patients taking regularly scheduled albuterol vs. 424 L/min in those taking as-needed albuterol. The 2 treatment groups were also comparable in peak flow variability, FEV_1, amount of supplemental albuterol required, asthma symptoms, quality of life, and airway responsiveness to methacholine. Differences in evening peak flow and in short-term response to inhaled albuterol were statistically but not clinically significant.

Conclusions.—Using inhaled albuterol on a regularly scheduled basis provides no benefit for patients with mild asthma than that achieved by using the medication on an as-needed basis. Neither does regular use have any apparent deleterious effects. Patients with mild ashtma should be prescribed inhaled albuterol on an as-needed basis only.

▶ Because treatment with either regular or as-needed therapy of albuterol was equivalent, the authors make the recommendation that either be used, depending on the feelings of the practitioner and the patient. In some cases, the investigators were punished by having too mild and well-controlled patients in their study. Really, the best approach patients with mild asthma, as with all patients with asthma, should be adequate teaching by the phy-sician. Unfortunately, medical schools do not prepare doctors for a teaching role. Of course, the as-needed β-agonist costs less money, which is quite good in this particular time and place in American history.

M. Weintraub, M.D.

Salmeterol Versus Theophylline in the Treatment of Asthma

Pollard SJ, Spector SL, Yancey SW, et al (Allergy and Asthma Associates, Louisville, Ky; Allergy Research Found Inc, Los Angeles; Glaxo-Wellcome Inc, Research Triangle Park, NC)
Ann Allergy Asthma Immunol 78:457–464, 1997   5–5

Objective.—Although oral β_2-agonists and theophylline are equally effective in reducing the airway obstruction and symptoms of asthma, they are not ideal. Theophylline has a narrow therapeutic index and oral β_2-agonists are not as effective as inhaled β_2-agonists. Combined results of 2 multicenter, randomized, double-dummy, parallel-group, placebo-controlled, 12-week studies comparing twice daily inhaled salmeterol with twice daily dose-titrated theophylline in asthmatic patients were presented.

Methods.—Either salmeterol (42 µg) by metered-dose inhaler (MDI) plus placebo tablets, oral extended-release theophylline plus placebo MDI, or placebo tablets plus placebo MDI were administered for 12 weeks to 484 theophylline-tolerant patients aged 12 years or older. The theophylline dose was adjusted in an open-label theophylline titration period for as long as 2 weeks to a serum concentration of 10 to 20 mg/L. Patients' forced expiratory volume in 1 second (FEV_1) and serum theophylline levels were assessed monthly. Patients measured their peak expiratory flow (PEF) rates daily in the morning and before bedtime. Efficacy results for the groups were compared statistically.

Results.—Eighty patients did not complete the study. During the titration period, the mean theophylline levels were 12.4 mg/L in the placebo group, 12.5 mg/L in the salmeterol group, and 12.7 mg/L in the theophylline group. During the treatment period, at 12 hours after dosing, serum theophylline levels at all time points averaged 7.9 mg/L, 7.7 mg/L, and 7.6 mg/L, respectively. Compared with placebo and theophylline, salmeterol significantly improved morning and evening PEF, significantly reduced night-time wakenings, and significantly decreased asthma symptoms at all time points. Compared with placebo, salmeterol significantly improved FEV_1 at all time points. There were no significant differences in FEV_1 between salmeterol and theophylline or between theophylline and placebo. Salmeterol patients required significantly less albuterol than either placebo or theophylline patients. The Physician-Rated Global Assessment was significantly higher for salmeterol patients than for theophylline or placebo patients at all time points. Significantly more theophylline-treated patients reported adverse gastrointestinal events. Patient satisfaction was significantly higher in the salmeterol group than in the theophylline or placebo groups.

Conclusion.—Salmeterol (42 µg twice daily) is significantly more effective than twice-daily, dose-titrated theophylline for relieving asthma symptoms and improving pulmonary function. Salmeterol users experienced fewer gastrointestinal complaints than did theophylline users.

▶ Salmeterol, which is a long-acting bronchodilator and, thus, not useful in the short-term treatment of asthma symptoms, was superior to theophylline in this study. Actually, theophylline, although a valuable agent, is more trouble to use, has a narrow therapeutic window, and requires both individualization of therapy and regular monitoring of serum levels. Hence, if possible, it should be avoided whenever other medications can be given.

M. Weintraub, M.D.

A Comparison of Ipratropium and Albuterol vs Albuterol Alone for the Treatment of Acute Asthma

Karpel JP, Schacter EN, Fanta C, et al (Albert Einstein College of Medicine, Bronx, NY; Harvard Med School, Boston; Boehringer Ingelheim Pharmaceuticals Inc, Ridgefield, Conn)

Chest 110:611–616, 1996   5–6

Background.—Although inhaled anticholinergic bronchodilators are known to be effective in the treatment of chronic obstructive pulmonary disease, their efficacy in the treatment of acute asthma is not established. The efficacy of ipratropium bromide in combination with albuterol in the treatment of acute asthma exacerbations was evaluated in a multicenter, double-blind, controlled study with a parallel group design.

Methods.—A total of 384 patients seen in the emergency department with acute asthma were randomly assigned to treatment with either 0.5 mL of 0.5% albuterol plus 2.5 normal saline solution or 0.5 mL of 0.5% albuterol plus 2.5 mL of 0.02% ipratropium bromide. The medication was administered twice, 45 minutes apart. Spirometry was performed before and 45 minutes after each treatment. Venous blood samples were obtained before treatment and after 90 minutes, and serum potassium levels were measured.

Results.—There were no statistically significant differences in spirometric values between the 2 treatment groups at either 45 or 90 minutes. However, there were more responders at 45 minutes in the group receiving combination therapy; this difference was no longer significant at 90 minutes. There were no significant differences between the groups in the decline in potassium levels or in the frequency of adverse events.

Conclusions.—Treatment of acute asthma exacerbations with combined inhaled ipratropium bromide and a β-agonist does not appear to confer a significant advantage over treatment with a β-agonist alone. Further study is needed to determine the efficacy of combination therapy in patients initially unresponsive to inhaled β-agonists alone.

▶ This is another study that has a negative outcome, but is important because of the large number of patients (384) and the participant population, which is a group of inner-city patients. Poorer patients, patients of color, and, therefore, inner-city patients are of interest because of their particular and serious problems with asthma. In fact, the death rate is higher in these patients. In any case, we have to hope that these negative trials continue to be published so that, once having been done, they will not have to be repeated.

M. Weintraub, M.D.

Effectiveness of the Leukotriene Receptor Antagonist Zafirlukast for Mild-to-Moderate Asthma

Suissa S, Dennis R, Ernst P, et al (Royal Victoria Hosp, Montreal; Montreal Gen Hosp; McGill Univ, Montreal; et al)

Ann Intern Med 126:177–183, 1997   5–7

Introduction.—Leukotriene receptor antagonists interfere with the action of leukotrienes, which are implicated in bronchoconstriction and formation of airway edema in patients with asthma. One of these agents, zafirlukast, is now being evaluated in randomized, double-blind trials. A multicenter study assessed the clinical and economic effectiveness of zafirlukast in patients with mild-to-moderate asthma.

Methods.—Participants in the trial were 146 patients aged 12 years or older with a forced expiratory volume in 1 second (FEV_1) at least 55% of predicted value and bronchial hyperresponsiveness. Eligibility required a smoking history of less than 10 pack-years and no smoking during the previous 6 months. Forty-three patients were randomized to placebo and 103 to zafirlukast (20 mg twice daily). Inhaled β-agonists were used according to need. Outcome data were gathered from medical examinations, patient questionnaires, and daily diaries.

Results.—The 2 groups were similar in baseline characteristics, except that the mean percent predicted FEV_1 at baseline was significantly lower in the zafirlukast group (74.2%) than in the placebo group (83.7%). During

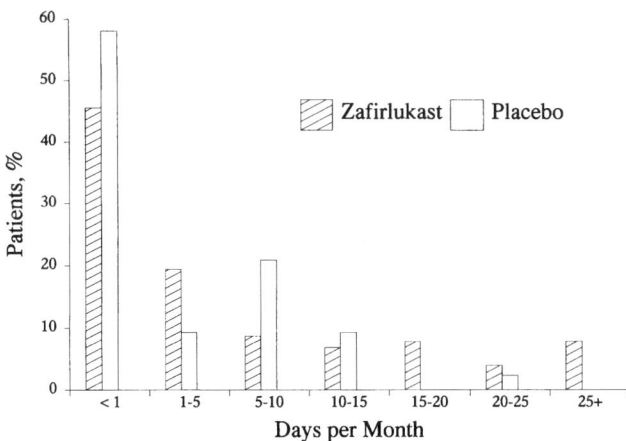

FIGURE.—Days without symptoms per month during the 13-week follow-up, by treatment group. No placebo recipients lacked symptoms on days 15 to 20 and day 25+. (Courtesy of Suissa S, Dennis R, Ernst P, et al: Effectiveness of the leukotriene receptor antagonist zafirlukast for mild-to-moderate asthma. *Ann Intern Med* 126:177–183, 1997.)

the 13-week trial, patients in the zafirlukast group had significantly more time without symptoms (Figure), without the use of β-agonists, and without episodes of asthma. Patients in the zafirlukast group also had 55% fewer health care contacts and 55% fewer days of absence from school or work. Compared with those assigned to placebo, patients treated with zafirlukast used 17% fewer canisters of inhaled β-agonists and 19% less nonasthma medication.

Conclusion.—Daily use of the leukotriene receptor antagonist zafirlukast together with as-needed inhaled β-agonists was more effective than β-agonists alone in the treatment of mild-to-moderate asthma. Because zafirlukast reduced the use of health services and absenteeism rates, the agent also had significant economic benefits.

▶ In this morning's paper there was another report of a young, otherwise healthy, asthmatic who died. Such deaths are all too common. Many of us have had friends, even physicians, who have died of an asthma attack, even though they should have known that they were seriously ill and getting worse and needed help. Therefore, this study of the efficacy and economic aspects of the leukotriene antagonists, such as zafirlukast, is helpful.

The investigators looked at a whole bunch of things that are not usually measured in clinical trials except for asthma. They include the number of days without symptoms, without limitation of activity, without use of β-agonists, without sleep disturbance, and without episodes of asthma. As shown in the figure, the percentage of patients having days per month without symptoms was heavily weighted toward the zafirlukast. When you add the decrease in absenteeism from school or work and the reduced use of health services resulting from zafirlukast use we can really see how helpful preventive therapy can be. This drug has recently been approved by the Food and Drug Administration.

M. Weintraub, M.D.

Acute and Chronic Effects of a 5-Lipoxygenase Inhibitor in Asthma: A 6-Month Randomized Multicenter Trial
Liu MC, and the Zileuton Study Group (Johns Hopkins Asthma and Allergy Ctr, Baltimore, Md)
J Allergy Clin Immunol 98:859–871, 1996   5–8

Background.—Leukotrienes are believed to mediate many of the pathologic effects of asthma, particularly inflammatory events and bronchoconstriction. Thus, inhibiting leukotrienes may improve airway function in patients with asthma. In a randomized, double-blind, placebo-controlled, parallel-group study, the effects of zileuton, an inhibitor of 5-lipoxygenase, on symptoms of mild-to-moderate asthma were evaluated.

Methods.—Patients were between ages 18 and 62 and were weaned from other medications (except for a β-agonist inhaler, albuterol sulfate). Patients were randomly allocated to receive 4-times-a-day dosing with 600 mg of zileuton (n = 122–123 [range provided because of dropouts, missing data, etc.]), with 400 mg of zileuton (n = 119–120), or with placebo (n = 120–122). Over the 6 months of the study, forced expiratory volume in 1 second (FEV_1), forced vital capacity (FVC), peak expiratory flow rate, how often the patient used a β-agonist inhaler, how often rescue corticosteroids were needed, how often the patient had acute exacerbations of asthma, and asthma symptoms were evaluated regularly.

Findings.—Zileuton showed acute and significant increases in FEV_1 and FVC at almost all time points up to 6 hours after dosing. Both doses of zileuton improved trough FEV_1 by the first visit after dosing, and the improvement was maintained throughout the study. Compared to baseline, over the course of the study, the FEV_1 and the peak expiratory flow rate were significantly improved in the 600-mg zileuton group compared to the placebo group. Patients taking zileuton at either dose reported fewer adverse effects and better symptom scores than patients taking placebo. The placebo group used significantly more corticosteroids and more puffs from the inhaler than either zileuton group. Finally, the percentage reductions in eosinophils were greater in the zileuton groups than in the placebo group.

Conclusions.—Zileuton resulted in a significant reduction in bronchodilator effect within 2 hours of dosing and this improvement was maintained up to 6 hours. Even by the first visit, zileuton improved spirometry results significantly, and again this effect persisted over 6 months. Patients reported fewer symptoms and fewer adverse effects while taking the drug. The decrease in peripheral blood eosinophils with active drug indicates a possible antiinflammatory action.

▶ Inhibitors of the production of 5-lipoxygenase substrates in the pathway of arachidonic acid metabolism were not shown to be as valuable as the inhibitors of the leukotrienes on the receptors. Once one medication, such as zafirlukast, has gone through the process, and been approved, frequently you can expect to see second and third ones.

M. Weintraub, M.D.

6 Blood Disorders

A Multiparameter Analysis of Sickle Erythrocytes in Patients Undergoing Hydroxyurea Therapy

Bridges KR, Barabino GD, Brugnara C, et al (Brigham and Women's Hosp, Boston; Children's Hosp, Boston; Massachusetts Gen Hosp, Boston; et al)
Blood 88:4701–4710, 1996   6–1

Background.—Patients with sickle cell disease with a large fraction of F cells (20% fetal Hb [HbF] and 80% HbS) tend to have milder disease. Hydroxyurea has been used to stimulate HbF synthesis as a form of therapy for sickle cell disease. Whether the clinical improvement seen with hydroxyurea results solely from changes in F-cell production or is related to other vaso-occlusive parameters was investigated.

Methods.—Three patients with sickle cell disease underwent therapy with hydroxyurea for 24 weeks. Red blood cell (RBC) parameters were measured, including F-cell and F-reticulocyte profiles, delay-time distributions for intracellular polymerization, sickle erythrocyte adherence to human umbilical vein endothelial cells (laminar flow chamber), RBC phthalate density profiles, mean corpuscular hemoglobin concentration and cation content, reticulocyte mean corpuscular hemoglobin concentration, ^{1}H-nuclear MR transverse relaxation rates of packed RBCs, and band 3 and glycophorin plasma membrane lateral and rotational mobilities.

Results.—The fraction of cells with delay times sufficiently long to escape the microcirculation before polymerization occurred was increased by hydroxyurea (Fig 1). This may have been possible because, after only 2 weeks of hydroxyurea treatment (before HbF levels had increased), high pretreatment adherence of sickle RBCs to human umbilical vein endothelial cells decreased to normal. Several biochemical and biophysical parameters were shifted toward those typical of the milder hemoglobin sickle cell disease.

Conclusions.—These data suggest that hydroxyurea, which is the only drug proven to decrease the frequency of pain crises in patients with sickle cell disease, alters certain RBC characteristics independently of its ability to induce HbF synthesis. Decreased numbers of reticulocytes and perhaps changes in the intrinsic adhesiveness of the cells could be involved.

▶ The delay times of intracellular polymerization in 3 patients over 24 weeks of treatment is shown in the figure. As can be seen, the fraction of cells

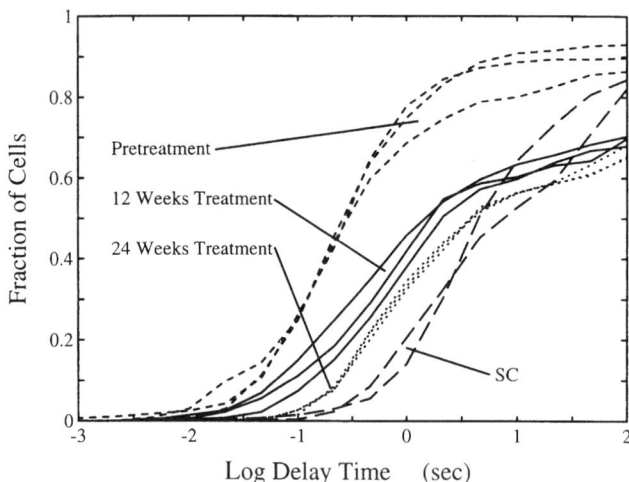

FIGURE 1.—Fraction of sickling cells as a function of time after initiating intracellular polymerization by complete photodissociation of CO. The fraction of cells with delay times shorter than a given time is plotted vs. the logarithm of the time. For each patient, 3 curves are shown. (*short dashes*), pretreatment control; (*solid line*), 12 weeks after beginning hydroxyurea treatment; and (*dotted line*), 24 weeks after beginning hydroxyurea treatment. Also shown are the results for 2 (untreated) patients with HbSC disease (*long dashes*). *Abbreviation:* SC, sickle cell. (Courtesy of Bridges KR, Barabino GD, Brugnara C, et al: A multiparameter analysis of sickle erythrocytes in patients undergoing hydroxyurea therapy. *Blood* 88:4701–4710, 1996.)

undergoing intracellular polymerization is prolonged in these patients. In patients with hemoglobin sickle cell disease, the delay in the polymerization of the cells is markedly prolonged in comparison with sickle cell red blood cells. The era of counting sickle cells may have been bypassed, as illustrated by this study. Not only are we seeing changes in smaller and smaller molecules, but we are able to tell so much more about what is going on in the sickle cell process. Measuring dense cells is another relatively simple, yet sophisticated, way of tracking the progress of sickle cell disease. All I can say is "More power to you." Hydroxyurea has been a revolutionary treatment. I certainly hope that we can find other treatments in the future.

M. Weintraub, M.D.

Cost-effectiveness of Interferon Alfa in Chronic Myelogenous Leukemia
Liberato NL, Quaglini S, Barosi G (Lab of Med Informatics, Pavia, Italy; Univ of Pavia, Italy)
J Clin Oncol 15:2673–2682, 1997   6–2

Background.—Research shows that interferon-alfa (IFN-α) induces karyotypic remission, delays disease progression, and prolongs overall survival, compared with conventional chemotherapy in patients with chronic myelogenous leukemia. However, the advantages of IFN-α are limited by its adverse effects and high cost. The cost-effectiveness of IFN-α treatment in patients with chronic myelogenous leukemia was compared with that of conventional chemotherapy.

Methods.—A decision–analysis model was developed to estimate the expected cost and quality-adjusted life expectancies for 2 cohorts of patients. The following 2 IFN-α strategies were used in the model: (1) prolonged therapy for patients achieving a hematologic response and (2) therapy only for patients achieving a cytogenetic remission in a 2-year period (designated scenarios A and B, respectively). Data for the analysis were obtained from studies identified in a MEDLINE search. Adjustments for quality of life were based on expert panel judgment.

Findings.—Therapy with IFN-α increased the quality-adjusted life expectancy by 15.5 and 12.5 months in scenarios A and B, respectively, compared with conventional chemotherapy. The marginal cost-effectiveness was found to be $89,500 and $63,500 per quality-adjusted life-year (QALY) gained. Reducing IFN-α dose would decrease the marginal cost-effectiveness to less than $20,000.

Conclusions.—Interferon-alfa therapy is markedly better than conventional chemotherapy in quality-adjusted survival. However, at currently used doses, the range of marginal cost-effectiveness was about $50,000 to $100,000 for each QALY gained.

▶ Only a minority of patients with chronic myelogenous leukemia who might benefit from bone marrow transplants can be so treated, for a variety of reasons. As a result, most of these patients now get either hydroxurea, busulfan, or IFN-α. IFN-α obviously provides benefits, but it produces unpleasant side effects and costs a lot more than conventional chemotherapy.

This study suggests therapeutic superiority for IFN-α, but with a high price tag. How much is a year of life worth?

L. Lasagna, M.D.

Treatment of Polycythemia Vera: Use of ³²P Alone or in Combination With Maintenance Therapy Using Hydroxyurea in 461 Patients Greater Than 65 Years of Age
Najean Y, for the French Polycythemia Study Group (Hôpital Saint Louis, Paris)
Blood 89:2319–2327, 1997   6–3

Background.—Despite myelosuppression, elderly polycythemic patients have a high risk of vascular complications. After 12 years, the leukemic risk exceeds 15%. The current study determined whether the addition of low-dose maintenance therapy with hydroxyurea (HU) after radiophosphorous (^{32}P) myelosuppression can reduce these complications.

Methods.—Four hundred sixty-one patients were assigned randomly to receive low-dose HU, 5 to 10 mg/kg/d, after the first ^{32}P-induced remission or no HU treatment. The patients were followed up through June 1996 or until they died.

Findings.—Maintenance therapy significantly prolonged the duration of ^{32}P-induced remissions and decreased the annual mean dose to one third. However, 25% of the patients had an excessive platelet count despite maintenance. In addition, the rate of serious vascular complications was not reduced, except in the most severely affected patients with short-term polycythemia relapse. Also, the leukemia rate was increased significantly beyond 8 years, and a significant excess of carcinoma was noted. Continuous HU use did not reduce the risk of progression to myelofibrosis. Except in the patients with the most severe cases, life expectancy was shorter. In most patients in whom the duration of the first ^{32}P-induced remission exceeded 2 years, the introduction of HU maintenance did not decrease the vascular risk (Fig 1).

Conclusions.—Though HU maintenance therapy substantially reduced the mean dose of ^{32}P received, this treatment significantly increased the

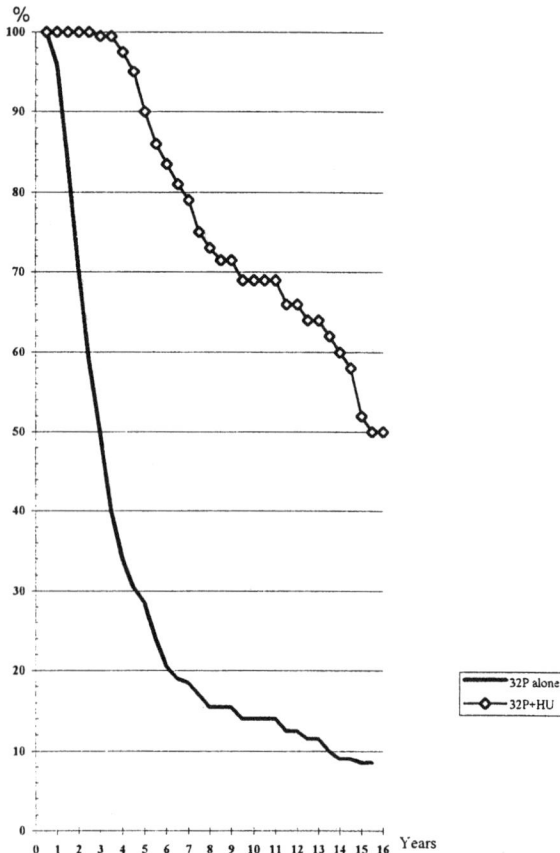

FIGURE 1.—Actuarial chance to remain in first remission after initial ^{32}P infusion. (Courtesy of Najean Y, for the French Polycythemia Study Group: Treatment of polycythemia vera: Use of P alone or in combination with maintenance therapy using hydroxyurea in 461 patients greater than 65 years of age. *Blood* 89:2319–2327, 1997.)

leukemia and cancer risks and decreased life expectancy by 15%. In patients with more rapid recurrence, however, maintenance therapy reduced the vascular risks, moderately prolonging survival. Thus, maintenance therapy with HU is only justified in these patients.

▶ ³²P is a splendid treatment for polycythemia in elderly patients, inducing lengthy survival with an excellent quality of life. Radiotherapy-chemotherapy combination doesn't seem to do much good, and even increases the risk of cancer and leukemia.

L. Lasagna, M.D.

A Randomized Controlled Study of Iron Supplementation in Patients Treated With Erythropoietin
MacDougall IC, Tucker B, Thompson J, et al (St Bartholomew's Hosp, London)
Kidney Int 50:1694–1699, 1996   6–4

Introduction.—Patients receiving recombinant human erythropoietin have been known to have problems with iron deficiency. To support erythropoiesis in such patients, large amounts of iron are required; however, the value of iron supplementation and the optimum route have never been assessed in a controlled clinical trial. The effects of using 3 different regimens of iron treatment were compared in a study of iron supplementation in iron-replete patients receiving erythropoietin therapy.

Methods.—Over a 12-month period, 38 patients who were iron-replete and in renal failure, and were beginning treatment with recombinant human erythropoietin, were randomly separated into 3 groups receiving iron dextran 5 mL every 2 weeks, oral ferrous sulfate 200 mg 3 times daily, or no iron. All the patients had a hemoglobin concentration of less than 8.5 g/dL and an initial serum ferritin level of 100 to 800 µg/L. Every 2 weeks for the first 4 months, measurements were taken of the hemoglobin concentration, reticulocyte count, serum ferritin level, transferrin saturation, and recombinant human erythropoietin dose.

Results.—In the group receiving IV iron, the hemoglobin response was significantly greater than in the other 2 groups. The IV iron group had a hemoglobin response of 7.3±0.8 to 11.9±1.2 g/dL. The oral iron group had a hemoglobin response of 7.2±1.1 to 10.2±1.4 g/dL. The no-iron group had a hemoglobin response of 7.3±0.8 to 9.9±1.6 g/dL. Patients receiving IV iron had serum ferritin levels that remained constant (345±273 to 359±140 µg/L). In the other 2 groups, the ferritin levels fell significantly. The oral iron group had values of 309±218 to 116±87 µg/L. The no-iron group had values of 458±206 to 131±121 µg/L. In the IV iron group, dosage requirements of recombinant human erythropoietin were lower than in the other groups. The IV iron group had a dosage requirement of 1,202±229 U/kg/16 wk; the oral iron group had a dosage requirement of 1,294±314 U/kg/16 wk and the no-iron group had a dosage requirement of 1,475±311 U/kg/16 wk.

Conclusion.—Compared with patients receiving oral iron and no iron supplementation, even iron-replete patients given supplementary IV iron have an enhanced hemoglobin response to recombinant human erythropoietin, with better maintenance of iron stores and lower dosage requirements of recombinant human erythropoietin.

▶ From the earliest clinical trials of erythropoietin, it has been suggested that such patients do better with iron supplementation. This is the first prospective controlled trial to address the issue and—guess what?—even in so-called iron-replete patients, supplementation with IV iron confers all sorts of benefits. A low serum ferritin level indicates iron deficiency, but a "normal" level does not mean that a patient will be able to mobilize iron adequately from body stores. Unfortunately, none of the other available laboratory tests has proved ideal either. So, what do do? Routine IV iron supplementation involves money, time, labor, and inconvenience, plus the (small) risk of serious adverse effects (e.g., anaphylaxis). At the very least, however, a poor response to erythropoietin in the absence of identifiable cause should lead to a consideration of adjuvant parenteral iron therapy.

L. Lasagna, M.D.

Erythropoietin Reduces Anemia and Transfusions After Chemotherapy With Paclitaxel and Carboplatin
Dunphy FR, Dunleavy TL, Harrison BR, et al (Saint Louis Univ, Mo; Belleville Otolaryngology Associates, Ill)
Cancer 79:1623–1628, 1997   6–5

Background.—Paclitaxel is a common cytotoxic agent in the treatment of cancer. Anemia has not been reported as a major side effect of paclitaxel when used alone. Anemia has been reported as a common side effect of carboplatin alone and of paclitaxel and carboplatin combined. The authors have noted cumulative anemia in patients with advanced head and neck cancer during preoperative treatment with paclitaxel and carboplatin. Recombinant human erythropoietin (rHuEpo) was added in later patients to lower the rate of surgical transfusions.

Methods.—Evaluations were made in 36 patients with advanced head and neck cancer after preoperative treatment with paclitaxel and carboplatin. There were 14 patients in group 1 who were treated with rHuEpo, 150 U/kg 3 times per week for 3 weeks. Patients who did not respond were given increased doses of 300 U/kg and 450 U/kg. There were 22 patients in group 2 who were not given rHuEpo.

Results.—A response to rHuEpo was defined as a lower decrease in hemoglobin during preoperative chemotherapy and less need for surgical transfusion. During preoperative treatment, the mean decrease in hemoglobin was 0.5 g/dL in group 1 and 3.3 g/dL in group 2; the difference was statistically significant. In group 1, none of 14 patients had packed red blood cell transfusions. In group 2, 4 of 22 patients had packed red blood cell transfusions; this was not statistically significant.

Discussion.—In patients with advanced head and neck cancer, preoperative treatment with paclitaxel and carboplatin resulted in a significant decrease in hemoglobin. Recombinant human erythropoietin appeared to prevent anemia and result in fewer surgical transfusions when administered with chemotherapy. Caution is advised when drawing conclusions from this uncontrolled study of a small population.

▶ Combination therapy with paclitaxel and carboplatin has been observed to cause anemia. Erythropoietin clearly helps to prevent this anemia and, thus, reduces the need for packed red blood cell transfusions. Chalk up another victory for erythropoietin!

L. Lasagna, M.D.

Anemia of Cancer: Pathogenesis and Treatment With Recombinant Erythropoietin
Mittelman M (Tel Aviv Univ, Israel)
Isr J Med Sci 32:1201–1206, 1996   6–6

Introduction.—Cancer-associated anemia (CAA) occurs in about 60% of patients with advanced cancer. Patients with cancer have decreased erythropoietin levels that are believed to be related to inflammatory cytokines. The effect of treatment with recombinant erythropoietin was described.

Treatment of CAA.—Transfusion of red blood cells is typically used to treat symptomatic anemia, but it is associated with risks that could affect prognosis in patients with cancer. The first patients to benefit from treatment with recombinant human erythropoietin (rHuEpo) were patients with end-stage renal failure and anemia. From 1990 to 1996, 20 trials of 870 patients with various neoplasms were conducted to test the efficacy of rHuEpo in treating CAA or to test rHuEpo in the prevention of anemia resulting from chemotherapy. About half the patients responded with significant increases in hemoglobin level, decreases in blood transfusion requirements, and improved performance status and quality of life.

Adverse Effects.—Minimal adverse effects are observed with rHuEpo administration and it is usually well tolerated. Elevated blood pressure and venous thrombosis have been significant only in patients with renal hypertension.

Conclusion.—Many questions need to be addressed regarding rHuEpo administration, including optimal dosage, duration of treatment, erythropoietin resistance, and the possibility of predicting the response.

▶ Although recombinant erythropoietin only helps the anemia of a bit over 50% of all patients with cancer, its contributions to these lucky patients are impressive: less transfusions and improved performance status and quality of life.

L. Lasagna, M.D.

The Duration of Oral Anticoagulant Therapy After a Second Episode of Venous Thromboembolism

Schulman S, and the Duration of Anticoagulation Trial Study Group (Karolinska Hosp, Stockholm; Huddinge Hosp, Sweden; Danderyd Hosp, Sweden; et al)
N Engl J Med 336:393–398, 1997   6–7

Introduction.—Two recent multicenter trials have shown that extending the duration of orally given anticoagulant therapy after a first episode of venous thromboembolism can reduce the rate of recurrence. Because the optimal duration of prophylactic orally given anticoagulant treatment after a second episode has not been determined, a multicenter trial compared the benefits of treatment for 6 months with indefinite treatment.

Methods.—During the 3-year enrollment period, 227 patients were randomly assigned to the 2 treatment groups. Eligible patients were at least 15 years of age and had a second episode of acute pulmonary embolism or deep vein thrombosis in the leg, the iliac veins, or both. Initial treatment consisted of heparin for at least 5 days; orally given anticoagulation with warfarin sodium or dicumarol was usually started at the same time as heparin therapy. The target chosen for the international normalized ratio was 2.0–to 2.85. Patients in the 6-month group discontinued orally given anticoagulant without tapering at their 6-month evaluation. Principal end points of the study were major hemorrhage, recurrent venous thromboembolism, and death.

Results.—There were 26 recurrences of venous thromboembolism during the 48 months of follow-up. Only 3 (2.6%) of the recurrences were in the indefinite therapy group, compared to 23 (20.7%) in the 6-month group. No recurrence took place during anticoagulant therapy (the 3 patients in the indefinite therapy group had prematurely discontinued therapy). When compared with therapy of indefinite duration, the relative risk of recurrence in the group assigned to 6 months of orally given anticoagulant therapy was 8.0. Thirteen major hemorrhages occurred, 3 (2.7%) in the 6-month group and 10 (8.6%) in the indefinite treatment group. The relative risk of major hemorrhage in the 6-month group was 0.3.

Discussion.—The risk of major hemorrhagic complications has been a deterrent to the long-term use of orally given anticoagulant therapy after a second episode of venous thromboembolism. There was a trend toward an increased risk of major hemorrhage with indefinite duration of therapy, but this was offset by a much lower rate of recurrent thromboembolism.

▶ Episodes of venous thromboembolism routinely lead to the initiation of orally given anticoagulant therapy, but how long to have such patients receive anticoagulant is controversial. It would seem that some patients probably need to receive the drugs indefinitely, but the price is the risk of major hemorrhage. This is further evidence that God is a Puritan, and exacts a price for every benefit.

L. Lasagna, M.D.

Prevention of Thromboembolism With Use of Recombinant Hirudin
Eriksson BI, Ekman S, Lindbratt S, et al (Univ of Göteberg, Sweden; Gentofte Hosp, Hellerup)
J Bone Joint Surg Am 79A:326–333, 1997   6–8

Objective.—The prevalence of deep vein thrombosis after total hip replacement ranges from 21% to 55% even after treatment with heparin or warfarin. Inhibition of thrombin is a new preventive technique that has been shown to be effective at preventing deep vein thrombosis. Results are presented of a randomized, double-blind study assessing the efficacy and safety of 15 mg desirudin as compared with heparin, administered subcutaneously as fixed doses to patients having elective hip surgery.

Methods.—Either desirudin (approximately 12,000 thrombin-inhibiting units/mg of protein, produced by recombinant DNA technology) or heparin was administered twice daily for an average of 9 days, to 445 total hip replacement patients in 11 centers in 2 Scandinavian countries. The number of thromboembolic events occurring during the treatment period was recorded. Deep vein thrombosis was confirmed by bilateral venography read by 2 independent radiologists. Pulmonary embolism was confirmed by angiography or ventilation-and-perfusion scan.

Results.—Of the 351 patients assessable for efficacy, 13 in the desirudin group ($n = 174$) and 41 in the heparin group ($n = 177$) had confirmed deep vein thrombosis ($P < 0.0001$). The reduction in relative risk was 68%. Compared with the heparin group, the desirudin group had a significant 79% reduction in the prevalence of proximal deep vein thrombosis (6 vs. 29). Four heparin-treated patients had a pulmonary embolus during the follow-up period. Two heparin-treated patients died during the follow-up period. Blood loss, transfusion requirements, bleeding complications, and incidence of side effects were similar between groups.

Conclusion.—Compared with heparin, administration of a fixed dose of desirudin, a thrombin inhibitor, twice daily for an average of 9 days, in patients having a total hip replacement significantly reduces the incidence of thromboembolic events with no increased incidence of bleeding complications and side effects.

▶ Hirudin appears to be a direct inhibitor of thrombin activity in humans. This study was clearly positive as it was analyzed for this publication. However, there is 1 nagging doubt. The patients who did not enter into the analysis and some who did not have a second venogram may have led to different results because, fortunately, no pulmonary emboli occurred in either of the treatment groups. So, the intent-to-treat analysis was not real because it required a repeat venogram. Some statisticians believe that the intent-to-treat population is 1 of the least biased ways of looking at the results. I see it as just another way, although quite important. Also, in some ways, the "by-protocol" analysis, as in this report, is really the only way to come up with a good answer to the question, "Did the medication help the patients?"

M. Weintraub, M.D.

Determinants of Compliance With Anticoagulation: A Case-Control Study

Arnsten JH, Gelfand JM, Singer DE (Harvard Med School, Boston; Harvard School of Public Health, Boston)
Am J Med 103:11–17, 1997   6–9

Introduction.—There has been a sharp increase in the number of patients receiving long-term anticoagulation therapy. Patient compliance is essential for safe and beneficial anticoagulation, yet there are no data on the barriers to compliance with anticoagulation. Poor compliance can be a particular problem among the elderly. Barriers to compliance with anticoagulation were assessed in a case-control study.

Methods.—The study included 43 case patients discharged from an anticoagulation therapy unit because of noncompliance and a random sample of 89 compliant control patients. The noncompliant patients had either stopped taking warfarin against medical advice or were still taking it but not complying with recommended monitoring of international nor-

TABLE 3.—Measures of Patient Satisfaction*

Variable	Cases (n = 43) n (%)	Controls (n = 89) n (%)	Odds Ratio (95% CI)	P Value
No regular physician	12 (28)	3 (3)	11.1 (3.6, 50.0)	<0.0001
Quality of information from physician rated as excellent or very good†	24 (77)	73 (86)	0.6 (0.2, 1.6)	NS
Skill and competence of physician rated as excellent or very good‡	25 (81)	81 (95)	0.2 (0.1, 0.8)	0.013
Willingness of physician to listen to patient concerns rated as excellent or very good	22 (71)	75 (87)	0.4 (0.1, 1.0)	0.04
Patient feels physician is not very concerned about them§	12 (39)	14 (17)	3.1 (1.2, 7.8)	0.01

*For assessments of patient satisfaction with physicians, only patients who reported that they had a regular physician were included (*n* = 117).
†Data missing on one subject.
‡Data missing on one subject.
§Data missing on three subjects.
(Reprinted by permission of the publisher from Arnsten JH, Gelfand JM, Singer DE: Determinants of compliance with anticoagulation: A case-control study. *Am J Med* 103:11–17, 1997. Copyright 1997 by Excerpta Medica, Inc.)

TABLE 4.—Perceived Benefits and Barriers to Anticoagulation

Variable	Cases (n = 43) n (%)	Controls (n = 89) n (%)	Odds Ratio* (95% CI)	P Value
Taking warfarin benefits my health	23 (53)	71 (80)	0.3 (0.1, 0.6)	0.002
Taking warfarin prevents blood clots	30 (70)	74 (83)	0.5 (0.2, 1.1)	0.08
Taking warfarin protects my future health	28 (65)	76 (85)	0.3 (0.1, 0.7)	0.008
Taking warfarin affects my lifestyle	23 (53)	28 (31)	2.5 (1.2, 5.3)	0.015
I worry about bleeding while taking warfarin	21 (49)	27 (30)	2.2 (1.0, 4.6)	0.04
Taking warfarin restricts my physical activity	13 (30)	13 (15)	2.5 (1.1, 6.0)	0.03
Regular blood tests to monitor warfarin are a problem	26 (60)	30 (34)	3.0 (1.4, 6.3)	0.004

*Odds ratios are for two group comparisons ("some/a great deal" vs. "not at all/don't know").
(Reprinted by permission of the publisher from Arnsten JH, Gelfand JM, Singer DE: Determinants of compliance with anticoagulation: A case-control study. *Am J Med* 103:11–17, 1997. Copyright 1997 by Excerpta Medica, Inc.)

malized ratio (INR) levels. Data from telephone interviews were analyzed to identify factors associated with noncompliance.

Results.—Mean age was 54 years for the noncompliant cases, vs. 69 years for the compliant controls. The noncompliant patients were more likely to be male (odds ratio [OR] 3.5) and nonwhite (OR 6.4). They were less likely to have a history of stroke or transient ischemic attack (OR 0.2). Twenty-eight percent of noncompliant patients reported having no regular physician, compared with 3% of compliant patients (Table 3). The noncompliant patients were less likely to see the benefits of taking anticoagulation, and more likely to find it burdensome (Table 4).

Conclusions.—Factors associated with noncompliance with anticoagulation therapy were identified. Many noncompliant patients are younger men who have not had a thromboembolic event. These patients may neglect monitoring of therapy or stop taking anticoagulation therapy altogether. Efforts to improve compliance could include improved patient education, physician involvement, and easier monitoring.

▶ Noncompliance with drug-dosing instructions is all too common. Sometimes physicians are aware of it, but often not. This study was an imaginative exploration of the reasons for failing to follow directions. Awareness of the reasons is the first step in correcting the problem. The perceived benefits and risks of anticoagulation are no surprise with regard to impact on behavior, but the data on "patient satisfaction" provide a lot of reasons for physicians to pay attention to *their* behavior as it may impact on patient performance.

L. Lasagna, M.D.

Intraoperative and Postoperative Bleeding Problems in Patients Taking Warfarin, Aspirin, and Nonsteroidal Antiinflammatory Agents: A Prospective Study

Billingsley EM, Maloney ME (Milton S Hershey Med Ctr, Hershey, Pa)
Dermatol Surg 23:381–385, 1997   6–10

Background.—Drugs that affect bleeding can lead to complications in patients undergoing major surgery, but few studies have examined the role of such medications in intraoperative and postoperative bleeding associated with cutaneous surgery. A prospective study evaluated the frequency of bleeding complications in patients undergoing Mohs surgery while being treated with warfarin, aspirin, or nonsteroidal anti-inflammatory drugs (NSAIDs).

Methods.—Data recorded for the 332 patients treated during the study period included age, sex, medication history, intraoperative bleeding, and postoperative data. Eighty-one patients (25.1%) had taken aspirin within 10 days of surgery, 12 had taken warfarin within 2 days of surgery, and 16 had taken NSAIDs within 1 day of surgery; 213 patients (66.1%) had taken no anticoagulant agent before surgery.

Results.—Intraoperative bleeding described as excessive occurred in 5 patients taking warfarin (41.7%), 9 taking aspirin (11%), 1 taking NSAIDs (6.2%), and 9 who had taken no anticoagulants (4.2%). Overall, 8 patients (2.5%) returned to the clinic before their scheduled appointment because of oozing or actively bleeding wounds. Five of these patients had not taken anticoagulants, 2 were taking aspirin, and 1 was being treated with warfarin.

Conclusion.—Few guidelines exist regarding the issue of discontinuation of anticoagulants before cutaneous surgery. Among these patients who were taking the most common anticoagulants, warfarin was associated with excessive intraoperative bleeding. The incidence of postoperative bleeding, however, did not differ between patients taking anticoagulants and controls. It may not be necessary to discontinue these agents for routine dermatologic surgical procedures.

► As time goes by and we learn more about the effects of surgery, including skin operations, the more confident we are that we do not need to stop a medication to perform a surgical procedure. In this case, the investigators felt no need to discontinue a group of platelet active agents and warfarin before dermatologic surgery. In the warfarin patients, there was excessive bleeding during the surgery with a significant *P* value as well. Thus, it comes down to an individual decision on how important anticoagulation is for the particular patient and whether the dermatologist can find a way of doing the surgery which will avoid excessive bleeding.

M. Weintraub, M.D.

A 14-Year Study of Heparin-induced Thrombocytopenia

Warkentin TE, Kelton JG (Hamilton Civic Hosps, Ont, Canada; Chedoke-McMaster Hosps, Hamilton, Ont; McMaster Univ, Hamilton, Ont, Canada)
Am J Med 101:502–507, 1996   6–11

Introduction.—The pathophysiology of heparin-induced thrombocytopenia has recently been defined. Patients produce antibodies, usually IgG, against a complex of heparin and platelet factor 4. The pathogenic IgG triggers platelet activation, which generates procoagulant platelet-derived microparticles. The clinical impact and natural history of this phenomenon is under debate. A 14-year retrospective analysis of a group of patients with serologically confirmed, immune-mediated, heparin-induced thrombocytopenia was conducted.

Methods.—The medical records of patients with evidence of new thrombotic events that occurred in association with the diagnosis of serologically confirmed, heparin-induced thrombocytopenia (group 1) or during the 30 days after recognition of isolated heparin-induced thrombocytopenia (group 2) were reviewed. Patients received heparin for therapeutic or prophylactic reasons.

Results.—Complete data were available for 127 patients with heparin-induced thrombocytopenia. Of those, 66.1% of the patients were from surgical services, most often orthopedic surgery. Surgical patients were significantly more likely to have heparin-induced thrombocytopenia than medical patients while receiving heparin for prophylaxis (88.1% vs.

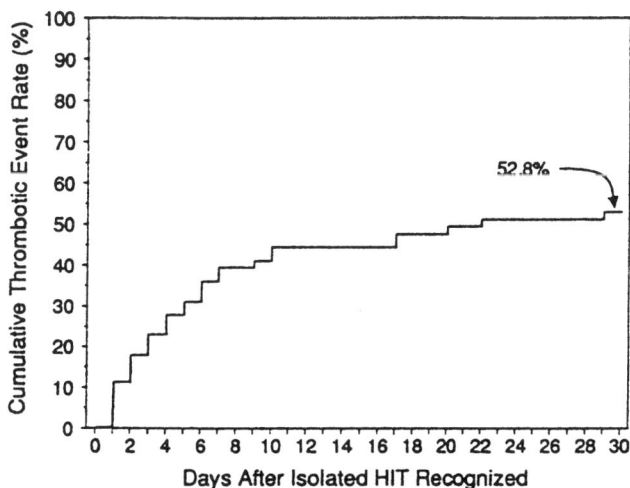

FIGURE.—Cumulative frequency of thrombosis in patients with heparin-induced thrombocytopenia who were first seen with isolated thrombocytopenia. Approximately 50% of patients with heparin-induced thrombocytopenia initially recognized with isolated thrombocytopenia had objective evidence for thrombosis during the subsequent 30-day period. *Abbreviation: HIT,* heparin-induced thrombocytopenia. (Reprinted by permission of the publisher, from Warkentin TE, Kelton JG: A 14-year study of heparin-induced thrombocytopenia. *American Journal of Medicine,* 101:502–507, Copyright 1996 by Excerpta Medica, Inc.)

44.2%). Heparin-induced thrombocytopenia was observed in 51.2% of group 1 patients after a thrombotic event associated with thrombocytopenia. These thrombi were typically venous, mostly proximal lower limb deep vein thrombosis and pulmonary embolism. Twenty-six group 1 patients experienced pulmonary embolism and 12 patients had arterial thrombotic events at the time of diagnosis of heparin-induced thrombocytopenia (Fig). Thirteen patients died during hospitalization. There were 62 group 2 patients in whom heparin-induced thrombocytopenia was identified because of isolated thrombocytopenia. The subsequent 30-day cumulative risk of thrombosis was 52.8% in this patient cohort. Overall, there were 78 venous thrombotic events and 18 arterial events associated with heparin-induced thrombocytopenia. Thirty-two of 127 patients (25.2%) had pulmonary embolism.

Conclusion.—These findings support the increasing evidence that immune-mediated, heparin-induced thrombocytopenia is a markedly prothrombic disorder. Venous thrombosis complicates heparin-induced thrombocytopenia more often than does arterial thrombosis. Conservative treatment approaches to patients with isolated heparin-induced thrombocytopenia may be associated with unacceptably high rates of subsequent thrombosis. Future investigation needs to address the efficacy of alternate anticoagulant agents in treating heparin-induced thrombocytopenia.

▶ Heparin-induced thrombocytopenia is important for 2 reasons—it is not uncommon and it is often associated with thrombotic events. This study suggests that venous thrombosis in such patients is more frequent than arterial thrombosis. What (if any) alternate anticoagulant approach is useful in this situation remains unclear.

L. Lasagna, M.D.

7 Cardiovascular Disorders

Pharmacists' Ability to Influence Outcomes of Hypertension Therapy
Erickson SR, Slaughter R, Halapy H (Wayne State Univ, Detroit)
Pharmacotherapy 17:140–147, 1997   7–1

Introduction.—Pharmacists have the ability to improve disease control through direct patient intervention. Such activities on the part of pharmacists are cost-effective and accepted by physicians and other health care providers. A controlled study was designed to measure the impact of pharmaceutical care on the outcomes of patients being treated for hypertension.

Methods.—Patients were recruited from an internal medicine clinic of a university health center. For those in the intervention group, pharmacists reviewed medical records, took a drug history, assessed patient-specific drug issues, provided information about hypertension and its treatment, monitored drug therapy, took and/or interpreted blood pressure measurements, and made recommendations to the physician. These activities took place during the patient's regularly scheduled clinic visits. Controls received regular care without these interventions. Health-related quality of life was evaluated for both groups using the SF-36 Health Survey.

Results.—The 2 groups of 40 patients each were comparable in mean age, racial and gender distribution, and baseline clinical variables. Over an average follow-up of 5 months, only the intervention group showed a significant decrease in mean blood pressures. The change in systolic pressure was more impressive than the change in diastolic pressure. None of the SF-36 score changes were significantly different between groups. The only change noted between baseline and final assessment was in the domain of physical functioning, which was reduced in the intervention group to a statistically significant degree.

Conclusion.—Blood pressure control was improved in patients with hypertension when they received interventions from the pharmacist. This beneficial effect occurred despite similar pharmacotherapy management in control and intervention groups and no appreciable changes in the number and type of antihypertensive agents prescribed from baseline to final assessment.

▶ Modern pharmacists unquestionably can play a very useful role in educating customers about drug usage, as this study shows, but they often fail to do so. Pouring capsules or tablets from a large container into a small one is hardly an appropriate end to years of pharmaceutical training.

L. Lasagna, M.D.

The Safety of Transdermal Nicotine as an Aid to Smoking Cessation in Patients With Cardiac Disease
Joseph AM, Norman SM, Ferry LH, et al (Univ of Minnesota, Minneapolis; Veterans Affairs Med Ctr, Kansas City, Mo; Veterans Affairs Med Ctr, Loma Linda, Calif; et al)
N Engl J Med 335:1792–1798, 1996   7–2

Introduction.—Smoking cessation benefits patients with cardiac disease by reducing symptoms of atherosclerotic disease and the rate of recurrence of acute cardiovascular events. Transdermal nicotine is known to aid smoking cessation, but its safety in patients with cardiac disease is controversial and some physicians consider underlying cardiac conditions in smokers an absolute contraindication to nicotine therapy. A randomized study examined the safety of transdermal nicotine in this setting.

Methods.—The 10-week, double-blind study randomized 294 patients to nicotine therapy and 290 to placebo. All smoked at least 15 cigarettes a day and had smoked for at least 5 years. Transdermal nicotine was given as a 21–mg patch for 6 weeks, a 14–mg patch for 2 weeks, and a 7–mg patch for 2 weeks. Patients were followed for a total of 14 weeks for cardiac events, side effects of therapy, and abstinence from smoking.

Results.—At least 1 of the primary end points (death; myocardial infarction; cardiac arrest; and hospital admission for increased severity of angina, arrhythmia, or congestive heart failure) was reached by 5.4% of the nicotine group and 7.9% of the placebo group. At 14 weeks, 21% of the nicotine group vs. 9% of the placebo group had stopped smoking. Abstinence rates were similar, however, at 24 weeks (14% vs. 11%). Side effects attributed to nicotine patches occurred as often in the placebo group as in the nicotine group.

Conclusion.—In this multicenter study, transdermal nicotine did not significantly increase cardiovascular events in high-risk outpatients with cardiac disease. Nicotine therapy is, thus, likely to be less dangerous than smoking for such patients. But among these patients, who had failed at least 2 previous attempts to quit smoking, the transdermal patch was not particularly effective.

▶ Cigarette smoking is often responsible for cardiovascular catastrophe, but the risks diminish if one can stop smoking, according to the Surgeon General. Transdermal nicotine has been proposed as an aid to such cessation, but because nicotine by itself is a threat, it is not clear how useful this approach is. This study provided good news and bad news. The good news is that transdermal nicotine does not pose much of a problem to cardiac patients. The bad news: it isn't much help in stopping this addiction.

L. Lasagna, M.D.

Reserpine: A Tragic Victim of Myths, Marketing, and Fashionable Prescribing
Fraser HS (Univ of the West Indies, Barbados)
Clin Pharmacol Ther 60:368–373, 1996   7–3

Introduction.—With each new advance in hypertensive drugs, the cost of treatment increases sharply. Today, almost 100 antihypertensive agents are in use. Massive overdosing and faulty science have occurred with the potent antihypertensive drug reserpine, an adrenergic antagonist with some central action. Its early doses were very high, and today the dose is one seventh to one third of doses first prescribed in the 1960s.

Ruined reputation.—Three perceived problems were associated with reserpine: depression, peptic ulceration, and breast cancer. With dosages up to 10 mg/d, suicides occurred; however, studies showed that the drug could not cause depression. Although reserpine was shown to stimulate the secretion of gastric acid, little or no effect was seen at dosages of 0.25 mg/d or less. The reputation of reserpine was ruined when it was erroneously linked with breast cancer; the drug was immediately replaced with clonidine. Reserpine was withdrawn from use in the United Kingdom but was used extensively in the United States because β-blockers were slow to gain acceptance.

Efficacy and Side Effects.—In several studies, reserpine has been found to be effective at low doses. One study recommended a dose of 0.2 mg with 100 mg of hydrochlorothiazide and 150 mg of hydralazine. In many studies reserpine with or without a diuretic, has been compared favorably with methyldopa; reserpine has also been shown to have efficacy equal to or greater than that of several β-blocker combinations. The effective dose range of reserpine has been found to be 0.05 to 0.25 mg, many times lower than the 1960s doses that led to the drug's undeserved poor profile. Side effects include nasal congestion, impotence, and lipid changes. However, poor compliance does not cause rebound hypertension, as is the case with other centrally acting drugs (such as clonidine and methyldopa).

Conclusion.—Reserpine, which has been shown to be effective in decreasing blood pressure and reducing morbidity and mortality, can cost as little as one fiftieth of the cost of most angiotensin-converting enzyme inhibitor–calcium-channel blocker combinations. In other words, 50 patients can be treated for the price of 1. Nevertheless, reserpine is out of fashion because of false information, a misled profession, and excessive early dose recommendations.

▶ This is a fascinating review of reserpine in all of its many guises as an antihypertensive agent. Certainly the dose was too high initially and was associated with serious adverse effects. Sometimes drugs such as reserpine don't die out. Their use continues, perhaps as in this case, because of their low price and effectiveness. Another drug whose dose initially was probably eight times too high was hydrochlorothiazide. I'd be really interested in how much time is devoted to reserpine in medical school curricula. With so many classes of antihypertensive agents available, more time may be spent on the different members of the class of angiotensin-converting enzyme inhibitors than on reserpine. Of course, the drugs that disappear are sometimes the ones that should go away. For example, α-methyldopa, guanethidine, and other drugs that I learned about in medical school, although they were falling into disfavor in those days, really don't belong in our therapeutic armamentarium anymore. However, with new information and articles (such as this article on reserpine), some of them should not pass away.

M. Weintraub, M.D.

The Effects of Replacing β-Blockers With an Angiotensin Converting Enzyme Inhibitor on the Quality of Life of Hypertensive Patients
Paran E, Anson O, Neumann L (Ben-Gurion Univ of the Negev, Beer Sheva, Israel)
Am J Hypertens 9:1206–1213, 1996   7–4

Introduction.—Most antihypertensive drugs control blood pressure without serious side effects, but these agents may adversely affect quality of life (QOL). Calcium channel blockers and angiotensin converting enzyme (ACE) inhibitors, however, appear to have less of an adverse impact on QOL than older β-blockers or central α-antagonists. To evaluate the results of a change from β-blockers to an ACE inhibitor, 149 patients with hypertension were randomized to receive captopril or continue with β-blocker treatment.

Methods.—All patients had mild-to-moderate hypertension. Sixty-nine were randomized to captopril (12.5 to 50 mg twice daily) and 80 to continue receiving β-blockers (Atenolol 25 to 100 mg once daily or Propranolol 10 to 80 mg twice daily). Hydrochlorothiazide (25 mg) was added in each group when required. Patients were followed for 6 to 12 months for blood pressure control, side effects of treatment, and QOL factors.

Results.—Sixteen patients in the captopril group were excluded from analysis because they received β-blockers during follow-up. Study and control groups were similar at baseline except that mean systolic blood pressure was higher in the captopril group. Both agents managed blood

TABLE 3.—Physical Quality of Life: Symptoms at Baseline and at Follow-Up

Symptom	Study Group (n = 53)			Control Group (n = 80)		
	T_1	T_2	Percent Change*	T_1	T_2	Percent Change*
Sleep						
Difficulties falling asleep	3.1	3.5	12.9	3.2	3.1	−3.1
Disturbed sleep	3.0	3.3	10.0	3.1	3.1	0
Nightmares	3.4	3.5	2.9	3.3	3.4	3.0
Difficulties getting up	3.5	3.4	−2.9	3.4	3.2	−5.9
Drowsiness‖	2.7	3.2	18.5	2.9	2.9	0
Gastrointestinal						
Abdominal pain	3.3	3.5	6.1	3.4	3.6	5.9
Loss of appetite	3.6	3.7	2.8	3.7	3.7	0
Dry mouth§	3.0	3.6	20.0	3.0	3.0	0
Change in taste	3.6	3.9	8.3	3.7	3.6	−2.7
Constipation‡	3.7	3.7	0	3.5	3.4	−2.9
Physical performance difficulties						
Weaker than usual	2.9	3.2	10.3	2.9	3.1	6.9
Climb stairs	2.5†	3.1	24.0	3.0†	2.9	−3.3
Usual walk	3.0	3.2	6.7	3.0	3.0	0
Physical work	2.8	3.2	14.3	2.9	2.8	−3.4
Usual work	2.9	3.2	10.3	3.3	3.1	−6.7
Cognitive functioning						
Difficulty concentrating‡	3.0	3.5	16.7	3.2	3.3	3.1
Forgetfulness	2.9	3.3	13.8	2.9	3.1	6.9
Sexuality						
Change in desire	3.1	3.8	22.6	3.4	3.8	11.8
Change in performance	3.3	3.8	15.2	3.3	3.8	15.2
Other symptoms						
Headache‡	2.6	3.1	19.2	3.0	3.0	0
Palpitation	3.1	3.5	12.9	3.0	3.3	10.0
Nocturia	3.1†	3.6	16.1	3.4†	3.5	2.9

Note: Mean response on a 4-point scale: 1, definitely yes; 4, not at all; i.e., the higher the score, the less one experiences the symptoms. T_1 refers to baseline; T_2 to follow-up.
*Change (%) from baseline (positive indicates improvement).
†Symptoms experienced more by the study group at T_1 vs. control group ($P < 0.05$).
‡The effect of treatment change is significant at $P < 0.05$.
§The effect of treatment change is significant at $P < 0.01$.
‖The effect of treatment change is significant at $P < 0.001$.
(Reprinted by permission of Elsevier Science Inc., courtesy of Paran E, Anson O, Neumann L: The effects of replacing β-blockers with an angiotensin converting enzyme inhibitor on the quality of life of hypertensive patients. *American Journal of Hypertension* 9:1206–1213. Copyright 1996 by American Journal of Hypertension, Inc.)

pressure equally well, but patients receiving captopril required a lower drug dose and showed improvement (Table 3) in several aspects of QOL (sleep-related, gastrointestinal, and physical activity-related symptoms). These benefits were not seen in controls.

▶ It is an old cliche that patients with hypertension are often symptom free until they start taking medication. Deterioration in QOL as a result of medications is both undesirable and likely to lead to poor compliance with dosing directions. These unfavorable consequences of drug-related adverse events are particularly important in a condition that requires life-long treatment. Studies like this one are important.

L. Lasagna, M.D.

Prevention of Heart Failure by Antihypertensive Drug Treatment in Older Persons With Isolated Systolic Hypertension

Kostis JB, for the SHEP Cooperative Research Group (UMDNJ-Robert Wood Johnson Med School, New Brunswick, NJ)
JAMA 278:212–216, 1997 7–5

Introduction.—More than 2 million persons are affected by heart failure in the United States. A common antecedent is hypertension, including isolated systolic hypertension. The incidence of total stroke was reduced by 36% and of major cardiovascular events by 32% in the Systolic Hypertension in the Elderly Program (SHEP), in which patients 60 years of age and older had antihypertensive stepped-care drug treatment with low-dose chlorthalidone. The occurrence of heart failure in active and placebo groups in the SHEP was studied among patients with a history of electrocardiographic evidence of myocardial infarction and compared with heart failure in the other patients.

Methods.—There were 4,736 persons aged 60 years and older with diastolic blood pressure below 90 mm Hg and systolic blood pressure between 160 and 219 mm Hg who received stepped-care antihypertensive drug therapy with chlorthalidone as the step 1 drug at 12.5 to 25 mg or matching placebo, and the step 2 drug as atenolol at 25–50 mg or matching placebo.

Results.—Fifty-five of 2,365 patients in the active therapy group had heart failure compared with 105 of 2,371 patients in the placebo group. A predictor of risk of fatal or hospitalized nonfatal heart failure was a history of ECG evidence of myocardial infarction at baseline. For the various heart failure end points examined, the risk reduction in the group with a history of ECG evidence of myocardial infarction at baseline ranged from 59% to 85%. A higher risk of heart failure development occurred among older patients, men, and those with higher systolic blood pressure or a history of electrocardiographic evidence of myocardial infarction.

Conclusion.—There was a strong protective effect in preventing heart failure among older persons with isolated systolic hypertension who received stepped-care treatment based on low-dose chlorthalidone. An 80% risk reduction was seen among patients with prior myocardial infarction.

▶ Heart failure has been estimated to affect over 2 million persons in the United States, with a resulting 1 million hospitalizations annually. It is the most common reason for hospitalization in persons 60 years of age or older and is the only cardiovascular disorder whose prevalence is increasing.

The SHEP study has previously shown that antihypertensive stepped-care treatment with low dose chlorthalidone reduces the incidence of stroke and of major cardiovascular events. The study abstracted here shows an impressive reduction in the occurrence of heart failure in persons 60 years of age or older with isolated systolic hypertension, as a consequence of such stepped-care antihypertensive treatment. To make the results even sweeter, chlorthalidone is inexpensive.

L. Lasagna, M.D.

Effect of Antihypertensive Drug Treatment on Cardiovascular Outcomes in Women and Men: A Meta-analysis of Individual Patient Data From Randomized, Controlled Trials
Gueyffier F and The INDANA Investigators (Claude Bernard Univ, Lyon, France; London School of Hygiene and Tropical Medicine; Bollington Med Ctr, England; et al)
Ann Intern Med 126:761–767, 1997   7–6

Objective.—Antihypertensive treatment reduces the relative risk for stroke and other cardiovascular events. Whether this treatment benefit is the same for men and women is not known. The Individual Data Analysis of Antihypertensive Intervention Trials Project (INDANA) analyzed the treatment effect on each sex and determined whether the treatment effect differed significantly between men and women.

Methods.—A subgroup meta-analysis was performed on data from 7 antihypertensive drug trials enrolling, between 1972 and 1990, 19,975 men (average age, 56.0 years) and 20,802 women (average age, 59.3 years). Data included fatal and nonfatal strokes, fatal coronary events, fatal and nonfatal major coronary events, cardiovascular-related mortality, major cardiovascular events, and total mortality. Antihypertensive drugs used were primarily β-blockers and thiazide diuretics.

Results.—In women, there was a significant treatment effect for both stroke and cardiovascular events. In men, there was a significant treatment effect for all outcomes. Whereas the rates of coronary events and total mortality for women were lower than for men, men and women had similar numbers of strokes. None of the studies compared the size of treatment benefit for men and women.

Conclusion.—The primary benefit of treatment for women was a decrease in risk of stroke. Benefits of treatment for men were observed for all cardiovascular outcomes.

▶ The ability of antihypertensive treatment to reduce cardiovascular risk is as great for women as for men, according to this meta-analysis. But for women the benefit is seen primarily for strokes, whereas in men the benefit is for coronary events as well as strokes. So, as usual, sex should not be ignored.

L. Lasagna, M.D.

Proteinuria in Mild-to-Moderate Hypertension: Results of the VA Cooperative Study of Six Antihypertensive Agents and Placebo

Preston RA, for the Department of Veteran Affairs Cooperative Study Group on Antihypertensive Agents (VA Med Ctr, Miami, Fla, et al)
Clin Nephrol 47:310–315, 1997   7–7

Background.—The prevalence and natural history of severe proteinuria in patients with mild-to-moderate hypertension have not been completely elucidated. Proteinuria was studied in hypertensive men enrolled in a double-blind prospective study of treatment with 6 antihypertensive agents and placebo.

Methods and Findings.—Of 1,635 hypertensive men screened, 1,292 with untreated diastolic blood pressures of 95 to 109 mm Hg were randomly assigned to single-agent therapy with hydrocholorothiazide, atenolol, captopril, clonidine, sustained-release diltiazem, prazosin, or placebo. Twenty-seven men found to have proteinuria exceeding 1,000 mg/24 hr were excluded from the study. Follow-up data were available on 19 of these men. One patient had focal segmental sclerosis that progressed to end-stage renal disease. In another 3 patients, severe chronic renal failure developed. One patient's serum creatinine level progressed from 1.4 to 2.2 mg/dL. However, the remaining 14 patients continued to have stable serum creatinine levels less than 2 mg/dL for 6 to 9 years of follow-up. Data were available for 93% of the whole group at the end of titration, for 87% at 1 year, and for 73% at 2 years. Proteinuria was significantly associated with obesity and higher systolic blood pressure. A trend toward a significant difference in mean 24-hour protein excretion rates at baseline was noted between black men and white men. No significant changes in urinary protein excretion/24 hr between or within the different treatment groups, including placebo, occurred. Active treatment was stopped in 18 patients because of proteinuria levels exceeding 1,000 mg/24 hr.

Conclusions.—Though the prevalence of severe proteinuria among hypertensive men is significant, it does not necessarily indicate a poor prognosis. The mean 24-hour urinary protein excretion rates did not vary in response to the different classes of antihypertensive agents. No drug-specific increase in proteinuria was detected.

▶ Severe and poorly controlled hypertension is often followed by progressive renal failure from hypertensive nephrosclerosis. Because most patients have milder degrees of hypertension, this study is a welcome addition to the literature. It indicates that the prevalence of severe proteinuria among patients with untreated hypertension is not trivial. On the other hand, severe proteinuria in these patients, even after 6 to 9 years of follow-up, was not generally associated with rapid deterioration of renal function. None of the drugs given to the patients in this study appeared to cause proteinuria. The authors suggest that the current labeling of angiotensin-enzyme–converting inhibitors as a possible cause of proteinuria should perhaps be reconsidered by the Food and Drug Administration.

L. Lasagna, M.D.

Effect of Long-acting and Short-acting Calcium Antagonists on Cardiovascular Outcomes in Hypertensive Patients
Alderman MH, Cohen H, Roqué R, et al (Albert Einstein College of Medicine, Bronx, NY)
Lancet 349:594–598, 1997   7–8

Introduction.—There is evidence that the use of short-acting calcium antagonists in patients with hypertension may lead to increased coronary artery morbidity, mortality, and noncardiovascular complications. Though short-acting calcium antagonists are recommended for the treatment of hypertension, the only approved formulations are the long-acting ones, along with short-acting verapamil. The effects of short-acting calcium antagonists on cardiovascular risk were assessed.

Methods.—The case-control study was nested in a prospective cohort of 4,350 patients participating in a systematic hypertension control program. The cases were 189 patients with hypertension who had an initial cardiovascular event — including cardiovascular deaths and hospitalizations for cardiovascular disease — over a 5-year period. The controls were 189 patients without such cardiovascular outcomes, matched for sex, ethnicity, age, previous antihypertensive treatment, year of entry into the study, and duration of follow-up. Information on prescription drugs taken on the day of the cardiovascular event was recorded for the cases, while drugs taken on the same date were noted for controls. Drug types were assessed to compare the incidence of cardiovascular events among patients taking long-acting vs. short-acting calcium antagonists.

Results.—One hundred thirty-six patients were taking long-acting calcium antagonists, while 27 were taking short-acting calcium antagonists. The risk of cardiovascular events was significantly increased for patients taking short-acting calcium antagonists, compared with patients taking β-blocker monotherapy (adjusted odds ratio 3.88). No such increase in risk was noted for patients taking long-acting calcium antagonists (adjusted odds ratio 0.76). On analysis of 38 matched pairs taking short-acting vs. long-acting calcium antagonists, the adjusted risk ratio for patients taking short-acting vs. the long-acting formulations was 8.56.

Conclusions.—Long-acting calcium antagonists do not carry the same risk of adverse cardiovascular events as short-acting calcium antagonists. The findings support the conclusions of previous studies questioning the safety of short-acting calcium antagonists. Trials currently under way will provide important data on the relative cardiovascular effects of different antihypertensive drugs.

▶ Criticism has come from various quarters regarding the use of calcium channel blockers in the treatment of cardiovascular disease. Long-acting drugs in this class appear safer than the short-acting ones.

L. Lasagna, M.D.

Withdrawal of Antihypertensive Medications
Froom J, Trilling JS, Yeh S-S, et al (State Univ of New York, Stony Brook)
J Am Board Fam Pract 10:249–258, 1997   7–9

Objective.—Drug treatment for patients with high blood pressure lowers the risk for stroke, congestive heart failure, renal failure, and death. However, it is unclear whether patients who start taking these medications need to continue taking them for life. A literature review and physician survey were performed to study the results of withdrawal of antihypertensive medications.

Methods.—A computerized literature search using relevant key words turned up few articles on withdrawal of antihypertensive medications. Therefore some articles known to the authors, and articles cited therein, were reviewed. Also, a random sample of family physicians was surveyed to find out how often physicians attempt withdrawal of antihypertensive medications.

Results.—The literature review included 18 studies of withdrawal of antihypertensive drugs. Twelve of these studies had an average success rate of 40% at 1 year's follow-up and 28% at 2 years. The other 6 studies included only elderly patients; their average success rate, at follow-up of 2 years or longer, was 26%. The various studies differed significantly in design, patient selection criteria, and follow-up. In the physician survey, 79% of respondents said they attempt to withdraw antihypertensive medications in patients whose blood pressure is under control and who are free of symptoms from medication.

Conclusions.—The available data suggest that withdrawal of antihypertensive medications can be safely carried out with benefits to the patient. The success rate of withdrawal is about one third. The authors call for further study to confirm the reported success rates, define the best technique of withdrawing medications, and identify those patients in whom withdrawal is most likely to succeed.

▶ "White coat hypertension" is a real entity and presumably does not require antihypertensive medications. For patients on such drugs, unpleasant side effects must impel at least some to stop medication on their own (with or without informing the physician). So, the question is: How do we try withdrawing antihypertensive drugs with a minimum of risk? Another key question is: What is the proper role for ambulatory self-measurement of blood pressure?

L. Lasagna, M.D.

Effect of Pharmacologic Lipid Lowering on Health-related Quality of Life in Older Persons: Results From the Cholesterol Reduction in Seniors Program (CRISP) Pilot Study
Santanello NC, for the CRISP Collaborative Study Group (Merck Research Labs, West Point, Pa)
J Am Geriatr Soc 45:8–14, 1997   7–10

Background.—The incidence of coronary heart disease events increases with age. Total cholesterol, low-density lipoprotein cholesterol, and high-density lipoprotein cholesterol are strong predictors of risk of coronary heart disease. There is little information regarding the effect of pharmacologic treatment of abnormal lipoproteins in older individuals with coronary heart disease.

Methods.—There were 431 patients with low-density lipoprotein levels greater than 159 mg/dL and less than 221 mg/dL. Most patients were aged 65 years or older. Patients with Mini-Mental State Examination Scores of less than 24 or chronic diseases likely to shorten survival were excluded. All patients were administered the National Cholesterol Education Program step 1 diet, then randomized to lovastatin, 20 mg/day; lovastatin, 40 mg/day; or placebo. Follow-up was at least 6 months in all patients and 12 months in some patients.

Results.—Evaluation of quality of life included physical functioning, sleep behavior, social support, depression, cognitive function, and health perception. In patients given lovastatin, 20 mg/day, total cholesterol decreased 17% and low-density lipoprotein cholesterol decreased 24%. In patients given lovastatin, 40 mg/day, total cholesterol decreased 20% and low-density lipoprotein cholesterol decreased 28%. Reports of side effects were similar in all 3 groups. At 6 months, there were no significant differences in mean change scores from baseline in the active treatment groups on measures of quality of life or global health perception.

Discussion.—In these older individuals, lovastatin, 20 mg/day and 40 mg/day, was well-tolerated, reduced total cholesterol and low-density lipoprotein cholesterol, and improved quality of life. The 2 doses of lovastatin produced similar effects. These findings from a relatively healthy cohort may not apply to individuals with comorbid conditions. The study was ended prematurely because of lack of funding.

▶ Like the Systolic Hypertension in the Elderly Program, the study in this paper shows — even though a pilot study — the value of an intervention in elderly people. The data indicate that the intervention did not have many adverse effects on patients' lifestyle and provided a pretty good outcome on their cholesterol. There have been a number of studies showing increases in accidents, suicides, violent crimes, etc., as well as cancer and other serious illnesses, with decreased cholesterol. Part of this was undoubtedly a "You can't beat city hall" type of response. However, it is always helpful to show that, at least at 6 months, there was no significant difference in the quality of life.

These elderly patients were very healthy and very few were in the "old" elderly group of over 85 years of age. Most of the adverse effects involved the occurrences of daily life among elderly patients. However, some of these effects could have been explained by the 40–mg, as opposed to the 20–mg, dose and, because the cholesterol responses were equivalent, the lower dose would be the one used for treatment. Still and all, when my father-in-law turned 80, he said that he was going to decrease his salmon intake and increase his hamburger intake. The change didn't seem to make a difference, but perhaps it did because the control of cholesterol in elderly patients does seem to improve cardiovascular disease while not causing a diminished quality of life.

There is one other thing regarding this particular study. Everybody calculates the cost involved in the disease in their particular study. In this case, the very large prevalence of coronary heart disease really does raise hospitalizations, outpatient visits, and direct medical care costs. However, if you really sat down and added up how the cost of everything raises the cost of everything else, you'd end up with hundreds and hundreds of billions of dollars involved. Probably more than the gross national product of the United States.

M. Weintraub, M.D.

Adverse Outcomes of Underuse of β-Blockers in Elderly Survivors of Acute Myocardial Infarction

Soumerai SB, McLaughlin TJ, Spiegelman D, et al (Harvard Med School, Boston; Harvard School of Public Health, Boston; Brigham and Women's Hosp, Boston)
JAMA 277:115–121, 1997   7–11

Purpose.—β-Blocker treatment is highly effective in reducing cardiovascular mortality and reinfarction after acute myocardial infarction (AMI). There are few data on how many and which patients receive β-blockers, however, especially among elderly patients living in the community. Levels, determinants, and outcomes of β-blocker treatment among elderly survivors of AMI were studied.

Methods.—The retrospective study used Medicare and drug claims data covering the years 1987 to 1992. It included a cohort of 5,332 elderly patients who survived for 30 days after AMI. Of these, 3,737 met eligibility requirements for β-blocker treatment. The analysis looked at the use of β-blockers and calcium-channel blockers in the first 90 days after hospital discharge. Mortality and cardiac hospital readmission rate were evaluated for the 2-year period after discharge, with adjustment for sociodemographic and baseline risk variables. Factors associated with underuse of β-blockers, and the consequences of that underuse, were assessed. The relative risks (RRs) of survival in patients taking β-blockers were compared with those from previously reported randomized controlled trials.

Results.—Throughout the period studied, just 21% of patients received β-blocker therapy. After AMI, prescription rates were nearly 3 times higher for calcium-channel blockers than for β-blockers. Older patients and those taking calcium-channel blockers were less likely to receive β-blockers. Mortality was significantly reduced (RR, 0.57) for patients receiving β-blockers, after adjustment for other survival predictors. β-Blockers significantly improved survival in all age groups—including those aged 85 years or older—as reported in the elderly subgroups of previous trials. Patients taking β-blockers were also less likely to be readmitted to the hospital (RR, 0.78). The risk of death was doubled (RR, 1.98) for patients receiving a calcium-channel blocker rather than a β-blocker. This was not because of any adverse effect of calcium-channel blockers, but rather because they were used instead of β-blockers.

Conclusions.—β-Blockers are not prescribed to elderly survivors of AMI as often as they should be, which leads to higher rates of adverse outcomes. β-Blockers can extend survival even for patients older than 75 years, who have been excluded from previous randomized, controlled trials. One reason for β-blocker underuse may be the mistaken belief than these drugs are potentially harmful for patients with left ventricular dysfunction or diabetes. The study is limited by the lack of information regarding life-style risk factors and patients who may have received β-blockers in the hospital but stopped taking them before discharge.

▶ We seem to have difficulty in discarding old clinical clichés about chronological cutoff points. "The elderly" are a heterogeneous group, and chronological age doesn't toll you much about the individual patient.

β-Blocker prophylaxis after AMI clearly decreases cardiovascular morbidity and mortality significantly and it is shameful that patients 65 years of age or older are so infrequently given the chance to profit from such β-blocker therapy.

L. Lasagna, M.D.

Final Outcome Results of the Multicenter Isradipine Diuretic Atherosclerosis Study (MIDAS)
Borhani NO, Mercuri M, Borhani PA, et al (Univ of California, Davis; Univ of Nevada, Reno; Bowman Gray School of Medicine, Winston Salem, NC; et al)
JAMA 276:785–791, 1996   7–12

Introduction.—Diuretic and β-blocker treatment can reduce the risk of stroke and coronary artery disease in patients with hypertension, but the effects of calcium-channel blocker treatment are uncertain. The dihydropyridine calcium antagonist isradipine has been found to have antiatherogenic properties in animals. Isradipine and hydrochlorothiazide were compared for their effects on progression of atherosclerosis in patients with hypertension.

Methods.—The Multicenter Isradipine Diuretic Atherosclerosis Study (MIDAS) included 883 patients with sustained hypertension from 9 clinics. Their mean baseline blood pressure was 150 mm Hg systolic and 97 mm Hg diastolic. The mean age was 58.5 years. The patients were assigned to receive 3 years of treatment with isradipine, 2.5–5.0 mg twice daily, or hydrochlorothiazide, 12.5–25.0 mg twice daily. Progression of atherosclerosis was assessed by means of quantitative β-mode ultrasonography to measure mean maximum intimal-medial thickness (IMT) of the carotid arteries at 12 carotid focal points. Other study outcomes were major vascular events, including myocardial infarction, stroke, congestive heart failure, angina, and sudden death, and nonmajor vascular events and procedures, including transient ischemic attack, dysrhythmia, aortic valve replacement, and femoropopliteal bypass grafting.

Results.—The rate of progression of mean maximum IMT over 3 years' treatment was similar in the 2 groups. The rate of major vascular events was significantly higher in the isradipine group than in the hydrochlorothiazide group, 5.65% vs. 3.17%. Nonmajor vascular events and procedures were also more frequent with isradipine, 9.05% vs. 5.22%. Both groups had a mean 13.0 mm Hg decrease in diastolic blood pressure after 6 months of treatment. The mean decrease in systolic blood pressure was 16.0 mm Hg with isradipine and 15.5 mm Hg with hydrochlorothiazide. The diastolic/systolic difference remained throughout the study period, but did not account for the difference in vascular event rates.

Conclusions.—In patients with sustained hypertension, progression of atherosclerosis—as reflected by the rate of progression of IMT in the carotid arteries—is similar with the calcium antagonist dihydropyridine and the diuretic hydrochlorothiazide. The risk of vascular events appears to be greater with isradipine. Prospective studies in progress will provide more information on whether calcium-channel blockers actually increase cardiovascular risk.

▶ A study with a great name like "MIDAS" should have come out proving its central hypothesis. Unfortunately, this well-run, yet difficult to do study, did not show a difference in the rate of progression of mean IMT. One of the main reasons for this study having a negative outcome is a common one in clinical trials. In the study, the patient population was based on a group of men who had hypercholesterolemia and in whom the carotid IMT was measured as a surrogate for atherosclerotic disease in general. That value was then used in a group of nonatherosclerotic, nonhypercholesterolemic patients. The different rate of IMT progression because of the different condition being treated was not realized before the study. One of the most important causes of concern over the use of isradipine is the increased vascular event rate between the 2 groups. This raises a very important issue of all calcium-channel blockers perhaps having a greater incidence of adverse effects. An excellent editorial[1] accompanied this article, which described many other faults in the study and many possible explanations for why the data turned out this way. The editorial recommended that we pay attention to the National Institutes of Health funded Anti-hypertensive and Lipid Lowering Treatment to Prevent Heart Attack Trial (ALLHAT), which will look at the effects, including long-term toxicity, of the long-acting calcium-channel blocker. The title is not any where near as interesting as MIDAS, but it will be an interesting study.

M. Weintraub, M.D.

Reference

1. Chobanian AV: Calcium channel blockers. Lessons learned from MIDAS and other clinical trials. *JAMA* 276:829–830, 1996.

A Clinical Trial Comparing Primary Coronary Angioplasty With Tissue Plasminogen Activator for Acute Myocardial Infarction
Ellis SG, for the Angioplasty Substudy Investigators (Cleveland Clinic Found, Ohio)
N Engl J Med 336:1621–1628, 1997   7–13

Introduction.—The goal of care for acute myocardial infarction is to restore coronary flow completely as soon as possible. Some centers can perform prompt coronary angioplasty, which has produced better coronary flow and 30-day survival than intravenous thrombolytic therapy with tissue plasminogen activator (t-PA). However, there are doubts as to whether this advantage would be maintained in general clinical practice. Newer techniques of thrombolytic therapy might further narrow the gap. A randomized clinical trial of primary coronary angioplasty vs. thrombolytic therapy for acute myocardial infarction is reported.

Methods.—The study was part of the larger Global Use of Strategies to Open Occluded Coronary Arteries in Acute Coronary Syndromes (GUSTO) trial. It included 1,138 patients with acute myocardial infarction from 57 hospitals in 9 countries. All patients were seen within 12 hours and showed ST-segment elevation at electrocardiography. They were randomized into 2 groups for initial management: primary angioplasty or accelerated thrombolytic therapy. In an additional factorial design, 1,012 patients were randomized to receive heparin or hirudin treatment. The patients were monitored for a composite 30-day study end point of death, nonfatal reinfarction, and nonfatal disabling stroke.

Results.—The primary end point was reached in 9.6% of the angioplasty group and 13.7% of the t-PA group (odds ratio, 0.67). In the angioplasty group, 5.7% of patients died, compared with 7.0% of those in the t-PA group. The reinfarction rate was 4.5% vs. 6.5%, and the rate of disabling stroke was 0.2% vs. 0.9%, respectively. By 6 months, there were no significant differences in outcome: the composite end point was reached by 14.1% of the angioplasty group and 16.1% of the t-PA group. The composite end point was reached by 10.6% of patients receiving heparin and 8.2% of those receiving hirudin.

Conclusions.—For patients with acute myocardial infarction, primary angioplasty provides some improvement in outcome over thrombolytic therapy with t-PA. The advantage is of small to moderate magnitude and is no longer apparent by 6 months' follow-up. When possible, prompt primary angioplasty is a valuable alternative technique for myocardial reperfusion. The most important consideration, however, is not to delay reperfusion.

▶ If we only had a definitive method for preventing reocclusion following angioplasty, then this study would be even more important. It appears that there may be some hope on the horizon for developing such a stenosis inhibitor with probucol. Of course, we really need to know whether competent angioplasty invasive cardiologists exist at an institution, and how much it really costs to carry out the angioplasty with x-ray exposure and dye exposure as parts of the procedure, which can be harmful. Still, it seems that angioplasty would be a reasonable approach in patients at risk for intracranial hemorrhage. Still, the authors make an excellent point, "not to delay in restoring myocardial reperfusion in suitable candidates with two attractive alternatives."

M. Weintraub, M.D.

Incidence and Predictors of Bleeding After Contemporary Thrombolytic Therapy for Myocardial Infarction
Berkowitz SD, for the Global Utilization of Streptokinase and Tissue Plasminogen Activator for Occluded Coronery Arteries (GUSTO) I Investigators (Duke Univ, Durham, NC; Univ of Massachusetts, Worcester; Thoraxcenter Erasmus Universiteit, Rotterdam, The Netherlands; et al)
Circulation 95:2508–2516, 1997   7–14

Background.—The benefits of thrombolytic treatment in decreasing mortality rates among patients with acute myocardial infarction are well established. The types of bleeding and risk factors for bleeding are less well documented.

Methods.—The baseline features, outcomes, and incidence of bleeding by location, severity, and treatment assigment were analyzed in 41,021 patients in the GUSTO-I (Global Utilization of Streptokinase and Tissue Plasminogen Activator for Occluded Coronary Arteries I) study of thrombolysis for acute myocardial infarction. Data on 40,903 patients were complete.

Findings.—Severe bleeding occurred in 1.2% of the patients, and moderate hemorrhage at a variety of sites occurred in 11.4%. Procedure-related sources of bleeding were most common. The thrombolytic regimen was highly correlated with the incidence of bleeding. More bleeding occurred with streptokinase plus IV heparin and the streptokinase and tissue plasminogen activator plus IV heparin combination. Older age, lower body weight, female sex, and African ancestry were the strongest independent predictors in a multivariate analysis, even when patients not undergoing invasive procedures were included. Serious hemorrhage was associated with other adverse outcomes, such as recurrent events, left ventricular dysfunction, arrhythmia, and stroke.

Conclusions.—In this population, important predictors of bleeding were advanced age, lower body weight, female sex, African ancestry, and having undergone invasive procedures. Other nonbleeding adverse clinical outcomes were correlated with moderate and severe bleeding, which was correlated with increased length of stay and 30-day mortality.

▶ Identification of risk factors for adverse drug events can at times improve therapy, but not always. In this case, at the very least an awareness of risk factors should help clinicians who want to weigh the possible hazards against the possible benefits.

L. Lasagna, M.D.

High-dose Streptokinase Therapy With Three Million Units in One Hour Significantly Improves Early Coronary Patency Rates in Acute Myocardial Infarction

Theiss W, Busch U, Renner U, et al (Universität München, Germany)
Am J Cardiol 78:1167–1169, 1996   7–15

Background.—Given at a dose of 1.5 million U over 1 hour, streptokinase has become a widely used treatment for acute myocardial infarction. However, this dosage and length of infusion were selected on the basis of little empiric evidence. The effects of a higher streptokinase dose and a faster or slower infusion time were evaluated in a randomized trial.

Methods.—A total of 46 patients with evidence of acute myocardial infarction were studied. All received 3.0 million U of streptokinase, given by continuous infusion over 1 or 2 hours. Heparin therapy was stated when the thrombin time decreased to less than 2 times normal and the fibrinogen concentration exceeded 80 mg/100 mL. Coronary angiography was performed 60, 90, and 120 minutes after the start of streptokinase therapy to evaluate the effects of infusion time on early coronary patency. Grade 2 or 3 TIMI (Thrombolysis in Myocardial Infarction) patency in the affected vessel was the definition of treatment success.

Results.—The success rates at 60 minutes were 52% in patients receiving infusion for 1 hour and 26% in those receiving infusion for 2 hours. No significant difference was seen at 90 or 120 minutes. One-hour infusion led to a faster and more pronounced decrease in fibrinogen concentration.

Conclusions.—A streptokinase at 3.0 million U — twice the conventional dose — leads to higher very early coronary patency rates in patients with acute myocardial infarction. More studies of this high-dose regimen are warranted. Prolonging the infusion over 2 hours offers no significant advantage.

▶ Dose–response studies are the hallmark of pharmacologic excellence but are done less frequently than might be desired. In this study, a doubling of the traditional dose of streptokinase yielded an impressive improvement in coronary patency without an increase in adverse events. Prolongation of the infusion to 2 hours (same dose) not only wasn't better, it was actually worse.

L. Lasagna, M.D.

Impact of an Aggressive Invasive Catheterization and Revascularization Strategy on Mortality in Patients With Cardiogenic Shock in the Global Utilization of Streptokinase and Tissue Plasminogen Activator for Occluded Coronary Arteries (GUSTO-I) Trial: An Observational Study
Berger PB, for the GUSTO-I Investigators (Mayo Clinic, Rochester, Minn; et al)
Circulation 96:122–127, 1997   7–16

Background.—Retrospective studies have demonstrated an association between survival and coronary angiography and angioplasty in patients with acute myocardial infarction complicated by cardiogenic shock. However, the extent to which bias in patient selection contributed to these findings is not known. The influence of an aggressive strategy of early angiography and coronary angioplasty or bypass surgery, if appropriate, on survival was investigated.

Methods and Findings.—Data on 2,200 patients in the Global Utilization of Streptokinase and Tissue Plasminogen Activator for Occluded Coronary Arteries (GUSTO-I) trial were obtained for analysis. All patients had acute myocardial infarction complicated by cardiogenic shock and survived for 1 hour or longer after the onset of shock. Attending physicians decided whether to perform revascularization. Shock was present in 11% of the patients on admission and developed thereafter in 89%. Mortality at 30 days was 38% in the patients undergoing early angiography, and they were referred within 24 hours for angioplasty, bypass surgery, angioplasty and bypass surgery, or neither, compared with 62% who did not undergo early angiography. However, these 2 groups differed in important baseline characteristics. After adjustment for these differences in a multivariate logistic regression analysis, an aggressive strategy was found to be associated independently with a reduced 30-day mortality.

Conclusions.—An aggressive strategy of early angiography and revascularization, when appropriate, markedly decreases 30-day mortality in patients with acute myocardial infarction and cardiogenic shock, receiving thrombolytic treatment, compared with a less aggressive strategy. The lower mortality in the aggressively treated patients could not be explained by differences in baseline clinical characteristics.

▶ Thrombolytic therapy for acute myocardial infarction reduces the risk of cardiogenic shock, but such shock still occurs, and there's no agreement about how to proceed when it does. The data summarized here suggest that such patients are best served with early angiography, followed by revascularization (when deemed appropriate) by either coronary angioplasty or bypass surgery.

L. Lasagna, M.D.

Magnesium in Cardioplegia: Is It Necessary?
Shakerinia T, Ali IM, Sullivan JAP (Victoria Gen Hosp, Halifax, Nova Scotia, Canada)
Can J Surg 39:397–400, 1996   7–17

Introduction.—After potassium, magnesium is the most plentiful intracellular cation. Its role in protecting the myocardium is not well understood. Administered intravenously, it may decrease the early death rate in patients with acute myocardial infarction. The clinical benefits of adding magnesium to the cardioplegic solution were evaluated in 50 patients undergoing coronary artery bypass grafting.

Methods.—All the patients had normal ejection fractions, normal preoperative serum magnesium levels, and no history of atrial or ventricular arrhythmias. Twenty-five patients each, respectively, were randomly assigned to receive magnesium sulfate (15 mmol/L) in the cardioplegic solution (group 1) or no magnesium sulfate in the cardioplegic solution (group 2). Outcome measures were serum magnesium levels, arrhythmias, infarctions, and cardiac-related deaths.

Results.—There were no cardiac-related deaths. Group 1 patients had significantly higher mean serum magnesium levels after operation, compared to group 2 patients. One patient from each group had a non–Q-wave myocardial infarction. Group 2 patients had significantly more global ECG changes than group 1 patients. Changes included T-wave inversion, depressed ST segment, and new bundle-branch block (right or left of any degree) appearing after completion of cardiopulmonary bypass and persisting 8 or more hours after operation. Group 2 patients had significantly more instances of ventricular arrhythmia than did group 1 patients. There was a nonsignificant higher occurrence of atrial fibrillation in group 2 patients, compared to group 1 patients.

Conclusions.—Findings support earlier reports recommending the addition of magnesium to the cardioplegic solution of patients undergoing coronary artery bypass grafting to decrease the incidence of perioperative ischemia and ventricular arrhythmias.

▶ Magnesium is a cofactor in literally hundreds of enzyme reactions and is acknowledged to be helpful in treating a variety of cardiac arrhythmias. Its utility in reducing mortality after acute myocardial infarction is debated, but the present study supports the recommendations of earlier workers that magnesium be added to a "cardioplegic" solution to reduce the incidence of myocardial ischemia and arrhythmias in patients undergoing coronary artery bypass grafting. *How* magnesium protects the heart is not clear.

L. Lasagna, M.D.

Failure to Prescribe Warfarin to Patients With Nonrheumatic Atrial Fibrillation
Antani MR, Beyth RJ, Covinsky KE, et al (Univ Hosps of Cleveland, Ohio; Cleveland Neighborhood Health Ctrs, Ohio; MetroHealth Ctr; et al)
J Gen Intern Med 11:713–720, 1996   7–18

Introduction.—Beginning in 1989, a number of randomized clinical trials reported the benefits of warfarin treatment for patients with non-rheumatic atrial fibrillation, an important cause of stroke. There is concern, however, that physicians infrequently prescribe the anticoagulant in this setting, particularly in older patients.

Methods.—A cross-sectional study examined how often warfarin is prescribed for patients with nonrheumatic atrial fibrillation. The medical records of inpatients at 2 teaching hospitals and outpatients at 5 neighborhood health centers were reviewed to obtain the study sample. Patients with nonrheumatic atrial fibrillation considered to be at high risk of stroke were age 75 years or older and had hypertension, diabetes mellitus, or a history of stroke. Three internists independently reviewed 189 consecutive patients for the appropriateness of warfarin therapy.

Results.—Warfarin was judged appropriate for 98 (52%) patients, but only 36 (37%) of these were prescribed the drug. Of the 44 (23%) patients who had been prescribed warfarin, only 11 were from the subgroup considered at high risk of stroke because of age and medical history. Multivariate analysis revealed that old age was independently associated with failure to prescribe warfarin. Patient characteristics significantly associated with warfarin prescription were under 75 years and the presence of another indicator for anticoagulant therapy.

Conclusion.—Despite the known benefits of warfarin therapy for older patients with chronic nonrheumatic atrial fibrillation, physicians infrequently prescribe warfarin in such cases. This practice suggests that many opportunities to prevent stroke are missed.

▶ Not knowing about the necessity for prescribing warfarin for patients with atrial fibrillation of a nonrheumatic cause is a very serious flaw. One explanation may be that since the study ended in 1992 the average physician may not have heard about its value in the prevention of stroke. We each have to think about our own lack of knowledge and understanding of things that passed us by. These may include aspirin for acute myocardial infarction, β-blockers for the prevention of second myocardial infarctions, statins for reduction of serum cholesterol and, perhaps, for primary prevention of myocardial infarction, and the list goes on. Hopefully, physicians reading this edition of the YEAR BOOK OF DRUG THERAPY will be well informed about some of the things that are of importance and interest to them and their patients.

M. Weintraub, M.D.

Why Isn't Warfarin Prescribed to Patients With Nonrheumatic Atrial Fibrillation?

Beyth RJ, Antani MR, Covinsky KE, et al (Univ Hosps of Cleveland, Ohio; Case Western Univ, Cleveland, Ohio; Cleveland Neighborhood Health Ctrs Inc, Ohio)
J Gen Intern Med 11:721–728, 1996   7–19

Introduction.—Warfarin can safely prevent two thirds of strokes in patients with nonrheumatic atrial fibrillation, but physicians seem to be reluctant to prescribe it for this patient cohort. A conceptual model was used that relates prescription of a drug to the prescribing physician's opinions regarding appropriate use of the drug, other characteristics of the physician, and clinical characteristics of the patient. This model was used to survey physicians regarding their use of warfarin in patients with nonrheumatic atrial fibrillation.

Methods.—Eighty physicians who had treated 189 consecutive patients with nonrheumatic atrial fibrillation were surveyed regarding their experience with and opinions about warfarin therapy through the use of 8 vignettes. Each vignette used 1 of 8 unique combinations of 3 clinical characteristics: age (65 years or 85 years); 2 risk factors for bleeding (renal insufficiency and a history of a 3–unit gastrointestinal hemorrhage 1 year earlier — both present or both absent); and a history of recent stroke (present or absent).

Results.—Seventy-three percent of physicians queried responded to the questionnaire. Ninety percent of physicians recommended warfarin for at least 1 vignette. There was no significant relationship between the number of vignettes for which physicians recommended warfarin and physician gender, years since graduation from medical school, specialty, or primary practice site. Physicians reporting good or excellent experience in using anticoagulation in patients with chronic nonrheumatic atrial fibrillation recommended warfarin for a mean of 4.5 vignettes, compared with physicians reporting satisfactory experience (mean, 2.8 vignettes) or bad or little experience (mean, 1.8 vignettes). Even physicians who reported good experience and favorable opinions did not in actuality prescribe warfarin in half of their patients for whom warfarin was independently judged to be appropriate.

Conclusion.—Despite compelling evidence of the efficacy of warfarin in treating patients with nonrheumatic atrial fibrillation, physicians did not prescribe warfarin to half of their patients in whom it would have been an appropriate treatment. Targeted, multicomponent interventions may be necessary to influence the appropriate use of warfarin in patients with nonrheumatic atrial fibrillation.

▶ As the King of Siam would say, "Is a puzzlement!" This survey finds physicians holding favorable opinions in theory about the benefits of warfarin in patients with atrial fibrillation, describing good personal experiences with it but not prescribing the anticoagulant to half of their patients for whom warfarin was independently judged appropriate. Older patients and patients with bleeding risk factors are particularly likely not to receive warfarin.

L. Lasagna, M.D.

8 Ear, Nose, Throat, and Eye Disorders

Extended Use of Topical Nasal Decongestants
Yoo JK, Seikaly H, Calhoun KH (Univ of Texas, Galveston)
Laryngoscope 107:40–43, 1997   8–1

Introduction.—The widely used topical nasal decongestants carry a risk of rebound swelling when applied for more than 3 to 5 days. Long-acting topical agents can be used beyond 5 days without the development of rebound swelling, but adverse effects appear with extended periods of application. The topical nasal decongestant oxymetazoline (Afrin) was tested in 10 healthy volunteers for its effects when used nightly for 4 weeks.

Methods.—Study participants were instructed to use oxymetazoline (0.05% concentration) nightly at bedtime, with 1 spray in each nostril. The participants reported subjective airflow after the spray and were examined weekly by anterior rhinomanometry for shrinking of nasal mucosa.

Results.—None of the volunteers had active sinusitis, but 4 had a history of allergic rhinitis and 2 used topical nasal steroids. Nightly nasal obstruction developed in 8 of 10 participants a few hours before the evening dose; the obstruction was relieved with the nightly dose and resolved within 48 hours if no more oxymetazoline was applied. Rhinomanometric data indicated sensitivity of nasal mucosa to the topical decongestant.

Conclusion.—Patients with intermittent mucosal edema, particularly when it appears only at bedtime, may benefit from long-acting decongestants that are used once nightly. All participants in this study reported a subjective increase in airflow and had a visible shrinkage in nasal mucosa. Although these agents appear to be safe, close physician follow-up is needed to prevent their overuse and the risk of rhinitis medicamentosa.

▶ The results of this study should be checked by performing the trial in patients who need nasal decongestants and including a placebo. Nonetheless, this is an important message.

M. Weintraub, M.D.

Once-daily Mometasone Furoate Aqueous Nasal Spray (Nasonex™) in Seasonal Allergic Rhinitis: An Active- and Placebo-controlled Study

Hebert JR, Nolop K, Lutsky BN (Université Laval, Ste-Foy, Quebec, Canada; Schering-Plough Research Inst, Kenilworth, NJ)
Allergy 51:569–576, 1996

8–2

Background.—Seasonal allergic rhinitis is a common condition that can negatively affect an individual's quality of life and contribute to absenteeism from work and school. Seasonal allergic rhinitis is treated by drug therapy and avoidance of allergens. Recently, topical nasal corticosteroids have been developed. These agents are well tolerated and effective against nasal symptoms. Mometasone 17–furoate is a corticosteroid that can cause systemic side effects such as hypothalamic-pituitary-adrenal axis suppression in rare cases when applied topically. A nasal spray formulation of mometasone furoate has recently been developed to treat rhinitis.

Methods.—This study was conducted in 19 centers in Canada and Europe. All patients were older than 18 years and had allergy to at least 1 tree or grass aeroallergen. Most patients had moderate-to-severe seasonal allergic rhinitis. Patients were assigned to 1 of 4 regimens for 4 weeks: (1) mometasone furoate 100 µg once daily, (2) mometasone furoate 200 µg once daily, (3) beclomethasone dipropionate 200 µg twice daily, or (4) placebo spray.

Results.—Of 501 patients enrolled, 497 were evaluated for safety and 477 were evaluated for efficacy. Physicians rated nasal symptom and total symptom scores, and physicians and patients rated overall condition and therapeutic response. The 3 active treatments were equally effective and significantly superior to placebo. Overall, mometasone furoate, 200 µg, was somewhat superior numerically, but not statistically, to mometasone furoate, 100 µg, at initial evaluation. At the end of treatment, 77% of patients who used mometasone furoate, 100 µg; 79% of patients who used mometasone furoate, 200 µg; 74% of patients who used beclomethasone dipropionate; and 54% of patients who used placebo had complete or significant relief. Both drugs were well tolerated.

Discussion.—In these adult patients, mometasone furoate aqueous nasal spray, 100 or 200 µg, administered once per day relieved moderate-to-severe symptoms of seasonal allergic rhinitis. Mometasone furoate is well tolerated and can be administered just once per day.

▶ Of course we need new nasal steroids for the treatment of allergic rhinitis. No drug is the best possible drug for all patients. In the United States, cromoglycate, a nonsteroid, has recently been made an over-the-counter drug and thus more available. One point about the clinical trial described in this report is that roughly the same number of patients received placebo, each dose, of the active therapy and the active control. In many cases in which the placebo response could be predicted well before the start of the study, all that the investigators needed to show was that their study was sensitive enough to show a difference between active drugs, such as the active therapy in this controlled study, and the placebo. Thus, they could have used something like half the number of patients they did to prove this point. Another important point is that even doubling the dose did not show a dose-response relationship. This is frequently true of drugs with a flat dose response, such as nonsteroidal anti-inflammatory agents (if they have a dose response), as well as many others.

M. Weintraub, M.D.

One-week Use of Oxymetazoline Nasal Spray in Patients With Rhinitis Medicamentosa 1 Year After Treatment
Graf P, Hallén H (Karolinska Inst, Stockholm)
ORL J Otorhinolaryngol Relat Spec 59:39–44, 1997   8–3

Background.—Once the effect of a nasal vasoconstrictor wears off, rebound congestion often leads to overuse of the drug in an effort to stop the stuffiness. The development of this condition, rhinitis medicamentosa (RM), calls for the immediate discontinuation of the drug until the nasal mucosa can recover. When and if patients with RM can start using nasal vasoconstrictors again was studied.

Methods.—Eight patients (4 men, 4 women) with chronic nasal obstruction and overuse of topical decongestants containing benzalkonium chloride were selected. Budesonide nasal spray eased their immediate withdrawal from the decongestant, and then patients were monitored for at least 1 year before entering the study. At study entry, patients had not been using budesonide for at least 2 weeks. Then, subjects began using a nasal spray containing benzalkonium chloride 3 times a day for 7 days. Rhinostereometry and histamine provocation were used to measure swelling of the nasal mucosa, and patients also estimated their degree of stuffiness on a visual analogue scale (1–100).

Findings.—Reinstitution of the nasal vasoconstrictor caused the mucosal surface position and the histamine challenge reactivity to increase significantly. After only 3 days of using the spray, patients reported that nasal stuffiness was significantly worse and stayed that way until the end of the study.

Conclusions.—For patients with RM resulting from overuse of nasal sprays containing benzalkonium chloride, even after a year of not using such sprays, another 7 days of dosing caused significant nasal mucosal hyperreactivity, swelling, and congestion. Such patients must be warned that rebound congestion can develop quickly should they start using such nasal sprays again.

▶ Perhaps the manufacturers of nasal vasoconstrictors should read this particular paper and search for a better preservative for their medications. It won't fix everything, but it may alleviate a large part of the negative effects.

M. Weintraub, M.D.

Can an Antihistamine Delay Appearance of Hay Fever Symptoms When Given Prior to Pollen Season?

Stern MA, Darnell R, Tudor D (Leicester Gen Hosp, England; Midlands Asthma and Allergy Research Assoc, Derby, England; Synthélabo Recherche, Bagneux, France)
Allergy 52:440–444, 1997   8–4

Background.—Mizolastine is a new antihistamine that provides adequate relief of symptoms without sedation in patients with allergic conditions. Whether mizolastine given before pollen season can delay the onset of hay fever symptoms in patients known to have seasonal allergic rhinoconjunctivitis symptoms was determined.

Methods.—Three hundred forty-two patients were enrolled in a double-blind, randomized study. Mizolastine, 10 mg, was given once daily to 115 patients; terfenadine, 120 mg, was given once daily to 116; and placebo was given to 111. Time to first hay fever crisis of the season, defined as the use of rescue medication, study withdrawal because of treatment failure, or total diary symptom score exceeding 18, was determined in each group.

Findings.—Both active treatments prolonged time to first crisis by about 1 week compared with placebo. The first crisis occurred at 55 days in mizolastine recipients, 57 days in terfenadine recipients, and 50 days in placebo recipients. Tolerability was satisfactory and similar in the 2 active treatment groups.

Conclusions.—Mizolastine is safe and effective in delaying and treating the symptoms of seasonal allergic rhinoconjunctivitis. Additional research is needed to determine whether a similar prophylactic effect can be obtained when mizolastin is taken only a few days before theoretically high pollen counts.

▶ With the availability of nonsedating antihistamines, taking these drugs prophylactically to prevent seasonal allergies has become an attractive idea. This study indicates that such usage can delay the onset as well as treat the symptoms of seasonal allergic rhinoconjunctivitis. Headache was the most frequent adverse event, but it occurred as often in the placebo group as in the drug groups.

L. Lasagna, M.D.

Methotrexate Management of Immune-mediated Cochleovestibular Disorders

Sismanis A, Wise CM, Johnson GD (Virginia Commonwealth Univ, Richmond; Dartmouth-Hitchcock Med Ctr, Lebanon, NH)
Otolaryngol Head Neck Surg 116:146–152, 1997   8–5

Background.—The traditional treatment of immune-mediated cochleovastibular disorders — corticosteroids and/or cyclophosphamide — can produce serious and occasionally life-threatening complications. Methotrexate is a less toxic immunosuppressive agent commonly used in patients with rheumatoid arthritis. One experience with methotrexate treatment of immune-mediated cochleovestibular disorders was reported.

Methods.—Twenty-five patients were treated for a mean of 12.9 months. The beginning dose of oral methotrexate was usually 7.5 mg/week. In most patients, this dose was increased to 12.5 to 15 mg/week to attain optimal response.

Outcomes.—Hearing was improved in 69.6% of the patients. In 80%, vestibular symptoms subsided or improved. Adverse reactions to methotrexate treatment, occurring in 8 patients, were acceptable and reversible. Nausea occurred in 4 patients, oral ulcerations in 2, transient rash in 1, and minimal alopecia in 1. Also, diffuse body rashes occurred in 2 patients shortly after treatment initiation, necessitating discontinuation.

Conclusions.—Treatment with methotrexate appears to be effective in a large proportion of patients with immune-mediated cochleovestibular disorders. The adverse effects associated with it are acceptable. The efficacy of methotrexate needs to be compared with that of other immunosuppressive agents in a prospective, randomized study.

▶ In this open study, hearing improved very dramatically in the patients with a variety of problems, including Meniere's disease. The low dose of methotrexate used in the study was based on that used in rheumatoid arthritis. It seemed to work, although, as with many aspects of methotrexate treatment, such as the duration, the diagnostic considerations and previous treatment with prednisone and/or cyclophosphamide will have to be decided on before undertaking the recommended prospective, randomized clinical trial that will be necessary to assess the value of this medication.

M. Weintraub, M.D.

Inhalod and Nasal Glucocorticoids and the Risks of Ocular Hypertension or Open-angle Glaucoma

Garbe E, LeLorier J, Boivin JF, et al (McGill Univ, Montreal; Université de Montreal)
JAMA 277:722–727, 1997   8–6

Purpose.—Topical corticosteroids provide the therapeutic benefits of corticosteroids while reducing the adverse effects. However, as higher doses of inhaled and nasal steroids are prescribed, there is growing concern regarding the possibility of systemic adverse effects. Two recent case reports have suggested that ocular hypertension and open-angle glaucoma may occur in patients taking inhaled and nasal glucocorticoids. A case-control study was performed to evaluate this risk.

Methods.—The study used data regarding elderly patients from a Canadian universal health insurance database. The study group included 9,793 ophthalmology patients who had newly diagnosed borderline or open-angle glaucoma or had started a new course of treatment for ocular hypertension or glaucoma between 1988 and 1994. The controls were a random sample of 38,325 patients who made ophthalmologist visits in the same month and year as the study group. Conditional logistic regression analysis was used to evaluate the odds ratio (OR) of ocular hypertension or open-angle glaucoma among users vs. nonusers of inhaled or nasal glucocorticoids. Adjustments were made for other factors, such as age, sex, diabetes mellitus, systemic hypertension, use of ophthalmic and oral glucocorticoids, and pattern of health system utilization.

Results.—In general, users of inhaled and nasal glucocorticoids were not at increased risk of ocular hypertension or open-angle glaucoma. However, patients who had used high doses of inhaled corticosteroids for 3 months or longer were at significantly increased risk (OR, 1.44). Only 21 patients were in this category of continuous use of high-dose, nasal steroids. Risk was not increased for continuous users of low- to medium-dose inhaled steroids.

Conclusion.—The risk of ocular hypertension or open-angle glaucoma is increased for patients taking high doses of inhaled corticosteroids for an extended period. These patients may be candidates for intraocular pressure monitoring. Patients with newly diagnosed ocular hypertension and open-angle glaucoma should be asked about their use of inhaled steroids.

▶ Millions of prescriptions are written worldwide for nasal steroids because of their beneficial impact on many types of rhinitis, especially those with an atopic basis. Inhaled corticosteroids for asthma grow more popular with each year. Recent case reports have suggested that systemic absorption of topical steroids may lead to ocular hypertension and glaucoma. This article suggests that prolonged use of high doses of inhaled corticosteroids only slightly increases the risk of such ocular complications.

L. Lasagna, M.D.

Effect of Intravenous Fenoldopam on Intraocular Pressure in Ocular Hypertension
Everitt DE, Boike SC, Piltz-Seymour JR, et al (Presbyterian Med Ctr, Philadelphia; Univ of Pennsylvania, Philadelphia; SmithKline Beecham Pharmaceuticals, Philadelphia)
J Clin Pharmacol 37:312–320, 1997   8–7

Background.—Fenoldopam mesylate, a postsynaptic dopamine-1 receptor agonist and potent systemic and renal vasodilator, has been successful in the treatment of accelerate hypertension and in increasing renal blood flow. The effect of IV fenoldopam on intraocular pressure in human beings has been studied previously. In the current study, the effects of intravenous fenoldopam on intraocular pressure, aqueous dynamics, and macular blood flow was studied under carefully controlled conditions in patients with established intraocular hypertension.

Methods.—Seven women and 5 men, aged 41 to 76 years, received fenoldopam doses titrated up to 0.5 µg/kg/min maximum. The main outcome variable was intraocular pressure, determined by pneumotonometry.

Findings.—During fenoldopam infusions, intraocular pressure increased from a mean baseline value of 29.2 mm Hg to a mean maximum of 35.7 mm Hg. During placebo infusions, mean pressure increased from 28.4 mm Hg at baseline to 29 mm Hg at the time corresponding to the mean maximum intraocular pressure on the day of intravenous fenoldopam administration, for a mean pressure difference of 6.7 mm Hg between the 2 study days. No apparent changes in macular blood flow, visual fields, or production or outflow of aqueous humor were associated with fenoldopam infusion.

Conclusions.—The rise in intraocular pressure occurring in these patients with ocular hypertension during fenoldopam infusion is consistent with fenoldopam-related increases in intraocular pressure reported previously in healthy persons and patients with accelerated systemic hypertension. Dopamine-1 receptors appear to play a role in intraocular pressure regulation.

▶ This drug has been studied just the way you'd expect it, from animals to healthy volunteers to patients with high blood pressure and now in patients with increased intraocular pressure. In patients with elevated ocular pressure, the study had to be stopped early before the titration to mean doses for hypertension could be achieved. Intraocular pressure was roughly 28 mm Hg at the start of the study and increased quite dramatically once the infusion was started to 34 mm Hg. Even though the intraocular pressure rose, the good news is that fenoldopam is going to teach us something about the mechanisms in the eye related to dopamine-1 receptors and their relation to aqueous humor production and outflow. So perhaps a new treatment will be revealed that is more specific to the eye than the dopamine-2 agonists such as bromocriptine or pergolide.

M. Weintraub, M.D.

9 Endocrine and Metabolic Disorders

NIDDM Patients' Fears and Hopes About Insulin Therapy: The Basis of Patient Reluctance
Hunt LM, Valenzuela MA, Pugh JA (Univ of Texas, Health Sciences Ctr, San Antonio; Audie L Murphy Mem Veterans Hosp, San Antonio)
Diabetes Care 20:292–298, 1997   9–1

Introduction.—Patients with non–insulin-dependent diabetes mellitus (NIDDM) are often hesitant to begin insulin injections after they have managed their disease with orally given agents. With the use of in-depth interviewing techniques, the attitudes of patients with NIDDM toward insulin therapy were studied.

Methods.—The participants, 44 Mexican American patients seen at 2 public clinics in Texas, were encouraged to be expansive in their responses to the interviewers. The group included 22 men and 22 women (mean age, 52.7 years); 54% had a disease duration of 6 or more years. Sixteen were current insulin users and about half were in good glucose control at the time of the interview.

Results.—Negative attitudes toward insulin were expressed far more frequently than positive ones (75% vs. 25%). Typical complaints were the inconvenience, expense, and discomfort of injections and hypoglycemic symptoms. More important, however, was the concern that insulin use meant that the disease had advanced to a very serious stage. Patients also feared that insulin itself would cause severe complications, including blindness. Those with positive attitudes tended to have had experience with insulin and to report themselves as active in self-care.

Conclusions.—The attitudes of these patients with NIDDM toward insulin were based on personal experience, others' observations, and interactions with health care providers. Some physicians use insulin as a "threat" against patients noncompliant with dietary control or orally given agents. Better patient education about the role of insulin in NIDDM may promote acceptance of the therapy.

▶ Some patients with NIDDM cannot control their metabolic problems with diet, exercise, or orally given hypoglycemics and can improve their lives with insulin. This article usefully explores the problem of negative attitudes toward insulin on the part of both patients and physicians, and how to cope with them.

L. Lasagna, M.D.

Can Insulin Therapy Delay or Prevent Insulin-dependent Diabetes Mellitus?
Kakka R, Koda-Kimble MA (Univ of California, San Francisco)
Pharmacotherapy 17:38–44, 1997   9–2

Background.—The prolonged prediabetic period that precedes clinical insulin-dependent diabetes mellitus (IDDM, type I) involves a slowly progressive immune process that reduces the number of functional pancreatic islet β-cells. Prophylactic therapy might disrupt the immune destructive process in patients identified as at risk for IDDM. Markers of risk include several antibodies directed against various islet cell antigens: glutamic acid decarboxylase and insulin autoantibodies. Animal and human studies have served as the basis for the NIH-sponsored diabetes prevention trial (DPT-1).

Immunotherapy.—Both immunosuppressive and immunomodulating agents are being investigated for their effectiveness in slowing progression toward IDDM. Cyclosporine, azathioprine, and nicotinamide were considered, but all have failed to bring about improvement in newly diagnosed IDDM. Although monoclonal antibodies helped to prevent IDDM in animal studies, adverse reactions to the murine components may limit their use in human beings. The DPT-1 is now studying the ability of insulin treatment to delay clinical onset of IDDM in first-degree relatives of individuals with the disease. Animal studies have helped to clarify the mechanism of insulin's action, and prophylactic insulin reduced the incidence of IDDM in experiments using mice.

Discussion.—The first human pilot study in which insulin was administered to prediabetic patients did not confirm that insulin prevents IDDM, but it strongly suggested that onset of clinical diabetes could be significantly delayed. No significant hypoglycemic events were reported. The projected number of enrollees in DPT-1 (more than 340) should provide adequate statistical power to detect a 35% difference in the yearly risk rate for IDDM onset. Many questions will have to be answered, however, including optimal dosage and the ideal time to start insulin treatment.

▶ Preventing the slow, progressive autoimmune process that destroy pancreatic islet β-cells is a noble idea. How effective prophylactic insulin will be awaits the results of the launched NIH trial. As these authors point out, a number of important questions deserve attention:

• How ethical are immune intervention trials in healthy subjects who may never develop diabetes mellitus?
• What is the ideal dose of insulin?

- What is the ideal time to start providing antigen?
- What is the best way to give insulin, and how do we monitor outcomes?

L. Lasagna, M.D.

Dexfenfluramine in Obese Chinese NIDDM Pateints: A Placebo-controlled Investigation of the Effects on Body Weight, Glycemic Control, and Cardiovascular Risk Factors
Chow C-C, Ko GTC, Tsang LWW, et al (The Chinese Univ of Hong Kong, Shatin)
Diabetes Care 20:1122–1127, 1997   9–3

Background.—Even a modest reduction in weight can result in significant improvements in diabetic control. However, long-term maintenance of weight loss is difficult. The safety, efficacy, and metabolic effects of dexfenfluramine were assessed in obese Chinese patients with NIDDM.

Methods.—Thirty-two patients with a mean body weight of 76.2 kg and body mass index of 31.1 kg/m² were included in the 2–phase, randomized study. Phase 1, beginning after a 2-week single-blind run-in period on placebo, was a randomized 3-month double-blind placebo-controlled trial during which dexfenfluramine or placebo was added to the existing regimens of diet with or without sulfonylureas without metformin. Phase 2 consisted of another 3-month single-blind trial, during which the placebo group received dexfenfluramine without the patients' knowledge. The active treatment group continued with active treatment. Twenty-seven patients were followed up for another 6 to 12 months after dexfenfluramine was withdrawn.

Findings.—At 3 months, mean body mass index changes were -1.2 kg/m² in the dexfenfluramine group and -0.1 kg/m² in the placebo group. The active treatment group also showed a significant improvement in hemoglobin A_{1c}. In phase 2, similar improvements in body weight and glycemic indices were seen in the group switched from placebo to active treatment. After dexfenfluramine was discontinued at 6 months, both groups had significant increases in body weight and glycemic indices, which returned almost to baseline values.

Conclusions.—Dexfenfluramine was a useful aid to weight loss in these patients, resulting in better glycemic control through a 3- to 6-month period. There was also a favorable impact on cardiovascular risk factors.

▶ It is now abundantly clear that dexfenfluramine can achieve (and maintain) weight loss in obese patients. Because obesity is a chronic disease, long-term weight reduction measures are crucial; short-term losses followed by regain of weight make no sense at all. There is good reason to suppose that effective weight loss should decrease the many undesirable health effects of obesity. Balanced against this not unreasonable expectation is the knowledge that primary pulmonary hypertension is a rare risk in patients treated with this agent (and possibly with other anorexiants as well).

The latest worry is the occurrence of abnormalities in the structure of cardiac valves, a phenomenon that has thus far not been observed carefully enough for us to be sure of either causal relationships or the magnitude of risk. Despite these uncertainties, dexfenfluramine has been withdrawn from the market by its manufacturers.

L. Lasagna, M.D.

Glipizide-GITS Does not Increase the Hypoglycemic Effect of Mild Exercise During Fasting in NIDDM
Riddle MC, McDaniel PA, Tive LA, (Oregon Health Sciences Univ, Portland; Pfizer Inc, New York)
Diabetes Care 20:992–994, 1997   9–4

Introduction.—A concern that hypoglycemia may occur prevents some patients with non–insulin-dependent diabetes mellitus (NIDDM) from eating less or exercising more when taking sulfonylureas. A randomized study compared the effects of mild exercise and omission of breakfast on patients treated with extended-release glipizide (glipizide-gastrointestinal therapeutic system [G-GITS]) and patients not taking an oral hypoglycemic agent.

Methods.—Study participants were 25 patients with NIDDM. All were moderately obese and had had 3 months of treatment with a sulfonylurea. Randomization was to placebo or G-GITS taken before breakfast daily. Seventeen patients received G-GITS and 8 were given placebo. The 2 groups were similar in age, duration of diabetes, and relative body weight at entry. Doses of G-GITS were 20 mg daily for 10 patients, 15 mg for 3, 10 mg for 2, and 5 mg for 2. Nine weeks later, a fasting-exercise study was performed. Glucose, insulin, and C-peptide concentrations were measured before, during, and after exercise.

Results.—At 8 AM, fasting values for glucose were significantly lower for G-GITS than for placebo (153 vs. 241 mg/dL). Both fasting insulin and C-peptide were significantly lower for placebo than for G-GITS (84 vs. 159 pmol/L and 846 vs. 1,419 pmol/L, respectively). Decreases in glucose after exercise and after 2 hours of recovery were slight and equivalent in the 2 groups (Fig 1). Insulin and C- peptide concentrations did not change significantly from baseline. No participant experienced symptoms suggesting hypoglycemia.

Conclusion.—Mild hypoglycemia can occur in patients with NIDDM treated with sulfonylureas. Contributing factors include exercise, decreased calorie intake, and patterns of drug absorption. The findings of this study suggest that the risk of hypoglycemia is slight for patients who restrict calories and exercise moderately during acceptable glycemic control with G-GITS.

▶ The 25 patients who participated in this study were members of a larger group of patients evaluating the G-GITS medication. I realize that this study

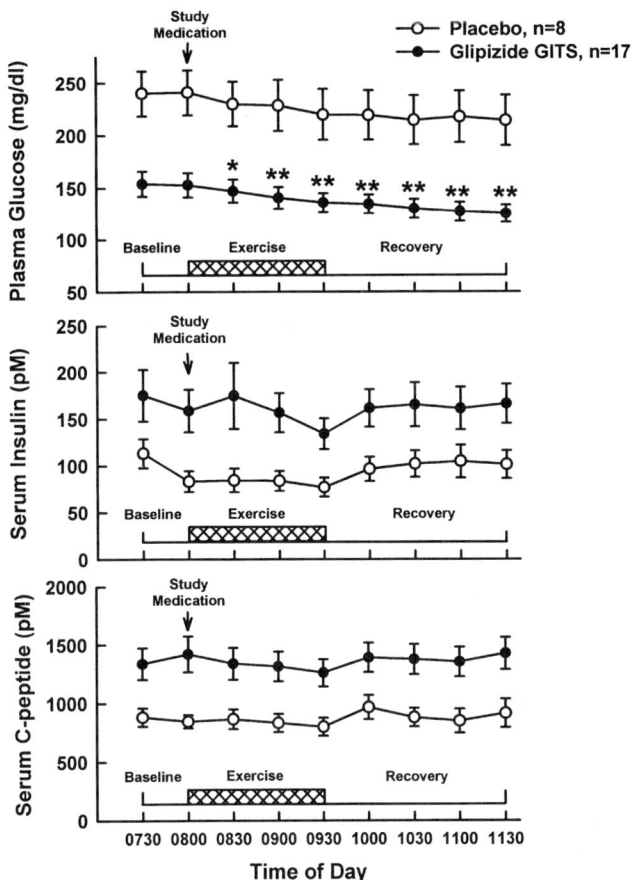

FIGURE 1.—Concentrations of plasma glucose, serum insulin, and serum C-peptide in the 2 treatment groups, measured before, during, and after exercise while fasting. Means ± standard error are shown. Significant declines from the 8 AM baseline value are indicated: *Asterisk* indicates *P* < 0.05; *Double asterisk* indicates P < 0.01. *Abbreviation: Glipizide G-GITS,* glipizide-gastrointestinal therapeutic system. (Courtesy of Riddle MC, McDaniel PA, Tive LA: Glipizide-GITS does not increase the hypoglycemic effect of mild exercise during fasting in NIDDM. *Diabetes Care* 20:992–994, 1997.)

was done in the Pacific Northwest at the Oregon Health Sciences University, but being able to walk on a treadmill for 90 minutes is a good test of your cardiovascular system, even if the treadmill is level and the speed of the treadmill is only 2½ miles per hour. As shown in the figure, there were no differences between placebo and G-GITS patients. Many investigators feel that they can get away with fewer patients because they cut the placebo group in half. That is often true, but you also pay a price for doing so because your power to demonstrate an effect between the active drug and the placebo may be seriously decreased.

M. Weintraub, M.D.

The Problem of Compliance to Cholesterol Altering Therapy
Insull W (Baylor College of Medicine, Houston)
J Intern Med 241:317–325, 1997   9–5

Introduction.—It is generally expected that patient compliance with cholesterol-altering drug regimens will be a major problem. This expectation is based on the concept that about 50% of patients will stop long-term treatment with all types of drugs after 1 year and about 85% of patients will stop after 2 years. It is assumed that these compliance rates also apply to patients taking medication to control cholesterol. The benefits of coronary heart disease prevention drug regimens depend on high levels of compliance. Current knowledge about patient compliance with long-term drug treatment for cholesterol in ambulatory, nonhospitalized patients was reviewed.

Risks of Discontinuation.—There is little reliable information on compliance rates in cholesterol-altering drug regimens in general practice. Estimates of compliance must rely on information from clinical trials and large patient groups treated in HMOs. The risk of discontinuation is summarized for 4 classes of lipid-altering drugs in 8 large clinical trials and 2 HMOs in Table 2. All studies show that the risk of discontinuing treatment increases with treatment time. Discontinuation risks for statin drugs may vary with treatment for primary and secondary prevention of heart disease. Discontinuation risks have also been shown to vary among different drugs depending on their benefits and side effects.

Levels of Compliance.—Electronic monitoring of compliance has revealed several dimensions of compliance behavior. Devices can record the date and time that a patient takes the medication. Four dimensions of noncompliance have been observed: missed doses, missed doses for a

TABLE 2.—Risks of Discontinuation of Drug Treatment for Cholesterol Reduction and Prevention of Coronary Heart Disease: Clinical Trials and HMOs

Trial/HMO	Drug	Number of patients	Period of risk	% Risk of discontinuation†
LRC-CPPT	Resin	1906	7.4 yr	27
CDP	Niacin	1119	5.0 yr	10.7
CDP	Clofibrate	1103	5.0 yr	7.4
HHS	Gemfibrozil	2051	5.0 yr	31.3
EXCELL	Lovastatin	6582	1.0 yr	16.5
4 S	Simvastatin	2221	5.4 yr	10.4
LIPID	Pravastatin	4007	4.0 yr	12
WOSCPS	Pravastatin	3302	4.9 yr	29.6
CARE	Pravastatin	2081	5.0 yr	6.0
HMO	Resin	1335*	1.0 yr	33.9
HMO	Niacin	729*	1.0 yr	44.6
HMO	Lovastatin	537*	1.0 yr	12.7
HMO	Gemfibrozil	435*	1.0 yr	28.0

*Number of courses of therapy with estimated annual risk of discontinuation.
†Percent risk of discontinuation during the treatment period.
(Courtesy of Insull W: The problem of compliance to cholesterol altering therapy. *J Intern Med* 241:317–325, 1997. Publisher, Blackwell Science Ltd.)

number of consecutive days, extra doses, and deviation from the prescribed dose time. The rate of partial compliance to the prescribed day and time may be high and may be more common in clinical practice than in clinical trials. Management of compliance must include evaluation of compliance to the total dose, to the day, and to the time of dose.

Risk Factors for Partial Compliance and Noncompliance.—Major risk factors include number of daily doses, number of medications, side effects, and compatibility with the patient's daily routine. Minor risk factors include the patient's knowledge of the disease and treatment, attitude toward drug treatment, strength of the patient-physician relationship, the patient's psychological state, and access to the physician. In general, age, gender, marital status, education, religion, ethnicity, and socioeconomic status are not significant risk factors.

Compliance Aids.—The major behavioral and physical aids to help compliance are identification of a cue in the patient's daily routine for taking medication, a written description with instructions, a daily medication record, medication containers with compartments for each daily dose, medication containers with timers or alarms, and electronic monitoring devices.

Discussion.—The concepts and information presented may help clinicians and their patients who take cholesterol-altering drugs. Other topics discussed in this extensive article include definitions, assessment, management, and prediction of compliance; costs of partial compliance and noncompliance; standards for compliance performance; the epidemiology of compliance; and training staff in compliance management.

▶ Effective medications are not effective if patients don't take them. As Insull shows in this report, the discontinuation risk for cholesterol-lowering drugs taken chronically ranges from 6% to 45%, with the results being better in the clinical trial data than in the HMO data. (The latter data are probably more like "real life" than are the clinical trial data.)

The reasons for noncompliance are multiple and are nicely discussed by Insull. The challenge is clear—how do we decrease the likelihood of noncompliance for drugs that will provide benefit if taken properly?

L. Lasagna, M.D.

Relative Effectiveness of Niacin and Lovastatin for Treatment of Dyslipidemias in a Health Maintenance Organization
O'Conner PJ, Rush WA, Trence DL, et al (HealthPartners Group Health Found, Minneapolis)
J Fam Pract 44:462–467, 1997   9–6

Background.—Niacin and the HMG-CoA reductase inhibitor lovastatin both effectively reduce low-density lipoprotein (LDL) cholesterol levels. However, they differ significantly in mechanism or action, dosing, and cost. The relative efficacy of niacin and lovastatin in the treatment of dyslipidemias in patients enrolled in an HMO was assessed in a historical cohort study.

Methods.—Adults initially treated with niacin or lovastatin in 1992 and 1993 were identified from pharmacy databases. Patients with a fasting lipid panel done before treatment initiation and a second fasting lipid panel done 9 to 15 months after treatment initiation were included. Two hundred forty-four patients given niacin and 160 given lovastatin met the eligibility criteria. The lovastatin recipients had higher baseline mean cholesterol and LDL cholesterol levels and higher rates of diabetes mellitus and heart disease than niacin recipients.

Findings.—Lovastatin was associated with a mean 25.8% reduction in LDL cholesterol levels; and niacin was associated with a mean 17.5% reduction. With niacin, high-density lipoprotein (HDL) cholesterol levels improved by 16.3%, compared with a 1.5% improvement with lovastatin. Triglyceride levels were improved by 18.4% and 8% in the niacin and lovastatin groups, respectively. The groups had similar LDL/HDL ratio differences before and after treatment. Forty-six patients treated with either agent reached their treatment goals. Treatment was discontinued in 73% of the niacin group and in 52% of the lovastatin group at follow-up (mean, 10.7 months in each group).

Conclusions.—Niacin and lovastatin are both effective in treating dyslipidemic patients. In this series, physicians appropriately used lovastatin more often for patients with higher baseline LDL levels and more comorbid conditions.

▶ Niacin and lovastatin are both helpful in correcting dyslipidemia. Their effects (both good and bad) are not identical, however, and their costs differ substantially. Not very encouraging were the very high discontinuation rates — 73% for niacin and 52% for lovastatin.

L. Lasagna, M.D.

The Efficacy of Lovastatin in Lowering Cholesterol in African Americans With Primary Hypercholesterolemia
Fong RL, Ward HJ (Drew Med Ctr, Los Angeles)
Am J Med 102:387–391, 1997   9–7

Objective.—Whereas previous studies have validated the risks of high cholesterol as a cause of coronary heart disease (CHD), the study populations have been white. As a result, little is known about the efficacy in African Americans (AA) of lipid-lowering drugs. The efficacy of lovastatin in AA patients with risk factors for developing CHD was investigated in a randomized, double-blind, placebo-controlled study.

Methods.—A total of 47 high-risk patients were recruited from the Hypertension, Family Practice, and General Medicine Clinics in Los Angeles and randomly allocated to receive placebo (n=19, 4 men) or 20 mg/dL lovastatin (n=22, 8 men) for 10 weeks. Height, weight, and blood pressure were measured at the first and last visits, lipid levels were determined at the first and last visits, and after 4 weeks on study. Patients were given a low-fat, low-cholesterol diet and received dietary counseling at 2 visits.

Results.—Lovastatin treatment significantly reduced total cholesterol by 14.7% and low-density lipoprotein by 20.0% and nonsignificantly reduced triglycerides by 10.5% and the total cholesterol/high-density lipoprotein (HDL) ratio by 10.5%. The same measures increased nonsignificantly in the placebo group. The side effects were minor, but tended to be more common in the lovastatin group. Aspartate aminotransferase, alanine aminotransferase, and creatinine phosphokinase values increased nonsignificantly in the lovastatin group.

Conclusion.—Lovastatin significantly reduced total cholesterol and LDL cholesterol in AA at high risk for CHD.

▶ In this study, the participants did not have a trial of diet alone prior to instituting the therapy with lovastatin as recommended by the National Cholesterol Education Program II guidelines. I think that they should have been tried on a diet for a period of time to weed out those who could respond pretty easily to a change in their intake. However, you rarely get much more than a 10% fall in cholesterol, and it's difficult to maintain for a long period of time. The real point of this study was to show that there is no difference in the response to statins in the African American population. Actually, there were probably African Americans in all of the preapproval studies, but it's relatively hard to tease them out. In the current study, it was relatively clear that the drugs would be effective in all subgroups tested. However, the magnitude was assessed and the response to various cholesterol subgroups measured. The fall in HDL was a little bit worrisome. Since the population started off with a relatively high HDL (in the 50s), the danger wasn't too great. If one could separate the patients with low HDLs who are at somewhat higher risk for heart attacks and put them in a separate group, I think we would have gotten more important data, not just for the African American population, but for the population in general.

M. Weintraub, M.D.

A Comparison of 20 or 40 mg Per Day of Carbimazole in the Initial Treatment of Hyperthyroidism
Page SR, Sheard CE, Herbert M, et al (City Hosp, Nottingham, England; Univ Hosp, Nottingham, England; Derby City Gen Hosp, England)
Clin Endocrinol (Oxf) 45:511–515, 1996   9–8

Background.—Although carbimazole (CBZ) has been used in the treatment of hyperthyroidism for about 50 years, the optimal dosage has not been established definitively. The early clinical and biochemical responses of patients with hyperthyroidism to 20 and 40 mg/day were compared.

Methods.—Sixty-three patients were enrolled in the prospective, randomized multicenter trial. Measures of serum total and free thyroid hormones, serum thyrotropin (TSH), and sex hormone binding globulin (SHBG) were obtained at baseline and at 4 and 10 weeks after treatment initiation. At 6 and 12 weeks, weight and pulse were monitored, and a symptom questionnaire was completed.

Findings.—Patients receiving a starting dosage of 40 mg/day of CBZ had lower total and free thyroxine (T4) levels as well as total and free triiodothyronine (T3) concentrations at 4 weeks than those given 20 mg/day. Clinical responses and SHBG concentrations at 6 and 12 weeks were comparable. At 4 and 10 weeks, drug-related hypothyroidism was less likely to occur in patients initially receiving 20 mg/day. However, this dosage less effectively controlled hyperthyroidism in patients with more severe hyperthyroidism with baseline total thyroxine (TT4) exceeding 260 nmol/L.

Conclusions.—A CBZ dosage of 20 mg/day is effective, convenient, and safer than 40 mg/day in the treatment of mild and moderate hyperthyroidism. Patients with severe hyperthyroidism will require higher dosages.

▶ Here is a dose-response relationship attempt which showed again that the higher dose of CBZ, really was unnecessary except for patients with severe hyperthyroidism. We have to look at the slope of the changes caused by the different drugs. We'd like to see, in many cases, a more gradual slope. We'd like to see things done gently rather than precipitously. We are learning that in many areas of therapeutics. Certainly in anticoagulation and the treatment of obesity, we have seen that a slow, gentle slope of drug effect seems preferable.

M. Weintraub, M.D.

Glucocorticoid Replacement Therapy: Are Patients Overtreated and Does it Matter?
Peacey SR, Guo C-Y, Robinson AM, et al (Northern General Hosp, Sheffield, England)
Clin Endocrinol (Oxf) 46:255–261, 1997   9–9

Background.—Adequately assessing patients on glucocorticoid replacement treatment is very important to avoid the consequences of undertreatment or overtreatment. However, no simple test is currently available for this. The adequacy of glucocorticoid replacement in hypoadrenal patients was determined, serum cortisol concentrations were correlated with 24-hour urine free cortisol excretion, and the effect of glucocorticoid dose optimization on markers of bone formation and resorption was assessed.

Methods and Findings.—Thirty-two consecutive patients receiving replacement glucocorticoid treatment were studied. Eighty-eight percent needed a change in treatment. Seventy-five percent required a decrease in total dose; 56%, a change in replacement therapy regimen or drug; and 44%, both. The mean daily hydrocortisone dose was decreased from 29.5 to 20.8 mg. Peak cortisol was significantly associated with 24-hour urine free cortisol-creatinine levels. After a decrease in hydrocortisone dose, median osteocalcin rose from 16.7 to 19.9 µg/L, with no change in the N-telopeptide of type I collagen/creatinine ratio.

Conclusions.—A high percentage of patients receiving conventional corticosteroid replacement treatment are overtreated or receiving inappropriate replacement regimens. Corticosteroid replacement should be determined individually and overreplacement avoided to decrease the long-term risk of osteoporosis.

▶ This article, like the one that follows by Howlett (Abstract 9–10), argues quite logically that to treat every patient in the same way is guaranteed to result in suboptimal treatment for some.

L. Lasagna, M.D.

An Assessment of Optimal Hydrocortisone Replacement Therapy
Howlett TA (Leicester Royal Infirmary, England)
Clin Endocrinol (Oxf) 46:263–268, 1997   9–10

Background.—Although hydrocortisone is now the standard form of glucocorticoid replacement in patients with primary and secondary adrenal insufficiency, there is still no agreement on the appropriate dose, timing, or monitoring of such therapy. The use of hydrocortisone replacement therapy at 1 center was reviewed.

Methods.—The case notes of 210 patients who had been treated with hydrocortisone were reviewed. One hundred thirty patients whose records contained the findings of at least one valid hydrocortisone day curve were identified. Data on 174 day curves were therefore analyzed.

Findings.—Optimal replacement was achieved in only 15% of the patients on twice-daily hydrocortisone regimens, compared to 60% on thrice-daily regimens. The mean overall "quality scores" for these regimens were 2.72 and 3.49, respectively. In 66% of the patients, 10 mg/5 mg/5 mg (on rising, at lunch, and in the evening) achieved optimal replacement. The mean quality score in these patients was 3.62. By contrast, doses of 10 mg/10 mg/5 mg and of 20 mg/–10 mg achieved optimal replacement in 50% and 10%, respectively, with corresponding quality scores of 3.32 and 2.48.

Conclusions.—Optimal replacement is achieved with thrice-daily hydrocortisone regimens. An appropriate starting dose is 10 mg/5 mg/5 mg, with subsequent individual adjustments based on simple hydrocortisone day curves.

▶ Although glucocorticoid replacement in patients with adrenal insufficiency is accepted by everyone, there is no universal agreement about optimal dose, timing, and monitoring of response.

This study suggests that thrice-daily dosing offers the best chance for optimal replacement, rather than the traditional twice-daily dosing. Howlett suggests an appropriate starting dose, with subsequent modification based on hydrocortisone day curve measurements so as to achieve individualized regimens. Sounds rational.

L. Lasagna, M.D.

Use of Postmenopausal Hormone Replacement Therapy: Estimates From a Nationally Representative Cohort Study

Brett KM, Madans JH (Natl Ctr for Health Statistics, Hyattsville, Md)
Am J Epidemiol 145:536–545, 1997   9–11

Introduction.—Although the use of postmenopausal hormone replacement therapy (HRT) has fluctuated since its approval in the 1940s, these drugs are now among the most commonly prescribed medications in the United States. To describe trends in HRT use by demographic, lifestyle, and heart disease risk factors, data obtained from the Epidemiologic Followup Study to the First National Health and Nutrition Examination Survey were analyzed.

Methods.—The survey cohort was followed up from the mid-1970s until 1992. Included in the analyses were a variety of sociodemographic, health behavior, and heart disease predictor variables. The study sample included 5,602 women who had become menopausal by their last follow-up interview.

Results.—By the last interview, the average age of the study cohort was 66.4 years; the mean reported age at menopause was 45.9 years. The use of HRT was found to increase with year of birth. An estimated 45% of women born between 1897 and 1950 and who were menopausal by 1992 had used HRT for at least 1 month, and 20% continued use for at least 5 years. These percentages increased by 32% and 54%, respectively, for younger members of the cohort. Throughout the study period, women most likely to use HRT were those who had undergone bilateral oophorectomy. Women who were white, more highly educated, and lived in the West also had a higher probability of HRT use; less likely users were women who were overweight or who abstained from alcohol. The median length of HRT use was 6.6 years.

Conclusions.—In this nationally representative cohort of women who provided self-reports of HRT use, approximately 20% who experienced menopause between 1970 and 1992 used HRT for at least 5 years. Acceptance of HRT was associated with sociodemographic factors. Although overall use of HRT is increasing, women tend to discontinue use within several years.

▶ Postmenopausal HRT has had a roller-coaster ride in the United States as a function of "good news–bad news" and the introduction of combined estrogen-progestin therapy in the 1980s. The data in this study shed light on some of the factors that affect the likelihood of such use.

L. Lasagna, M.D.

Menopausal Hormone Therapy: Physician Awareness of Patient Attitudes

Ghali WA, Freund KM, Boss RD, et al (Boston Med Ctr)

Am J Med 103:3–10, 1997   9–12

Objective.—Because women's opinions about the use of menopausal hormone therapy (HT) vary widely, physicians need to tailor their counseling to each patient. Results are presented of a cross-sectional survey of physicians' awareness of patients' attitudes toward menopause and general health beliefs; physicians' estimates of their patients' degree of concern about risk for certain diseases or conditions; and whether certain physician characteristics predict greater awareness of patient attitudes.

Methods.—Women (n = 182), ages 50–70, attending an outpatient primary care facility of an academic medical center were surveyed about sociodemographic factors, health behaviors, menopausal health history, and use of HT. On a 4–point scale, patients were to rate their knowledge of the risks and benefits of HT use and their degree of concern about the risk of heart disease, breast cancer, hip fracture, endometrial cancer, severe hot flashes, urinary incontinence, and vaginal dryness. Patients' general health beliefs and attitudes about menopause, as well as desire for autonomy and information were assessed. Physicians' knowledge of risks, benefits, and physiologic effects of HT and their awareness of patients' attitudes were assessed.

Results.—Faculty and fellows knew more about HT than interns and residents did. Whereas physicians were aware of patients' need for autonomy, they significantly underestimated patients' need for information, concerns about using HT, and degree to which women thought of menopause as a health problem. This lack of awareness was greater for male physicians than for female physicians, and for interns/residents than for faculty/fellows. Male physicians and interns/residents were also less knowledgeable about HT. Physicians significantly overestimated patients' concerns about heart disease and breast cancer and underestimated their concerns about incontinence. Predictors of HT use were white race, alcohol intake, hysterectomy, oophorectomy, no family history of breast cancer, recent menstruation, menstrual symptoms, and knowledge of HT.

Conclusion.—Physicians, particularly those who are male, less experienced, and less knowledgeable about HT, underestimated patients' information needs and concerns about HT and incontinence and overestimated patients' concerns about heart disease and breast cancer.

▶ At least at this Boston academic center, informational gaps (or errors) about menopausal hormone therapy were found among both patients and physicians. Factual knowledge doesn't guarantee wise judgments but should be a goal in any case (unless one espouses paternalism and materialism, as opposed to libertarianism).

L. Lasagna, M.D.

Risk of Venous Thromboembolism in Users of Hormone Replacement Therapy

Daly E, Vessey MP, Hawkins MM, et al (Univ of Oxford, England; Radcliffe Infirmary, Oxford, England; Childhood Cancer Research Group, Oxford, England)

Lancet 348:977–980, 1996   9–13

Background.—Studies that have shown an increased risk of venous thromboembolism with the use of estrogen have studied young women using oral contraceptives. It is not generally believed that hormone replacement therapy also raises the risk of venous thromboembolism in postmenopausal women. None of the studies of hormone replacement therapy have found a significantly higher risk of venous thromboembolism in users of hormone replacement therapy, but they have lacked the power to detect important risks. The *British National Formulary* lists active thrombophlebitis or thromboembolic disorders as contraindications to hormone replacement therapy. Whether there is an association between current use of hormone replacement therapy and venous thromboembolism was investigated in a hospital-based, case-control study.

Methods.—The study participants were 103 women between 45 and 64 years old with idiopathic venous thromboembolism; 22 were studied retrospectively. The control subjects were 178 women with disorders of the eye, ear, skin, repiratory and alimentary tracts, kidneys, bones, and joints, or who had trauma; 32 were studied retrospectively. Information was gathered on medical and gynecologic history; use of hormone replacement therapy, oral contraceptives, and other drugs; height and weight; and use of tobacco and alcohol.

Results.—There were 44 study subjects and 44 controls who were current users of hormone replacement therapy. The adjusted odds ratio for venous thromboembolism among current users of hormone replacement therapy compared to that of nonusers was 3.5; nonusers included those who had never used hormone replacement therapy and those who had used it in the past. There was no association between past use of hormone replacement therapy and risk of venous thromboembolism. The risk was highest among subjects who had used hormone replacement therapy for a short period of time.

Discussion.—There appears to be a higher risk of venous thromboembolism in current users of hormone replacement therapy. This risk seemed to be greatest in women who used hormone replacement therapy for a short period of time. No association was observed in those who had used hormone replacement therapy in the past. The risk of venous thromboembolism was similar in users of oral and transdermal therapy, and in users of unopposed estrogen and combined estrogen-progestogen therapy.

▶ As with oral contraceptives, hormone replacement therapy (HRT) carries with it a very slight risk of venous thromboembolism. This has to be weighed against the benefits of HRT — fewer fractures and less coronary disease.

L. Lasagna, M.D.

Effect of Three Years of Oral Alendronate Treatment in Postmenopausal Women with Osteoporosis
Tucci JR, for the U.S. Alendronate Phase III Osteoporosis Treatment Study Group (Roger Williams Hosp, Providence, RI; Fletcher Allen Health Care, Burlington, Vt; Reading Hosp and Med Ctr, Pennsylvania; et al)
Am J Med 101:488–501, 1996   9–14

Background.—Oral alendronate sodium specifically inhibits bone resorption mediated by osteoclasts. The efficacy and safety of this potent agent in postmenopausal women with osteoporosis were investigated.

Methods.—Four hundred seventy-eight women were enrolled in the 3-year, randomized, double-blind, multicenter trial. The women received alendronate, 5 or 10 mg/day for 3 years or 20 mg/day for 2 years followed by 5 mg/day for 1 year (20/5), or placebo. In addition, all received 500 mg mg/day supplemental calcium.

Findings.—After 3 years of treatment, alendronate 10 mg induced substantial increases in bone mineral density (BMD) at the lumbar spine, femoral neck, and trochanter. Bone mineral density at these sites declined in the women receiving placebo. The progressive increases were significant in the second and third years. Alendronate 10 mg also increased total body BMD. Though it prevented loss at the 1/3 forearm site, it did not increase BMD. The efficacy of alendronate 20/5 was not greater than that of the 10–mg dose. Alendronate 5 mg was significantly less effective than 10 mg at all sites. Bone turnover declined to a stable nadir during 3 months for resorption markers and during 6 months for formation markers. In alendronate recipients, mean loss of stature was reduced by 41%. Abdominal pain was reported by women given active treatment but was usually mild and resolved with continued treatment.

Conclusions.—Alendronate appears to be an important advance in the treatment of postmenopausal women with osteoporosis. It is a highly effective treatment with a safety profile comparable to that of placebo.

▶ Osteoporosis affects 30% to 50% of postmenopausal women and has been said to be the cause of 1.5 million fractures each year in the U.S. The search for remedies for this common and distressing ailment has come up with the bisphosphonates (previously called diphosphonates), one of which is alendronate, a selective inhibitor of osteoclast-mediated bone resorption.

This 3-year study is most encouraging with regard to both the efficacy and the safety of alendronate. Let's pray that the eventual fracture risk data are as encouraging.

L. Lasagna, M.D.

Efficacy of Pamidronate in Reducing Skeletal Complications in Patients With Breast Cancer and Lytic Bone Metastases

Hortobagyi GN, for the Protocol 19 Aredia Breast Cancer Study Group (Univ of Texas, Houston; Saint Thomas Hosp, Nashville, Tenn; Saint Vincent Med Ctr, Los Angeles; et al)

N Engl J Med 335:1785–1791, 1996   9–15

Introduction.—Most women with advanced breast cancer have bone metastases. Osteoclast-induced bone resorption causes the destruction of bone in these lesions, and cytotoxic chemotherapy or hormone therapy is the treatment most often preferred. However, this therapy causes progressive skeletal destruction, which leads to immobility and more pain. Potent inhibitors of osteoclastic bone resorption are biophosphonates, which are effective in treating cancer that has metastasized to bone. Skeletal complications may be reduced by pamidronate disodium, a second-generation bisphosphonate. A randomized, double-blind study was conducted to compare monthly infusions of pamidronate (90 mg) with a placebo to prevent skeletal complications.

Methods.—Placebo or pamidronate at 90 mg were given to 380 women with stage IV breast cancer as a 2-hour intravenous infusion monthly for 12 cycles. The women also were receiving cytotoxic chemotherapy and had at least one lytic bone lesion. Each month, an assessment was made to determine of the patient had skeletal complications, including pathologic fractures, the need for radiation to bone or bone surgery, spinal cord compression, and hypercalcemia (a serum calcium concentration above 12 mg per dL [3.0 mmol per liter] or elevated to any degree and requiring treatment). Evaluations were also done on bone pain, performance status, use of analgesic drugs and quality of life.

Results.—There was a greater length of time for the occurrence of the first skeletal complication among the women receiving the pamidronate (13.1 months) than in the group receiving placebo (7 months). In the pamidronate group, 43% of women had skeletal complications compared to 56% of women in the placebo group. In the pamidronate group, there was significantly less increase in bone pain and deterioration of performance status than in the placebo group. The women tolerated the pamidronate well.

Conclusion.—Women with stage IV breast cancer who have osteolytic bone metastases are more protected against skeletal complications with monthly infusions of pamidronate as a supplement to chemotherapy.

▶ In this excellent study, the patients were really quite advanced and had at least 1, (usually a lytic) metastatic bone lesion of a certain diameter. Thus, the investigators called this palliative treatment. Perhaps if it were started earlier, it would not be just palliative but might be considered preventative or, in fact, treatment for bone lesions which had not yet even appeared. The next study should perhaps be done in a group of patients who have apparently normal bones.

M. Weintraub, M.D.

Biochemical and Radiologic Improvement in Paget's Disease of Bone Treated With Alendronate: A Randomized, Placebo-controlled Trial

Reid IR, Nicholson GC, Weinstein RS, et al (Univ of Zuckland, New Zealand; Univ of Melbourne, Australia; Univ of Arkansas for Med Sciences, Little Rock; et al)

Am J Med 101:341–348, 1996   9–16

Background.—The potent bisphosphonates are very promising in the treatment of Paget's disease of the bone. However, in most countries these agents are only available in parenteral preparations. Alendronate, a new oral aminobisphosphonate, has shown promise in preliminary studies of patients with Paget's disease.

Methods.—Fifty-five patients with Paget's disease were enrolled in a double-blind, randomized comparison of oral alendronate, 40 mg/day, and placebo. Treatment was given for 6 months.

Findings.—Alendronate recipients had an 86% decrease in N-telopeptide excretion and a 73% reduction in serum alkaline phosphatase. These measures were unchanged in the placebo group. Previous bisphosphonate therapy did not affect responses. In 48% of the patients, alendronate normalized alkaline phosphatase. Radiologic improvement in osteolysis was seen in 48% of patients in the alendronate group, compared with only 4% in the placebo group. None of the patients had a worsening of osteolysis. Bone histomorphometric analysis indicated that alendronate tended to normalize turnover indices. Twelve alendronate recipients underwent bone biopsy, none of which showed evidence of abnormal mineralization. Alendronate was tolerated well.

Conclusion.—Oral alendronate appears to be effective and safe in the treatment of Paget's disease. Healing of lytic bone lesions was observed.

▶ This study is interesting and important because it tried to establish new surrogate markers for Paget's disease. One of them was N-telopeptide excretion, which decreased by an amazing 86%. Of course, the authors also investigated serum alkaline phosphatase, which decreased by 73% in patients receiving alendronate. Although pain was not an outcome criterion, it declined in both groups to a nonsignificant degree. The authors caution against using pagetic pain as an outcome criterion because of the possibility that it can respond to placebo.

One problem with this study is that 19 of 55 patients had received other therapy before the onset of the trial. Unfortunately, the authors never told us what happened to those patients and whether they were, in fact, better responders or were not evenly distributed between treatment groups. We need to know what happened in the study population because that helps us to understand what would be more likely to happen with our patients.

M. Weintraub, M.D.

Nitric Oxide May Mediate the Hemodynamic Effects of Recombinant Growth Hormone in Patients With Acquired Growth Hormone Deficiency

Böger RH, Skamira C, Bode-Böger SM, et al (Hannover Med School, Germany)

J Clin Invest 98:2706–2713, 1996   9–17

Introduction.—Patients with hypopituitarism are at increased risk of death from cardiovascular causes, but the relationship between growth hormone deficiency and cardiovascular disease is unclear. Decreased biological activity of nitric oxide (NO) is associated with atherosclerosis and hypertension, and recent experimental studies suggest that NO release may be involved in the beneficial cardiovascular effects of growth hormone therapy. A study of growth hormone-deficient patients measured the effects of recombinant growth hormone on systemic NO formation.

Methods.—The 30 patients had adult-onset hypopituitarism and had not started growth hormone therapy. Randomization was to recombinant human growth hormone (r-hGH; 2.0 IU/d) or placebo for 12 months. The study continued for another 12 months with both groups receiving r-hGH. Urine and plasma samples were collected at regular intervals. Plasma IGF-1 levels were determined and urinary nitrate and cyclic guanosine monophosphate measured as indices of systemic NO production. Patients underwent echocardiography at 1, 12, and 24 months for evaluation of cardiac output.

Results.—Patients randomized to r-hGH exhibited a 4–fold increase in plasma IGF-1 concentrations after the first month of treatment. Indices of NO production, which were low at baseline in growth hormone-deficient patients, were significantly increased with r-hGH treatment after both 12-month periods. Treatment with r-hGH also significantly increased cardiac output (by 30% to 40%) and decreased total peripheral resistance by about one-third. Systolic and diastolic blood pressure showed no significant changes with active treatment. At the end of the second study year, when all patients had received r-hGH, the 2 groups were similar in plasma IGF-1, urinary nitrate, cyclic guanosine-monophospate excretion, and hemodynamic parameters.

Conclusion.—Production of NO is impaired in adult patients with untreated growth hormone deficiency, and treatment with r-hGH significantly increases NO formation and cardiac output. This effect of r-hGH supports the view that increased NO formation contributes to the improved cardiovascular performance of patients during r-hGH therapy for hypopituitarism.

▶ When a new mediator appears, we look for all kinds of effects. At first, we seek explanations of well-known phenomena, later, we look for its effects where we have no explanation of standard medications. Certainly, that's what happened in this study, which showed that systemic nitric oxide formation was decreased in growth hormone deficient people and that the treatment normalized it as well as the cyclic guanosine monophosphate excretion. We'll have to wait and see whether this study's hypothesis holds true, and learn what other amazing things nitric oxide can do.

M. Weintraub, M.D.

Effects of Physiologic Growth Hormone Therapy on Bone Density and Body Composition in Patients With Adult-onset Growth Hormone Deficiency: A Randomized, Placebo-controlled Trial
Baum HBA, Biller BMK, Finkelstein JS, et al (Massachusetts Gen Hosp, Boston; Maine Med Ctr, Portland)
Ann Intern Med 125:883–890, 1996   9–18

Introduction.—Adult-onset growth hormone deficiency is associated with reduced bone density and increased fat mass. Treatment with high-dose growth hormone may reduce body fat. However, the effects of physiologic doses of growth hormone remain unclear. A randomized, controlled trial was undertaken to assess the effects of physiologic doses of growth hormone on bone density and body composition in patients with adult-onset growth hormone deficiency.

Methods.—The trial included 32 men with adult-onset growth hormone deficiency (median age, 51 years). They were assigned to 18 months of treatment with growth hormone or placebo. Growth hormone treatment started at a dose of 10 µg/kg, with a 25% dose reduction in case of elevated levels of insulin-like growth factor-1. Every 6 months, dual-energy x-ray absorptiometry was performed to assess body composition and bone mineral density in the lumbar spine, femoral neck, and proximal radius. Bone turnover markers were assessed during the first year of treatment.

Results.—Patients assigned to growth hormone had a mean 5% increase in bone mineral density in the lumbar spine, and a 2% increase in the femoral neck. These patients also had significant increases in certain markers of bone turnover, including osteocalcin, urinary pyridinoline, and urinary deoxypyridinoline. The growth hormone group had a significant reduction in percentage of body fat—from 32% to 28%—and a significant increase in lean body mass—59.0 to 61.5 kg. All of the changes were significant, compared with those in the placebo group.

Conclusion.—In physiologic doses adjusted to serum levels of insulin-like growth factor-1, growth hormone treatment is beneficial in men with adult-onset growth hormone deficiency. Treatment can increase bone density and stimulate bone turnover while reducing body fat and increasing lean body mass. The long-term significance of these changes remains to be seen. The incidence of side effects is low.

▶ Use of growth hormone has traditionally been restricted to children with deficiency of this hormone. But growth hormone deficiency can occur in adults as well. This study suggests that benefits, with regard to both bone and fat, can accrue from treatment with growth hormone.

L. Lasagna, M.D.

Adult Height in Growth Hormone (GH)-Deficient Children Treated With Biosynthetic GH

Blethen SL, for the Genentech Growth Study Group (State Univ of New York, Stony Brook)

J Clin Endocrinol Metab 82:418–420, 1997   9–19

Background.—Children with growth hormone deficiency (GHD) will have short stature unless treated with growth hormone (GH). The advent of GH prepared by recombinant DNA technology has permitted children to receive larger doses of human GH for longer periods. The results of treatment of 121 GHD children with recombinant GH until near adult height (AH) were determined.

Methods.—The study group consisted of 49 girls and 72 boys aged 4.2 to 17.2 years at the time the study began. Of the 121 participants, 84 were treated with methionyl-GH and 37 were treated with GH with the same amino acid sequence as human pituitary GH. All received 0.3 mg/kg each week in either daily or thrice-weekly doses. The children were examined every 3 months until 1991 and were then examined every 6 months. Height, weight, and pubertal status were noted at each visit. Near AH was defined on the basis of a growth rate of 2.0 cm/yr or less over at least a 6-month period and by age.

Results.—Of the 121 children in the study group, 87.6% reached AH within 2 SD of the normal average for American adults. The average final height for males was 171.6 cm, and for females it was 158.5 cm. This 13-cm difference in AH is comparable to that between males and females in the general population. When AH was expressed as standard deviation score, there was no difference in outcome between males and females. The cause of GHD and spontaneous puberty did not affect outcome. Adult height was positively affected by initial height, treatment duration, and growth rate during the first year. It was negatively affected by age at start of treatment, bone age delay, and gender.

Conclusion.—In this series of children with GHD, treatment with re-combinant human growth hormone significantly increased AH in both boys and girls beyond predicted adult height. Early diagnosis and long-term treatment with large doses of recombinant human growth hormone should improve outcome in children with GHD.

▶ The use of GH originally isolated from human cadaver pituitaries to increase AH in short-statured GHD children was hampered by inadequate supplies and the delayed risk of Creutzfeld-Jakob disease. Biosynthetic GH has seemingly solved both these problems. This study suggests that GH therapy should be started early and used continuously in adequate dosage if a more normal height is to be achieved.

L. Lasagna, M.D.

Long-term Pharmacotherapy in the Management of Obesity
National Task Force on the Prevention and Treatment of Obesity (Tufts Univ, Boston; HEALTH WATCH, New York; Univ of Colorado, Denver; et al)
JAMA 276:1907–1915, 1996   9–20

Background.—Much confusion exists about the role of medications in the management of obesity. Long-term pharmacotherapy in the treatment of obese individuals was investigated in the current literature review.

Methods.—English-language articles on the role of medications in the treatment of human obesity and studies of their safety and efficacy (for at least 24 weeks) were identified through electronic database and manual searches. Experts in nutrition, obesity, and eating disorders evaluated the reports.

Findings.—Net weight loss achieved with medication use appears to be modest, ranging from 2 to 10 kg. However, patients receiving active agents were more likely to lose 10% or more of their initial body weight. Weight remains at less than baseline throughout treatment, with loss tending to plateau by 6 months. Some studies, however, report partial weight regain, despite continued drug treatment. Although most side effects are mild and self-limiting, serious outcomes occur rarely.

Conclusions.—When combined with behavioral approaches aimed at changing diet and physical activity levels, pharmacotherapy can help some obese patients lose weight and maintain weight loss for 1 year or more. Little justification exists for the short-term use of anorexiant agents. More studies are needed before pharmacotherapy can be recommended for routine use in obese individuals, although it may be helpful in carefully selected individuals.

▶ Actually, this article is a review. However, the subject is of great interest and it's a good collection of studies and information gathered by the National Institutes of Health, National Task Force on the Prevention and Treatment of Obesity.

M. Weintraub, M.D.

Dementia and Subnormal Levels of Vitamin B_{12}: Effects of Replacement Therapy on Dementia
Teunisse S, Bollen AE, van Gool WA, et al (Univ of Amsterdam)
J Neurol 243:522–529, 1996   9–21

Background.—Routine screening of patients with dementia includes determination of serum vitamin B_{12}. Some authorities believe that a vitamin B_{12} deficiency is a cause of reversible dementia. Several studies have reported beneficial effects of vitamin B_{12} replacement therapy in patients with dementia who have subnormal levels of this vitamin.

Methods.—In a prospective, longitudinal study of 170 consecutive patients, 65 years of age or older, with dementia, serum vitamin B_{12} levels were determined. The treatment group consisted of patients with subnormal levels of serum vitamin B_{12}, and the reference group consisted of patients with normal levels. The effects of vitamin B_{12} replacement therapy on cognitive impairment, disability in activities of daily living, behavioral changes, and the burden experienced by caregivers were examined.

Results.—Subnormal serum vitamin B_{12} values were found in 26 of the 170 patients. All but 1 patient met the criteria for possible Alzheimer's disease. The effect of cobalamin supplementation was analyzed after 6 months in all patients. Functioning did not improve after replacement therapy after taking into account the size and pattern of individual change scores and the mean change scores on all instruments. The change scores of the treatment group were compared with those of patients with Alzheimer's disease. This comparison showed that replacement therapy did not slow the progression of dementia.

Discussion.—These findings suggest that subnormal serum vitamin B_{12} levels are not an important cause of reversible dementia. The study used standardized and comprehensive evaluations of cognitive impairment, disability in activities of daily living, behavioral changes, and the burden experienced by caregivers.

▶ Too bad. It would be so nice if Alzheimer's dementia could be slowed by vitamin B_{12}. This disease does not seem to be a reflection of B_{12} deficiency.

L. Lasagna, M.D.

10 Gastrointestinal Disorders

Omeprazole and Clarithromycin With and Without Metronidazole for the Eradication of *Helicobacter pylori*
Chiba N (McMaster Univ, Hamilton, Canada)
Am J Gastroenterol 91:2139–2143, 1996   10–1

Objective.—The ideal treatment regimen for eradication of *Helicobacter pylori* infection remains unclear. "Omeprazole plus" regimens may help to reduce side effects and improve compliance compared with triple therapy of bismuth, metronidazole, and tetracycline. Omeprazole plus clarithromycin is better than omeprazole plus amoxicillin but still is not as good as triple therapy. Two "omeprazole plus" regimens for the eradication of *H. pylori* were compared for safety and efficacy.

Methods.—The randomized, open trial included 65 patients with confirmed *H. pylori* infection. One group of patients received twice-daily treatment with low-dose omeprazole, 20 mg, and clarithromycin, 250 mg, (OC). The other group received OC plus metronidazole, 500 mg, (OCM). Gastric biopsy specimens were obtained at least 4 weeks after treatment to determine whether *H. pylori* had been eradicated.

Results.—Efficacy was significantly greater with OCM than with OC. This was so by both intention-to-treat analysis (82% vs. 58%) and per protocol analysis (93% vs. 62%). Side effects were common, occurring in more than 60% of each group. However, most side effects were mild, and patients in both groups took 97% of their pills. Only 1 patient withdrew (from the OC group) because of side effects.

Conclusion.—The OCM combination is more effective in eradicating *H. pylori* than is OC alone. Although side effects are common, there are no serious adverse events and compliance is good. The OCM regimen may prove especially useful as more family practitioners treat *H. pylori* infection in patients with ulcer, without referral to a gastroenterologist.

▶ We know how to cure *H. pylori* infection, but the "gold standard" originally described (bismuth, metronidazole, and tetracycline) required that a lot of pills be taken 4 times a day, with frequently troublesome side effects. The triple therapy described in this article requires only 6 pills a day given on a twice-daily schedule. The cure rate is high, and the compliance is good.

L. Lasagna, M.D.

Ethnic and Genetic Determinants of Omeprazole Disposition and Effect
Caraco Y, Lagerstrom P-O, Wood AJJ (Vanderbilt Univ, Nashville, Tenn)
Clin Pharmacol Ther 60:157–167, 1996   10–2

Introduction.—Ethnic origin affects the ability of an individual to metabolize endogenous compounds and xenobiotics. Race-related differences at the phenotypic level may be explained by this phenomenon. Acid secretion by the parietal gastric mucosa cells is inhibited by omeprazole, a proton pump inhibitor. Although the plasma half-life of omeprazole is short, after a single oral dose of 20 mg, gastric acid output is suppressed for 24 hours. In poor metabolizers of mephenytoin, the increased omeprazole plasma concentrations might be expected to result in markedly diminished acid secretion and marked elevations in plasma gastrin levels. The central role of CYP2C19 has been shown in omeprazole metabolism. The pharmacokinetics and dynamics of omeprazole were compared in white and Chinese individuals.

Methods.—The study included 7 Chinese non-smoking extensive metabolizers of mephenytoin and debrisoquin and 8 white males. Blood samples were obtained after the 8th omeprazole dose at 40 mg/day over 24 hours in the double-blind, 2-stage study. From the respective plasma concentration-time curves, omeprazole, omeprazole sulfone, and hydroxyomeprazole pharmacokinetics were calculated. From the respective plasma gastrin concentrations, 12- and 24-hour integrated plasma gastrin levels were calculated. A determination was made of the activities of CYP2D6, CYP2C19, and CYP3A4 a week before omeprazole administration was initiated.

Results.—In the white individuals, omeprazole concentrations were significantly lower and oral clearance of the drug was greater than in the Chinese individuals. Whites had an omeprazole concentration of 7.53 ± 1.21 µmol/hr/L^{-1} and Chinese individuals had a concentration of 12.80 ± 2.13 µmol/hr/L^{-1}. The oral clearance for the whites was 319 ± 60 mL/min, and for the Chinese it was 183 ± 35 mL/min. Omeprazole and omeprazole sulfone integrated plasma gastrin values were well correlated with the S/R mephenytoin ratio, and with urinary 4'-hydroxymephenytoin. Fasting gastrin and 12–and 24-hour integrated plasma gastrin levels were significantly greater in the chinese males than in the white males. The Chinese had fasting gastrin values of 30 ± 6.4 pmol and the whites had values of 14.4 ± 1.2 pmol. The Chinese had 12-hour integrated plasma gastrin values of 661 ± 114 pmol/hr/L^{-1} and the whites had values of 334 ± 38 pmol/hr/L^{-1}. The Chinese had 24-hour integrated plasma gastrin values of $1,414 \pm 228$ pmol/hr/L^{-1} and the whites had values of 747 ± 99 pmol/hr/L^{-1}. The extent of omeprazole-induced hypergastrinemia was correlated with the S/R mephenytoin ratio and omeprazole integrated plasma gastrin.

Conclusions.—There is a genetic determination and ethnic dependency in the metabolism of omeprazole and the rise in gastrin concentration after its administration. Further evaluation is necessary to determine the need for dosage adjustment in patients with diminished CYP2C19 activity and in patients of Chinese ancestry.

▶ Ethnic differences in metabolizing and eliminating drugs are not uncommon, but are not often deemed to be clinically important by physicians. The present study suggests that Chinese patients may need less omeprazole than non-Chinese patients for a given effect. Because omeprazole is a very safe drug, the described findings may be more important for non-Chinese patients, a percentage of whom (perhaps 15% to 20%) are considered to be nonresponders to 20 mg of omeprazole per day. If this is not due to noncompliance, a higher dose should be tried in such refractory cases.

L. Lasagna, M.D.

Determination of CYP2C19 Phenotype in Black Americans With Omeprazole: Correlation With Genotype
Marinac JS, Balian JD, Foxworth JW, et al (Univ of Missouri-Kansas City; Georgetown Univ, Washington, DC)
Clin Pharmacol Ther 60:138–144, 1996   10–3

Introduction.—To assign metabolic phenotype in specific populations, probe drugs for polymorphic enzymes have been used, and have been helpful in evaluating potential metabolic predisposition for scleroderma, bladder cancer, and eosinophilia-myalgia. Omeprazole has been shown to be useful for measuring the activity of CYP2C19. Some of the drugs that metabolize through this pathway include clomipramine, mephobarbital, diazepam, chloroguanide hydrochloride, and lansoprazole. The distribution of CYP2C19 phenotypes and genotypes in a large population of healthy adult black Americans was determined using omeprazole as the probe.

Methods.—One hundred healthy, black adults, aged 18 to 50 years, who were receiving no medications participated in this single-dose, open-label outpatient study. For phenotype determination, baseline omeprazole and 2-hour post-ingestion omeprazole and 5'-hydroxyomeprazole concentrations were measured. $CYP2C19_{m1}$ genotypes were identified using polymerase chain reaction.

Results.—Among the 72 women and 28 men for whom results were obtained, 98 were phenotypically extensive metabolizers and 2 were poor metabolizers. Of the 2 who were poor metabolizers, 1 was a man and the other a smoker. They were both also homozygous for a single base pair mutation of exon 5 of CYP2C19, according to genotype determination. In the extensive metabolizer group, 28 were heterozygous and the remaining 70 were homozygous. There were no reports of side effects.

Conclusions.—In this healthy black population, the 2% prevalence rate of poor CYP2C19 metabolizers is similar to that reported in whites and in the Shona population of Zimbabwe; however, it is much less than that reported in an Asian population. A safe and specific probe of the CYP2C19 enzyme system, omeprazole correlates well with genotype. Further evaluation could study the 15% of patients with reflux esophagitis who fail to respond to conventional omeprazole dosing, and to determine whether poor metabolizers of omeprazole are at greatest risk for long-term omeprazole toxicity.

▶ The cytochrome P-450 enzyme system has long been known to be important in drug metabolism, and genetic polymorphism with regard to P-450 helps to explain some differences between individuals in therapeutic or toxic response. Someone should study those patients (a not insubstantial minority) with reflux esophagitis who fail to respond to conventional omeprazole dosing.

L. Lasagna, M.D.

Efficacy and Safety of Lansoprazole in the Treatment of Erosive Reflux Esophagitis

Castell DO, Richter JE, Robinson M, et al (Graduate Hosp, Philadelphia; Cleveland Clinic Found, Ohio; Univ of Oklahoma, Oklahoma City; et al)
Am J Gastroenterol 91:1749–1757, 1996   10–4

Objective.—Treatment of reflux esophagitis involves diminishing the acidity and quantity of reflux material. A randomized, double-blind, parallel-group, multicenter safety and efficacy comparison of lansoprazole, omeprazole, and placebo in the treatment of erosive reflux esophagitis is presented.

Methods.—Either lansoprazole (15 mg, $n = 218$, or 30 mg, $n = 421$), omeprazole (20 mg, $n = 431$), or placebo $(n = 213)$ was administered once daily for 8 weeks before breakfast to 1,284 patients with erosive reflux esophagitis. Endoscopic evaluations were performed at baseline and after 2, 4, 6, and 8 weeks of therapy. Patients kept a daily diary of dosing information, frequency of antacid use, episodes of heartburn, and any missed doses. Gastrin concentrations were determined. Symptoms, gastrin concentrations, and adverse events were compared statistically.

Results.—A total of 1,226 patients were assessable. Healing rates for assessable patients at 2, 4, 6, and 8 weeks were 65.3%, 83.3%, 89.4%, and 90.9% for lansoprazole, 30 mg; 56.3%, 74.6%, 80.3%, and 78.8% for lansoprazole, 15 mg; 60.9%, 82.0%, 89.7%, and 90.7% for omeprazole; and 23.9%, 32.8%, 36.6%, and 40.0% for placebo. Lansoprazole, 30 mg, and omeprazole had similar healing rates, and both had healing rates significantly higher than lansoprazole, 15 mg, during the study period. Patients receiving lansoprazole, 30 mg had significantly less day and night heartburn during the first day and week than did patients receiving omeprazole. All regimens were well tolerated. Common adverse reactions were headache, diarrhea, and nausea. Patients receiving lansoprazole (15 mg) reported significantly more side effects than did patients in the other treatment groups. All patients in active treatment groups had significantly higher increases in gastrin secretion than did patients in the placebo group.

Conclusion.—Both lansoprazole (30 mg) and omeprazole (20 mg) were safe and similarly effective for treating erosive reflux esophagitis. The drugs were well tolerated and side effects were mild. Lansoprazole, 30 mg, was significantly more effective than lansoprazole, 15 mg.

▶ Lansoprazole is the second proton pump inhibitor. It is pharmacologically related to omeprazole and was recently approved by the Food and Drug Administration. The study described was important for several reasons. It was a head-to-head test of new and old drugs. It had a dose–response aspect to it. Finally, it was both long enough and placebo-controlled. We should say, "Good job" to the investigators.

The appearance of a second drug may result in a decreased price for either this drug or omeprazole itself. However, some drug companies maintain the price of the original drug because some physicians still prescribe it. What will happen with managed care on the scene is a new issue. We'll just have to wait and see about it.

M. Weintraub, M.D.

Lansoprazole Heals Erosive Reflux Esophagitis Resistant to Histamine H2–Receptor Antagonist Therapy
Sontag SJ, Kogut DG, Fleischmann R, et al (Veterans Affairs Hosp, Hines, Ill; Piedmont Gastroenterolgy, Statesville, NC; Metroplex Clinical Reseach Ctr, Dallas; et al)
Am J Gastroenterol 92:429–437, 1997   10–5

Introduction.—Although antacids can relieve the symptoms of gastro-esophageal reflux, these agents are unable to heal reflux esophagitis. High doses of histamine H2-receptor antagonists (H2-RA) are reported to heal erosive esophagitis in up to 80% of cases. The proton pump inhibitor, lansoprazole, has an even higher success rate and may benefit those resistant to H2–RA therapy. A multicenter trial examined outcome in patients switched to lansoprazole after failing to respond to H2-RA.

Methods.—The double-blind, randomized trial enrolled 159 patients aged 22 to 79 years. All had endoscopic evidence of at least grade 2 esophagitis that failed to heal after 12 continuous weeks of therapy with 1 or more H2–RAs given at no less than standard dosages. Endoscopic assessments took place at baseline and at weeks 2, 4, 6, and 8. Patients received ranitidine (150 mg b.i.d. for 8 weeks) or lansoprazole (30 mg for 4 weeks), followed by lansoprazole (30 mg or 60 mg) for another 4 weeks.

Results.—Patients in the 2 treatment groups were similar in baseline characteristics. At all evaluation times, healing rates were statistically significantly higher with lansoprazole than with ranitidine. By week 8, healing had occurred in 84% of those randomized to lansoprazole vs. 32% of the ranitidine group. Lansoprazole was also significantly superior in reducing the need for antacids and in providing relief of upper abdominal burning and daytime heartburn. Doubling the dose of lansoprazole in weeks 4 to 8 did not appear to influence healing but provided greater symptom relief. The incidence of adverse effects was similar in the 2 groups. Fasting serum gastrin levels were significantly higher in the lansoprazole group at weeks 4 and 8.

Conclusion.—Lansoprazole, taken for 8 weeks, was safe and effective in healing erosive reflux esophagitis in patients resistant to H2–RA therapy. Such patients benefit significantly by switching to lansoprazole rather than by continuing with ranitidine.

▶ The effect of lansoprazole was dramatically demonstrated in this very efficient clinical trial. The reason for its efficiency was that patients who had failed previously with ranitidine therapy were randomly allocated to the new therapy and again to the ranitidine therapy. Despite the fact that they had been taking ranitidine for 12 weeks some patients might have responded to a second course. In fact, many of them may have been late responders to the ranitidine, particularly in the setting of a clinical trial. However, that was not true for 68% of the patients randomized to receive ranitidine. Where there are treatments for a disease, I believe that clinical trialists should be using this very design more often. I don't think that the investigators needed the relatively large (150) number of patients in the study, although, for certain diseases, large numbers may be needed when the therapy that the patients had been receiving previously is continued and shows efficacy. Of course, in this study, the use of a higher dose of lansoprazole might have required the larger number of patients as well. Proper dose-response studies frequently require larger patient samples.

M. Weintraub, M.D.

Lansoprazole Prevents Recurrence of Erosive Reflux Esophagitis Previously Resistant to H2–RA Therapy
Sontag SJ, and the Lansoprazole Maintenance Study Group (Veterans Affairs Hosp, Hines, Ill; Piedmont Gastroenterology, Statesville, NC; Metroplex Clinical Research Ctr, Dallas; et al)
Am J Gastroenterol 91:1758–1765, 1996   10–6

Background.—If maintenance therapy is not continued, esophagitis recurs in as many as 80% of patients within 6 months of complete erosive reflux esophagitis (RE) healing with H_2-receptor antagonist (H_2-RA) or proton pump inhibitor therapy. Most patients with more severe disease need some type of maintenance therapy indefinitely. The efficacy of lan-

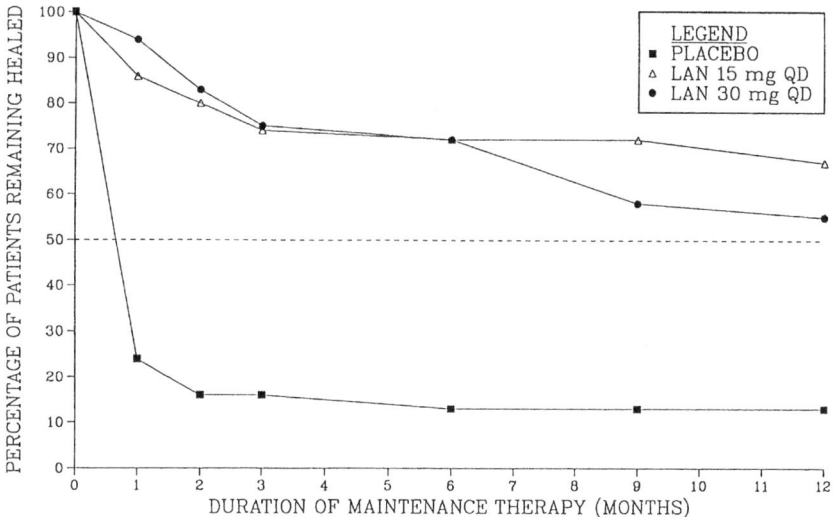

FIGURE 1.—Maintenance rates (in percentages) show the proportion of assessable patients remaining healed of erosions (endoscopy-proven) during the 1-year maintenance period. Lansoprazole (*LAN*) was significantly superior to placebo in preventing recurrence (*P* < 0.001). Within 1 month, 24% of the placebo group remained healed, compared with 86% of the lansoprazole 15–mg group and 94% of the lansoprazole 30–mg group. (Courtesy of Sontag SJ, and the Lansoprazole Maintenance Study Group: Lansoprazole prevents recurrence of erosive reflux esophagitis previously resistant to H2–RA therapy. *Am J Gastroenterol* 91:1758–1765, 1996.)

soprazole, a new proton pump inhibitor and substituted benzimidazole containing a novel trifluoroethyl group, was investigated in a randomized, double-blind study.

Methods.—One hundred sixty-three patients were enrolled in the trial. All had healed erosive RE resistant to healing with at least 3 months of H$_2$-RA treatment. One hundred forty-six patients were available for evaluation at the end of the study.

Findings.—At 1 year, 13% of placebo recipients remained healed, compared with 67% of those given 15 mg of lansoprazole and 55% of those giving 30 mg of lansoprazole. All patients given placebo were symptomatic by the end of the year, compared with only one third of the lansoprazole recipients. The 2 doses of lansoprazole were of comparable efficacy in maintaining healing and symptom control. Both doses were well tolerated. Fasting serum gastrin values rose significantly, to approximately 1.5 to 2 times the baseline values, during the first 2 months of lansoprazole therapy (Fig 1).

Conclusions.—Lansoprazole, once a day, is effective as maintenance therapy for erosive esophagitis resistant to standard treatment with H$_2$-RAs. Both doses tested were equally effective and well tolerated.

► One could question whether a placebo group would have been necessary, especially for the 1-year–long study. Fortunately, patients were treated upon their first relapse. As shown in the graph, the maintenance of healing rates was really very dramatic.

M. Weintraub, M.D.

Endoscopic Injection for Bleeding Peptic Ulcer: A Comparison of Adrenaline Alone With Adrenaline Plus Human Thrombin

Kubba AK, Murphy W, Palmer KR (Western Gen Hosp, Edinburgh, Scotland)
Gastroenterology 111:623–628, 1996   10–7

Background.—Endoscopic injection therapy has been shown to improve outcomes in patients with bleeding peptic ulcer. However, the optimal regimen has not been established.

Methods.—One hundred forty patients with significant peptic ulcer bleeding and active arterial bleeding or a nonbleeding visible vessel were studied. By random assignment, the patients were treated with an endoscopic injection of 1:100,000 adrenaline (group 1) or adrenaline plus 600 to 1,000 IU of human thrombin (group 2).

Findings.—Rebleeding occurred in 20% of group 1 patients and in 4.5% of group 2. Ten percent in group 1 died within 30 days of admission, compared with none in group 2. Two hundred ninety-seven units of blood were needed in group 1, compared with 219 units in group 2.

Conclusion.—Endoscopic injection of adrenaline plus human thrombin appears to be better than injection with dilute adrenaline alone in patients with bleeding peptic ulcer. Larger studies are needed to confirm these findings.

▶ This study, although very convincing, shows how difficult it is to prove that a treatment can not only be effective, but can save money as well. For example, there really was no change in the need for emergency surgery, transfusion requirements, or duration of hospital stay, although there was a statistically significant decrease in the patients rebleeding or dying. The authors believe that their study should be repeated, with particular checking for possible thrombotic complications, of course, and virus transmission.

M. Weintraub, M.D.

A Comparison of Omeprazole and Placebo for Bleeding Peptic Ulcer

Khuroo MS, Yattoo GN, Javid G, et al (Sheri Kashmir Inst, Soura, Srinagar, India)
N Engl J Med 336:1054–1058, 1997   10–8

Background.—The role of medical therapy in the treatment of bleeding peptic ulcers has not been established definitively. The effects of omeprazole and placebo were compared.

Methods.—Two hundred twenty patients with endoscopy-confirmed duodenal, gastric, or stomal ulcers and signs of recent bleeding were enrolled in a double-blind, placebo-controlled study. Arterial spurting was present in 26 patients, active oozing in 34, nonbleeding visible vessels in 35, and adherent clots in 125. Patients were randomly assigned to receive omeprazole, 40 mg orally every 12 hours for 5 days, or placebo.

Findings.—Eleven percent of the patients given omeprazole had continued or further bleeding compared with 36.4% of those given placebo. Surgery to control bleeding was required in 8 omeprazole recipients and 26 placebo recipients. Two patients given omeprazole and 6 given placebo died. Twenty-nine percent of the omeprazole group and 70.9% of the placebo group needed transfusions. In a subgroup analysis, omeprazole treatment was found to be associated with significant reductions in the rates of recurrent bleeding and need for surgery in patients with nonbleeding visible vessels or adherent clots but not in patients with arterial spurting or oozing.

Conclusions.—Omeprazole treatment reduces the rate of further bleeding and the need for surgery in patients with bleeding peptic ulcers and signs of recent bleeding. Length of hospital stay and the need for transfusion were also decreased in omeprazole recipients.

▶ Gastrointestinal bleeding causes a substantial number of hospital admissions and deaths each year. Effective medical therapy would be a boon, but histamine-2–receptor antagonists have been disappointing. Omeprazole seems a good choice, but the clinician may still need to institute endoscopic therapy or surgery.

L. Lasagna, M.D.

A Randomized, Placebo-controlled, Double-blind Trial of Mesalamine in the Maintenance of Remission of Crohn's Disease
Sutherland LR, and The Canadian Mesalamine for Remission of Crohn's Disease Study Group (Univ of Calgary, Alberta, Canada; Univ of Montreal, Quebec, Canada; Univ of Alberta, Edmonton, Canada)
Gastroenterology 112:1069–1077, 1997   10–9

Introduction.—Several recent reports suggest that mesalamine may reduce the risk of relapse after remission in patients with Crohn's disease. Not all trials, however, confirm the drug's clinical efficacy. The patients reported here took part in the largest randomized, placebo-controlled multicenter trial of mesalamine in the maintenance of remission of Crohn's disease.

Methods.—Patients were recruited during a 3-year period from 31 Canadian centers. All had at least 2 flare-ups of active disease within the last 4 years, 1 within the last 18 months, or a recent resection. None had ulcerative colitis, a history of cancer, or any other clinically significant disease. The 293 study participants were randomized to placebo or to mesalamine treatmemt (750 mg 4 times a day for 48 weeks) and classified according to type of remission (medical or surgical). Patients kept diary cards for calculation of Crohn's disease activity index (CDAI) and were assessed at 4, 12, 24, 36, and 48 weeks after baseline.

Results.—The final cohort consisted of 246 patients with at least 4 weeks of follow-up: 118 in the mesalamine group and 128 in the placebo group. Relapse, defined as a CDAI greater than 150 (+ 60 points over baseline), occurred in 25% of patients who received mesalamine and in 36% of those given placebo. Median time to relapse did not differ significantly between the 2 groups. Women treated with mesalamine had a far lower relapse rate (19%) than women given placebo (41%). Differences in the rate of relapse were also pronounced among patients with ileocolonic disease (21% with mesalamine vs. 41% with placebo).

Conclusion.—In this group of patients considered to be at high risk of recurrence of Crohn's disease, those treated with mesalamine tended to have fewer relapses. Men benefited less than women, and no benefit was shown for patients with disease confined to the terminal ileum.

▶ Unfortunately, this clinical trial, despite its being conducted in the correct fashion, was unable to demonstrate the effect of continuing mesalamine. One of the problems in this study may have been the compliance of the patients. If patients with serious diseases, including cancer, AIDS, and transplantations, are unable to comply with their medication regimen, could we expect better from patients with Crohn's disease? This is 1 clinical trial (mesalamine 750 mg given 4 times per day) in which the determination of compliance should not be trusted to pill counts to assess how well the patients took their medication, at what time they took their medication, if they took a day off, or if they threw their pills down the toilet. Some of the differences between the patient groups may have been diminished by the lack of the patients taking their medication and avoiding, in that case, hospitalization. Unfortunately, the answer is still not available. However, if left to our own devices, physicians can give the therapy, but they'll have to talk to the patients about the risks of increased relapses if the patient is noncompliant. We are not taught in medical school how to teach patients without scaring them. I don't know in what other way we can talk to patients effectively about compliance. It really is a self-, and perhaps mentor-, taught skill.

M. Weintraub, M.D.

5-Aminosalicylates, Sulfasalazine, Steroid Use, and Complications in Patients With Ulcerative Colitis
Walker AM, Szneke P, Bianchi La, et al (Epidemiology Resources Inc, Newton Lower Falls, Mass; Harvard School of Public Health, Boston; Proctor & Gamble Pharmaceuticals, Cincinnati, Ohio; et al)
Am J Gastroenterol 92:816–820, 1997   10–10

Introduction.—Sulfasalazine and 5-aminosalicylates (5-ASAs) have been the most important agents in the treatment of ulcerative colitis. The choice of sulfasalazine or 5-ASA often depends upon efficacy and tolerance in the individual patient. Differences in the rate of adverse events were compared in a large population of patients with ulcerative colitis. Also examined were rates of hospitalization and use of steroids.

Methods.—The study population was drawn from a database of patients of general practitioners in the United Kingdom. A computerized search performed for the period from January 1990 through October 1993 identified patients who received medical care on at least 2 occasions for diagnosed ulcerative colitis and those with a diagnosis on 1 occasion and a prescription of a drug specific to ulcerative colitis during the study period. The histories of 2,894 patients were categorized according to dose of 5-ASAs, sulfasalazine, steroids, and immunosuppressants and classified on the basis of disease activity.

Results.—Patient records contained few mentions of hepatic, pancreatic, renal, and hematologic events other than anemia, and there was no evidence of a preferential association of these side effects with any of the drugs. There were 380 references to anemia, including 127 instances among current users of sulfasalazine and 105 among current users of 5-ASA. Compared with nonusers of sulfasalazine, high-dose users had a relative risk of anemia of 3.2%. Rates of hospitalization for ulcerative colitis were generally similar for sulfasalazine and 5-ASA users. Low-dose maintenance therapy with either drug decreased the rate of hospitalization by 30% to 40% compared with no treatment. Drug choice did not affect discontinuation rates for prednisolone among established steroid users.

Conclusion.—Hospitalizations for the signs and symptoms of disease are approximately 100 times more common than hospitalization for adverse drug effects among patients with ulcerative colitis. Because serious adverse reactions are rare, the choice of therapeutic agent can be based primarily upon efficacy.

▶ Hurray! The analysis of a large database from a whole country (Britain) establishes that it's better to treat patients and not worry about adverse drug reactions than to not treat. In addition, we don't know what (presumably good) would have happened had the patients been treated with nicotine enemas in addition to the standard medications.

M. Weintraub, M.D.

Pharmacokinetics of Nicotine Carbomer Enemas: A New Treatment Modality for Ulcerative Colitis
Green JT, Thomas GAO, Rhodes J, et al (Univ Wales, Cardiff; New Cross Hosp, London; St Andrews Univ, Fife; et al)
Clin Pharmacol Ther 61:340–348, 1997   10–11

Introduction.—Largely a disease of nonsmokers, ulcerative colitis can be managed with transdermal nicotine patches in addition to conventional treatment with 5-aminosalicylic acid. Topical application of nicotine to large-bowel mucosa would circumvent the side effects caused by 15 mg of transdermal nicotine in up to two thirds of patients, particularly lifelong nonsmokers. Nicotine was combined with a polyacrylic carbomer for administration as an enema in patients with ulcerative colitis.

Methods.—After an enema in 8 healthy volunteers and 8 patients with active ulcerative colitis, serum levels of both nicotine and continine were measured and side effects were documented. All 16 patients were nonsmokers; mean ages were 33 years for the controls and 60 years for patients with ulcerative colitis. Five patients took oral prednisolone (median dosage, 12 mg/d), and all were taking 5-aminosalicylic acid compounds. The 100-mL enema consisted of 6 mg of nicotine complexed with 400 mg of carbomer 974P. Serial blood measurements were obtained over 8 hours.

Results.—No statistically significant differences were seen between groups; however, time until nicotine reached peak concentration was longer in patients (median time, 60 minutes) than in controls (45 minutes). In patients with active disease, the enema was retained without difficulty. The maximum nicotine concentration (8.1 ± 3.5 ng/mL) occurred after a median of 60 minutes; the maximum continued concentrations (60.4 ± 11.5 ng/mL) occurred after 4 hours. In 5 female patients who were lifelong nonsmokers and had low body weight, the mild or moderate side effects included nausea, headache, and lightheadedness.

Conclusion.—Substantial nicotine concentrations can be achieved at the site of disease with only modest increases in serum nicotine concentrations because the active ingredient of nicotine is converted to continine on the first pass through the liver. The side effects are caused by the increased serum concentrations of nicotine; continine has low pharmacologic activity. For distal ulcerative colitis, topical administration of nicotine may be useful. Modifications in concentrations of nicotine should overcome side effects in patients with lower body weights who achieve higher maximum concentrations.

▶ This study was done in patients with ulcerative colitis compared with normals. Most important, these patients were older and took 5-aminosalicylic acid compounds and oral prednisolone. I think that these factors should be included in a study in which the pharmacokinetics in patients is important. Of course, the most interesting aspect of this study really is that patients with ulcerative colitis tend to be nonsmokers and that the effect of the disease can be partially controlled with nicotine.

M. Weintraub, M.D.

Etidronate Versus Fluoride for Treatment of Osteopenia in Primary Biliary Cirrhosis: Preliminary Results Afer 2 Years
Guañabens N, Parés A, Monegal A, et al (Univ of Barcelona)
Gastroenterology 113:219–224, 1997   10–12

Introduction.—Osteopenia increases the risk of bone fractures in patients with primary biliary cirrhosis (PBC). There is no definitive treatment for osteopenia associated with PBC. The effects of intermittent, cyclical etidronate vs. sodium fluoride on bone density and mineral metabolism was evaluated in 32 women with PBC.

Methods.—Patients were randomly assigned to receive etidronate 400 mg/day for 14 days every 3 months or fluoride 50 mg/day. Bone mineral density of the lumbar spine and proximal femur were measured at baseline and every 6 months for 2 years.

Results.—Thirteen patients in the etidronate group and 10 patients in the fluoride group were available for final follow-up. The bone mineral density increased significantly in the lumbar spine and was unchanged in the proximal femur in the etidronate group. In the fluoride group, the lumbar bone mineral density was unchanged and femoral bone mass decreased, especially in the Ward's triangle. Two and no patients in the fluoride and etidronate groups, respectively, had new vertebral fractures. The number of nonvertebral fractures did not differ between groups. There was no evidence of impaired liver function or cholestasis in either group.

Conclusions.—Cyclical etidronate was more effective and better tolerated than fluoride in preventing bone loss in patients with PBC.

▶ The investigators were a little bit too enthusiastic about their own work. They claim that this preliminary 2-year study definitively proves that etidronate is superior to fluoride and should be used in the treatment of osteopenia in patients with PBC. In the next sentence, however, the authors make a very impressive point: that osteopenia in PBC should be treated with some bisphosphonate plus estrogen. That alone is worthy of a clinical trial giving the combination against the 2 medications independently. I don't think you need to use a placebo, based on the results of this study, but it's a bit much to recommend now that bisphosphonate therapy be used in all patients with PBC.

M. Weintraub, M.D.

Therapeutic Efficacy of L-Ornithine-L-Aspartate Infusions in Patients With Cirrhosis and Hepatic Encephalopathy: Results of a Placebo-controlled, Double-blind Study

Kircheis G, Nilius R, Held C, et al (Martin-Luther-Univ Halle-Wittenberg, Halle, Germany; Humboldt Univ, Berlin; et al)

Hepatology 25:1351–1360, 1997   10–13

Objective.—Approximately one quarter of patients with cirrhosis will experience an episode of hepatic encephalopathy (HE) within 5 years of diagnosis that will significantly lower the odds of survival. Because hyperammonemia is thought to be an important pathogenic factor in the development of HE, agents such as L-ornithine-L-aspartate (OA) that lower blood ammonia may have a favorable effect on HE. Results of a randomized, double-blind, placebo-controlled, multicenter trial to test the clinical efficacy of OA in the treatment of HE in cirrhotic patients with hyperammonemia and chronic (persistent) manifest HE or subclinical HE, as well as the influence of OA on the improvement of number connection test A (NCT-A) times and mental states, were presented.

Methods.—Placebo or 20 g OA in 5% fructose were administered daily over a 4-hour period for 1 week to 126 cirrhotic patients with HE. Placebo (n = 63) and treatment (n = 63) groups had similar mental states, NCT-A performance times, fasting venous blood ammonia levels, and Child-Pugh criteria at baseline.

Results.—The NCT-A score decrease after 7 days was significantly larger in the OA group than in the placebo group (19 vs. 7 seconds). The decrease in fasting venous ammonia concentration was significantly larger in the OA group than in the placebo group (17 vs. 6 µmol/L). Whereas mental state scores improved during treatment in the OA group, the values at 7 days were not significantly different from baseline. Compared with the placebo group, portal systemic encephalic index (PSEI) values were significantly improved and near normal in the OA group at day 7. Twelve OA patients had adverse events or adverse drug reactions necessitating discontinuation of treatment at 4 days (n = 2) or 2 days or less (n = 5).

Conclusion.—Treatment with OA significantly improved NCT-A times, mental state grades, and PSEI scores and decreased venous ammonia concentrations in patients with cirrhosis and HE or subclinical HE.

▶ The good news is that the long and convoluted history of OA infusions appears to have been settled, at least in the short term. The real remaining question is how to improve the administration of OA and decrease the time it takes (4 hours every day) to aid patients with HE. One could say that even though a patient's HE was improved, that patient had only, perhaps, 12 hours to enjoy the improvement because of the infusion. Perhaps administration at night or enteral methodology, or administration per rectum could be worked out to improve OA treatment.

M. Weintraub, M.D.

Thalidomide: A Novel Therapy for Microsporidiosis
Sharpstone D, Rowbottom A, Francis N, et al (Chelsea and Westminster Hosp, London; Charing Cross and Westminster Med School, London; London School of Hygiene and Tropical Medicine)
Gastroenterology 112:1823–1829, 1997   10–14

Background.—Microsporidiosis, a common cause of chronic diarrhea in HIV-seropositive patients, is often refractory to treatment. Because fecal tumor necrosis factor-α (TNF-α) is increased in microsporidiosis, the efficacy of treatment with thalidomide, an anti–TNF-α agent, was investigated.

Methods.—Eighteen patients with chronic diarrhea caused by *Enterocytozoon bieneusi* that was unresponsive to albendazole and 1 previously untreated patient with *Encephalitozoon intestinalis* were treated with thalidomide, 100 mg at night, for 1 month.

Findings.—Seven patients had a complete clinical response, assessed by stool frequency and body weight, and 3 had a partial response. Stool frequency was reduced significantly from 5.3 to 3.1 per day. Weight gain was a significant 1.2 kg. Thalidomide also significantly increased the villus height/crypt depth ratio and number of abnormal forms of microsporidia. Fecal TNF-α level declined from 17.9 to 8.9 U/mL, which was nonsignificant. All stages of the life cycle of *E. intestinalis* were apparently disrupted.

Conclusions.—Thalidomide may be an effective therapy for patients with diarrhea and weight loss caused by *E. bieneusi* that is unresponsive to conventional treatment. In this series, thalidomide objectively improved body weight and villus height/crypt depth ratios.

▶ This experimental study did not show a complete effect of thalidomide on the diarrhea and weight loss in AIDS patients. About half of them achieved a complete response. This may be one of those situations where a historical control is valid. It is unlikely that patients will get better spontaneously from microsporidiosis diarrhea, and all but one of the patients had received treatment with albendazole in the past without response. The next step may be to try treating the disease state in an active controlled trial. In such a study, one group would receive an active comparator and another group the thalidomide. That would tell us more about the response to thalidomide but not as much as a placebo group. Unfortunately, this is a bad complication of AIDS and occurs, often, late in the course.

M. Weintraub, M.D.

Are More Antiemetic Trials With a Placebo Necessary?

Kris MG, Cubeddu LX, Gralla RJ, et al (Mem Sloan-Kettering Cancer Ctr, New York; Central Univ of Venezuela, Caracas; Ochsner Cancer Inst, New Orleans, La; et al)
Cancer 78:2193–2198, 1996   10–15

Introduction.—Cisplatin predictably causes emesis, and has therefore been the standard stimulus of emesis in clinical trials of antiemetic drugs. The incidence and severity of cisplatin-induced vomiting in patients receiving placebo antiemetics is now well established; however, trials continue to use placebo-control arms. Data from previous studies of placebo antiemetics and cisplatin were reanalyzed in the hope of avoiding the need for further placebo-controlled trials for this indication.

Methods.—The analysis included 48 patients from 4 randomized trials who received a placebo antiemetic. The time and number of episodes of emesis were assessed, including episodes occurring after antiemetic "rescue" therapy.

Results.—All but 1 of the patients experienced emesis. The patients had a median of 6 episodes of emesis in the 24 hours after cisplatin therapy. More than three fourths of the patients continued to have emesis despite receiving "rescue" therapy. By these data, any treatment that prevented acute emesis in 8 of the 48 patients at a cisplatin dose of greater than 50 mg/m^2 was considered an active antiemetic.

Conclusion.—In patients receiving cisplatin, severe emesis predictably occurs even after rescue medication. The group of patients described in this study can serve as a control group for studies of new antiemetic treatments. Future studies of antiemetics should use active, not placebo, controls.

▶ Bioethicists periodically criticize the use of placebos in randomized controlled trials as unethical and not really answering the important question (How does the new drug compare with the old?), but rather addressing another question (Is the new drug any good at all?).

The present study suggests that vomiting after cisplatin is so predictable (and universal) that placebo controls are unnecessary, i.e, both questions stated above can be answered by comparing a new drug candidate with a standard antiemetic.

The presumption that "rescue" medication in the event of vomiting after placebo gets one off the horns of the ethical dilemma simply won't wash, because the goal of antiemesis therapy today is *prevention*, not treatment (which often fails).

L. Lasagna, M.D.

11 Genitourinary Tract Disorders

Efficacy and Safety of Finasteride Therapy for Benign Prostatic Hyperplasia: Results of a 2–Year Randomized Controlled Trial (The PROSPECT Study)
Nickel JC, and the PROSPECT Study Group (Queen's Univ, Kingston, Ont, Canada; Laval Univ, Sainte Foy, Que, Canada; Univ of Alberta, Edmonton; et al)
Can Med Assoc J 155:1251–1259, 1996
                                                    11–1

Objective.—Benign prostatic hyperplasia (BPH) results in impaired urine flow and symptoms of irritation that can lead to complications such as infection, urinary retention, and upper trace sequelae. Medications such as α-adrenergic blockers and 5α-reductase inhibitors have proved beneficial. A 2-year double-blind, prospective, placebo-controlled, randomized study investigated the safety and efficacy of the 5α-reductase inhibitor finasteride for treating BPH in men with moderate symptoms.

Methods.—After baseline values were obtained from 613 patients with BPH in 28 centers across Canada during a 1-month placebo period, patients were randomly allocated to receive 5 mg/day finasteride (n = 310) or placebo (n = 303) for 2 years. Patients were examined at baseline and at 1 and 2 years to measure urinary flow rates, prostate volume, and serum prostate-specific antigen. Patients filled out a questionnaire about symptoms.

Results.—There were 246 patients receiving finasteride and 226 receiving placebo who completed the study. Symptoms in both groups decreased for the first 8 months. After 8 months, symptoms in the finasteride group continued to decrease, but symptoms in the placebo group began to increase. Maximum urinary flow rate, prostate volume, urinary retention, incidence of urologic intervention, and prostate-specific antigen levels were significantly lower in the finasteride group than in the placebo group at all time points. The incidence of adverse events was similar for both groups (81.0% in the finasteride group and 81.2% in the placebo group), although specific rates of ejaculatory disorders and impotence were significantly higher in the finasteride group.

Conclusion.—Finasteride, as treatment for BPH in men with moderate symptoms, is safe, effective, and well tolerated.

▶ Benign prostatic hypertrophy is all too common, with troublesome symptoms either related to obstruction or to irritation. Mild symptoms can be tolerated, but as they increase in severity, the quality of life can be significantly impaired.

Surgery is associated with a considerable list of potential adverse events, so medical therapy deserves a trial first. Finasteride yields worthwhile benefit in some patients, but only modest effects in many. The mechanism of action is a decrease in prostatic size.

L. Lasagna, M.D.

The Efficacy of Terazosin, Finasteride, or Both in Benign Prostatic Hyperplasia
Lepor H, for the Veterans Affairs Cooperative Studies Benign Prostatic Hyperplasia Study Group (New York Univ; VA Med Ctr, Perry Point, Md; Massachusetts Gen Hosp, Boston; et al)
N Engl J Med 335:533–539, 1996   11–2

Purpose.—Two different types of drug therapy are now available for the treatment of benign prostatic hyperplasia (BPH). The 5α-reductase inhibitor finasteride works by reducing tissue androgen concentrations, whereas the α_1-adrenergic antagonist terazosin relaxes prostatic smooth muscle. These 2 approaches have not been compared directly. Terazosin, finasteride, and the combination of the 2 were compared for safety and efficacy in the treatment of BPH.

Methods.—The double-blind, placebo-controlled study included 1,229 men with symptomatic BPH. They were assigned to receive placebo; finasteride, 5 mg/day; terazosin, 10 mg/day; or a combination of finasteride and terazosin for 1 year. The results were assessed by American Urological Association symptom scores and peak urinary flow rates.

Results.—Symptom scores, on a 35-point scale, decreased by a mean of 2.6 points with placebo, 3.2 points with finasteride, 6.1 points with terazosin, and 6.2 points with combination therapy. Peak urinary flow rates increased by 1.4, 1.6, 2.7, and 3.2 mL/sec, respectively. By both assessments, terazosin alone and with finasteride was significantly better than finasteride alone or placebo. The rate of discontinuation because of adverse effects was 2% in the placebo group and 5% to 8% in the other 3 groups.

Conclusions.—Terazosin is an effective treatment for BPH but finasteride is not. Finasteride is not effective even in combination with terazosin. It may be that finasteride is effective only in men with very large prostates.

▶ Benign prostatic hyperplasia is certainly preferable to malignant prostatic hyperplasia, but the associated symptoms, including urinary retention, infection, and hematuria, can be exceedingly bothersome. Prostatectomy can relieve a lot of the trouble, but it is not risk free, so nonsurgical approaches are attractive.

Finasteride has been shown, in controlled trials, to ameliorate the symptoms of patients with prostatic enlargement, but the benefits are modest. Indeed, in this study, the effects of finasteride were indistinguishable from those of placebo, whereas terazosin *was* effective. The latter drug presumably helps by blocking adrenoceptors in the abundant prostatic smooth muscle.

Finasteride is thought to work by suppressing androgen formation. Perhaps what is needed is simultaneous suppression of both androgen *and* estrogen, because prostatic tissue seems to be sensitive to both.

L. Lasagna, M.D.

Doxazosin for Benign Prostatic Hyperplasia: Long-term Efficacy and Safety in Hypertensive and Normotensive Patients
Lepor H, for the Multicenter Study Group (New York Univ; Columbia Univ, New York; Pfizer Central Research, New York; et al)
J Urol 157:525–530, 1997   11–3

Objective.—The prevalence of benign prostatic hyperplasia (BPH) increases with age and is almost 50% in men 60 to 80 years old. A recent study showed that the antihypertensive drug doxazosin also increased urinary flow in normotensive and hypertensive men. Safety and sustained efficacy of doxazosin for long-term treatment of normotensive and hypertensive men with BPH were studied.

Methods.—There were 272 men with normotension and 178 men with mild to moderate hypertension enrolled in a 4-year, open-label, dose titration extension treatment of BPH. They received 1 mg/day doubling at 2-week intervals to 8 mg/day for normotensive and to as high as 16 mg/day for hypertensive, if warranted. Efficacy and safety data were evaluated and compared statistically with baseline values.

Results.—The mean daily doses were 4 mg for patients with normotension and 6.4 mg for patients with hypertension. Maximum and average urinary flow rates and symptoms improved significantly in the intent-to-treat group. Blood pressure and heart rate decreased significantly in both groups, with blood pressure readings decreasing more in the hypertensive group. The incidence of adverse reactions for the long-term study were similar to those for the shorter-term studies and included dizziness, fatigue, hypotension, edema, and dyspnea. Most adverse reactions were mild or moderate, and only 75 patients were withdrawn because of adverse events.

Conclusions.—Doxazosin, as treatment for BPH, was safe, effective, and well tolerated in men with normotension or hypertension for up to 48 months. The drug also significantly lowered heart rate and blood pressure in patients with hypertension.

▶ Selective α1–adrenoceptor antagonists such as doxazosin seem superior on average to prostatic 5α-reductase inhibitors.

L. Lasagna, M.D.

Transition Zone Ratio and Prostate-specific Antigen Density as Predictors of the Response of Benign Prostatic Hypertrophy to Alpha Blocker and Anti-androgen Therapy
Kurita Y, Masuda H, Suzuki K, et al (Hamamatsu Univ, Japan; Univ of Tokyo)
Br J Urol 80:78–83, 1997   11–4

Background.—Many elderly men have benign prostatic hypertrophy (BPH). The medical treatment of choice consists of α-blockers and anti-androgens. Whether clinical response to this treatment can be predicted by transrectal ultrasonography (TRUS) was investigated.

Methods.—One hundred twenty-eight patients with BPH were randomly assigned to 6 months of treatment with tamsulosin, a long-acting selective α_1-blocker, or allylestrenol, an antiandrogen. Transrectal US was used to determine the transition zone (TZ) volume, transition zone ratio (TZ ratio = TZ volume/total prostate volume), total prostate volume, and prostate-specific antigen density (PSAD).

Findings.—At 6 months, both treatment groups had a significantly improved American Urologic Association (AUA) symptom score, quality-of-life (QOL) score, and peak urinary flow rate (Q_{max}). In patients receiving tamsulosin, pretreatment PSAD was significantly negatively correlated with the percentage of change in Q_{max}. There was a positive correlation between PSAD and the percentage change in the AUA symptom score. Patients receiving allylestrenol showed a significant positive association between PSAD and percentage change in Q_{max} and a negative correlation between PSAD and the AUA symptom score.

Conclusions.—Patients with a high PSAD before treatment responded well to antiandrogen therapy, whereas those with a low PSAD responded better to α_1-blocker treatment. Transrectal US provides a simple way of assessing PSAD and the TZ ratio.

▶ This paper represents what I think is a very important application of research and thinking about a disease and its treatment. As we learn more about how to treat many diseases, we've got to know who will respond. In this particular study, the patients with a high pretreatment PSAD responded well to antiandrogens, whereas those with a low level responded to α_1-blocker therapy. Because there are few diseases with only one therapy, and because the diseases don't respond uniformly to any one intervention, use of these noninvasive methods for assessing BPH in assigning treatment may be a giant step forward.

M. Weintraub, M.D.

Estrogen Reduction by Aromatase Inhibition For Benign Prostatic Hyperplasia: Results of a Double-blind, Placebo-controlled, Randomized Clinical Trial Using Two Doses of the Aromatase-inhibitor Atamestane
Radlmaier A, Eickenberg HU, Fletcher MS, et al (Franziskus Hosp, Bielefeld, Germany; Gen Hosp, Brighton, England; Centre Hospitalier, Auxerre, France; et al)
Prostate 29:199–208, 1996

11–5

Background.—Benign prostatic hyperplasia (BPH), which increases the size of the prostate, often results in urinary outflow obstruction. The effect of selective reduction of estrogens using atamestane for 48 weeks on established BPH was investigated.

Methods and Findings.—Two hundred ninety-two patients with clinical symptoms of BPH were assigned randomly to placebo or atamestane, 100 or 300 mg/day, for 48 weeks. Both atamestane doses significantly decreased serum levels of estradiol and estrone and produced a slight dose-dependent counter-regulatory increase in concentrations of peripheral androgen. All 3 groups showed improvement in clinical symptoms. Active treatment was no more effective than placebo, even after 48 weeks. Overall, tolerance of 100 mg of atamestane was excellent. However, patients given the 300-mg dose had a slightly greater incidence of adverse effects than those given placebo.

Conclusions.—Treatment of symptomatic BPH with the selective aromatase inhibitor atamestane is well tolerated but no more effective than placebo. Because of the strong, long-lasting effect of placebo on clinical BPH, studies of different treatments of this condition must have a strict double-blinded design.

▶ This, like other studies, shows that placebo is in fact the best treatment for many of the signs and symptoms of BPH. In this case, even though the dose was tripled, the investigators were still unable to show an effect of the drug. Ah well, another negative study in the literature. However, these really do help us tell what's really important and prevent us from repeating some obviously negative studies.

M. Weintraub, M.D.

Second-line Hormonal Therapy for Advanced Prostate Cancer: A Shifting Paradigm

Small EJ, Vogelzang NJ (Univ of California, San Francisco; Univ of Chicago)
J Clin Oncol 15:382–388, 1997   11–6

Background.—Prostate cancer is the most common malignancy in men, but hormonal therapy produces a sustained response in only a small minority of patients with metastasis. Combined androgen blockade improves survival in some patients, but all patients with advanced prostate cancer treated with androgen deprivation will subsequently have progressive hormone-insensitive disease. Almost all deaths from prostate cancer result from hormone-refractory prostate cancer. The management of patients with advanced prostate cancer who do not respond to androgen deprivation has changed significantly in the last 2–3 years.

Methods.—Current reports of prostate-specific antigen and the value of secondary hormonal treatment after combined androgen blockade were reviewed.

Findings.—The use of prostate-specific antigen as an end point in studies of patients with prostate cancer who are refractory to hormonal therapy is becoming more common, but is still controversial. Using prostate-specific antigen as an end point, it is clear that various hormonal treatments can produce a response. In about 20% of patients, antiandrogen withdrawal is effective and is seen with the use of flutamide, bicalutamide, megestrol acetate, and other antiandrogens. Megestrol, bicalutamide, glucocorticoids, aminoglutethimide, and ketoconazole and other regimens retain activity in patients who do not respond to combined androgen blockade and flutamide withdrawal.

Discussion.—After treatment with combined androgen blockade is begun, additional hormonal treatment is effective in some patients with progressive disease. Antiandrogen withdrawal is now mandatory before attempting other treatment. Some patients will have a continued response to hormonal therapy even after antiandrogen withdrawal. Better understanding of the molecular basis of these responses may improve treatment.

▶ Prostate cancer, the most common malignancy in males, caused 41,000 deaths in the United States last year. Androgen deprivation, the standard first line of treatment for metastatic prostate cancer, produces benefit for about 18 months on average, and all such patients eventually have progressive, hormonally insensitive disease.

As this paper reports, second-line hormonal therapy has something to offer these patients, but is in a state of flux.

L. Lasagna, M.D.

Long-term Efficacy and Safety of Nilutamide Plus Castration in Advanced Prostate Cancer, and the Significance of Early Prostate Specific Antigen Normalization
Dijkman GA, Janknegt RA, De Reijke TM, et al (Univ Hosp Nijmegen, The Netherlands)
J Urol 158:160–163, 1997   11–7

Introduction.—The nonsteroidal antiandrogen nilutamide is effective when combined with castration for advanced prostate cancer. The long-term efficacy and tolerability of nilutamide with orchiectomy in patients with advanced prostate cancer were reported.

Methods.—A multicenter, double-blind, placebo-controlled investigation was conducted with 457 patients with stage D2 prostate cancer. After orchiectomy, patients were randomly assigned to receive placebo or 300 mg of nilutamide once daily for 1 month, then 150 mg once daily. Patients were followed up for 8.5 years. Progression-free and survival actuarial rates were calculated.

Results.—At long-term follow-up of 8.5 years, patients who underwent orchiectomy combined with nilutamide therapy had significant improvements in cancer survival, overall survival, and interval to progression, compared with patients who had orchiectomy and received placebo. Normalized prostate specific antigen (PSA) levels at 3 months from start of therapy were significantly greater in the nilutamide plus orchiectomy groups, compared with the placebo plus orchiectomy group (59% vs. 28%). Long-term treatment with nilutamide was well tolerated, with no increase in the incidence of drug-specific adverse events.

Conclusions.—Significant benefits in interval to progression and survival were observed at long-term follow-up in patients undergoing orchiectomy and long-term treatment with nilutamide, compared with patients undergoing orchiectomy and receiving placebo. Monitoring PSA levels early in therapy had prognostic value for survival and progression. It is possible that PSA may be considered a surrogate marker of efficacy.

▶ The real test in this Dutch study is of an antiandrogen plus castration. One of the most important aspects of the trial is that it has 8.5 years of follow-up. Such a long period enhances a positive treatment effect. Prediction of PSA decrease is also possible with this long-term follow-up. Patients with even advanced prostate cancer often die of other diseases before they die of their malignancy. Very often the therapy is only palliative for these patients with more advanced disease. Nonetheless, physicians have to be aware of the value of treatment and improving the quality of life of some of these patients. Because PSA is an adequate marker, if it doesn't go down by 3 months, perhaps further studies and treatment of the primary cancer are indicated.

M. Weintraub, M.D.

Bicalutamide for Advanced Prostate Cancer: The Natural Versus Treated History of Disease

Scher HI, Liebertz C, Kelly WK, et al (Mem Sloan-Kettering Cancer Ctr, NY; Cornell Univ, New York; Zeneca Pharmaceuticals, Wilmington, Del)
J Clin Oncol 15:2928–2938, 1997   11–8

Background.—Different hormones may play a role in different stages of prostate cancer. The optimal time of antiandrogen dosing with bicaluta-mide, a pure antiandrogen, was determined in patients with prostate cancer at various stages and after various treatments.

Methods.—Bicalutamide, 200 mg/day, was administered to 104 patients with progressive prostate cancer. Tumors were classified as androgen-dependent (serum testosterone greater than 35 ng/mL; n = 53) or andro-gen-independent (n = 51). Patients in the androgen-dependent group included 37 who had not received hormones before and 16 who were either being treated with an intermittent approach or who had been treated with neoadjuvant therapy before surgical or radiation treatment but who then stopped taking hormones. The androgen-independent group was subdivided into 4 groups: those who had a relapse after orchiectomy or gonadotropin-releasing hormone [GnRH] analogue monotherapy (first group, n = 13); those whose disease progressed despite androgen blockade with a GnRH analogue and flutamide, and who either responded (second group, n = 14) or did not respond (third group, n = 12) to flutamide withdrawal; and those whose disease progressed despite 2 hormone treat-ments exclusive of antiandrogen withdrawal (fourth group, n = 12).

Findings.—Bicalutamide had a much better effect on androgen-depen-dent tumors as measured by decreases in prostate-specific antigen (PSA) levels (88% vs. 10%, androgen-dependent vs. androgen-independent) (Fig 1), an improvement in bone scan (48% vs. 12%, respectively), and regres-sion of soft-tissue disease (37% vs. 0%, respectively). Bicalutamide results in the 2 subgroups of the androgen-dependent tumors did not differ significantly. In the androgen-dependent group as a whole, of 15 patients whose rising PSA levels were treated by a GnRH analogue, 5 had a greater than 80% decrease in PSA levels. Of those who did not respond to bicalutamide plus GnRH analogue, bicalutamide withdrawal caused a greater than 80% decrease in PSA levels in 3 patients.

In the patients with androgen-independent tumors, those in the first group (relapse) received only a modest benefit from bicalutamide, and those in the fourth group (2 previous hormones) showed no response at all. However, both groups 2 and 3 (previous exposure to flutamide) received benefit, as 38% experienced a greater than 50% decrease in PSA level (no significant difference between groups 2 and 3). Adverse effects in all patients included decreases in libido, difficulty in erections, hot flashes, and breast swelling or tenderness or both.

Conclusions.—Prior hormone exposure had a significant effect on the response to the antiandrogen, bicalutamide. The drug had more effect on androgen-dependent tumors and in those androgen-independent tumors

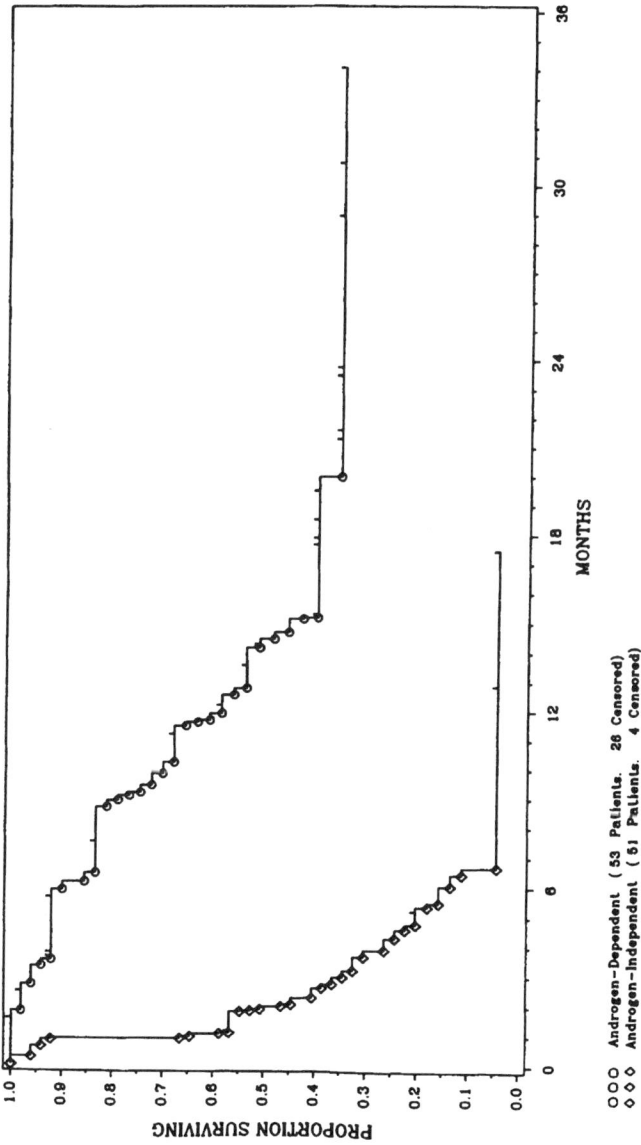

Tick mark(0) indicates last follow-up

○○○ Androgen-Dependent (53 Patients.   26 Censored)
◇◇◇ Androgen-Independent (51 Patients.   4 Censored)

FIGURE 1.—Time to progression based on prostate-specific (PSA) elevations for patients with androgen-dependent and androgen-independent progression. (Courtesy of Scher HI, Liebertz C, Kelly WK, et al: Bicalutamide for advanced prostate cancer: The natural versus treated history of disease. *J Clin Oncol* 15:2928–2938, 1997.)

that had been exposed to flutamide. Thus a patient's prior treatment history had a significant influence on response to therapy, and should be considered in individualizing patient management.

▶ As shown in the accompanying figure, the outcome of androgen-dependent patients is better almost regardless of what else is done with therapy. What I think the authors of this study were trying to tell us is that you have to know what happened in the past in order to better select therapies for the future. We have always known about the influence of past therapy, but it is becoming clear for some things that you wouldn't think would affect treatment. In cancer chemotherapy, we have been stressing the stratification of patients to the various treatment groups on the basis of their past history. In some cases, we have even done studies just in patients treated with x, y, or z. We will have to learn to follow individual patients and trace their courses on a new therapy based on what they have had in the past. It is going to be more and more difficult to do this, but we have got to get away from checking the "herd" response. We need to delineate responders. One way is to find out more about the influence of past treatment on current and future therapy.

M. Weintraub, M.D.

A Placebo-controlled Study of Intravesical Pentosanpolysulphate for the Treatment of Interstitial Cystitis
Bade JJ, Laseur M, Nieuwenburg A, et al (Univ of Groningen, The Netherlands)
Br J Urol 79:168–171, 1997   11–9

Background.—Previous research has provided the rationale for sodium pentosanpolysulphate (PPS), a heparin analogue, for the treatment of interstitial cystitis (IC). The efficacies of intravesical PPS and placebo were compared.

Methods.—Twenty patients with IC were enrolled in the double-blind, placebo-controlled trial. Ten were given intravesical PPS, 300 mg in 50 mL of 0.9% sodium chloride, twice a week for 3 months.

Findings.—Forty percent of the PPS recipients had significant symptomatic relief, compared with 20% of placebo recipients. Only the urodynamic bladder capacity was significantly increased in patients given PPS. Eighteen months after study initiation, symptoms were relieved in 80% of patients still receiving PPS and in 40% of those not being treated.

Conclusions.—Intravesical PPS is an effective option for the treatment of IC. The intravesical application of this agent is safe, with no serious side effects.

▶ This uncontrolled illness, interstitial cystitis, affects many people and makes their lives hellish. The amount of difficulty the patients experience is measured by the fact that they are willing to be catheterized twice a week for 3 months as the treatment described with PPS. One of the scientists working on interstitial cystitis had a quotation published in the newspaper, that "even if only a few patients can be helped with any specific treatment, they would be willing to keep trying things until they found something that might help them." The National Institutes of Health has described the symptoms and helped with the diagnosis by outlining the various aspects of the disease, such as bladder pain, symptoms of urgency and frequency, and sterile urine. I hope that the research undertaken helps some of the unfortunate people who are suffering with this illness.

M. Weintraub, M.D.

Quality of Life Effects of Alprostadil Therapy for Erectile Dysfunction
Willke RJ, Glick HA, McCarron TJ, et al (Pharmacia & Upjohn Inc, Kalamazoo, Mich; Univ of Pennsylvania, Philadelphia; AMGEN Inc, Thousand Oaks, Calif; et al)
J Urol 157:2124–2128, 1997   11–10

Objective.—Erectile dysfunction can result in severe quality of life problems. The short-term and long-term effects of therapy with intracavernosal injection with a new formulation of alprostadil sterile powder was investigated for its effects on patient satisfaction, psychological status, and overall quality of life for up to 18 months.

Methods.—Between 1992 and 1993, 579 patients aged 20 to 78 were entered into a self-injection trial using the drug 1 to 3 times a week for up to 18 months. Most (99%) patients reported an erection with the drug. Patients and partners reported satisfactory sexual activity 87% and 86% of the time. The Center for Marital and Sexual Health Sexual Functioning Questionnaire (CMSH-SFQ), which measures psychosocial and physical aspects of erectile dysfunction; the Brief Symptom Inventory, which measures mental health; and the Duke Health Profile, which measures quality of life; were self-administered at baseline, and at 3, 6, 12, and 18 months. Changes in quality of life were analyzed statistically. Reasons for discontinuing therapy were documented.

Results.—Patients were dysfunctional for an average of more than 4 years. All CMSH-SFQ and Brief Symptom Inventory responses showed significant improvements at 6 months. For the Duke Health Profile, mental health, anxiety, depression, and self-esteem improved significantly. Whereas general health and social health tended to improve, perceived health tended to decrease and pain increased. Most changes that occurred by 3 to 6 months persisted. The 203 patients who dropped out of the study did so mainly because of lack of firm erections (52.3%), pain during injection (40.9%), pain during erection (41.3%), and lack of spontaneity (38.5%).

Conclusion.—Sexual activity, sexual satisfaction, and psychosocial health improved after treatment with alprostadil for erectile dysfunction.

Reasons for discontinuing therapy included lack of firm erections and pain during injection and/or erection.

▶ Perhaps for the articles on quality of life or other softer endpoints, we should require some sort of higher standard that they have to fulfill to convince us that cost-effectiveness studies are correct. The higher standard could be several studies or perhaps even lower *p* values to be really acceptable. Of course, some studies are just so overwhelming, so telling, that we don't really need either replication or statistical correlates. We just know that they are correct.

M. Weintraub, M.D.

Ejaculation-retarding Properties of Paroxetine in Patients With Primary Premature Ejaculation: A Double-blind, Randomized, Dose-response Study
Waldinger MD, Hengeveld MW, Zwinderman AH (Leyenburg Hosp, The Hague, The Netherlands; Leiden Univ, The Netherlands)
Br J Urol 79:592–595, 1997   11–11

Background.—A previous placebo-controlled study reported that the selective serotonergic antidepressant, paroxetine, 40 mg/day, significantly delayed intravaginal ejaculation time in men with premature ejaculation. However, there were problems with fatigue and bursts of frequent, severe yawning. The effects of 20 mg/day and 40 mg/day doses of paroxetine on ejaculatory latency were compared in a randomized trial.

Methods.—The study included 34 men with primary premature ejaculation. For 1 week, all patients received a 20-mg dose of paroxetine daily. They were then randomly assigned to 7 weeks of treatment with 20 or 40 mg of paroxetine per day. Outcomes were assessed in double-blind fashion in separate interviews with the men and their female partners.

Results.—Twenty-seven patients completed the study. The results were unchanged by an intention-to-treat analysis. Both dose groups had a statistically significant improvement from baseline in ejaculation latency, as well as a clinically meaningful increase in ejaculation time. Median ejaculation times improved from 10 seconds to 4–5 minutes within 3 weeks, with no significant difference between groups. The improvement could not be explained by decreased anxiety. Side effects occurred in both groups, but became less intense during the trial.

Conclusions.—Paroxetine 20 mg/day is a clinically effective treatment for men with primary premature ejaculation. If the patient desires a further delay in ejaculation, it may be helpful to increase the dose to 40 mg/day. At either dose, failure of ejaculation is possible but rare.

▶ Fortunately, these investigators could build on a previous study that was done with a placebo. As we realize, premature ejaculation really has a high psychological etiology. In this study, the adverse effects were different.

Slight or moderate yawning, sweating, nausea, fatigue, and dry mouth occurred. Fortunately, they diminished as time passed. The authors recommend more research on the subtype of serotonin receptor involved. They use a very interesting word to characterize the field of which premature ejaculation is a part, i.e., neurosexology. It reminds me of how we can change language to suit our "agenda." A woman speaking at a large meeting referred to "non-women." Of course she meant "men."

M. Weintraub, M.D.

Priapism Following Ingestion of Papaverine Tablets
Prasad K, El-Sherif A (Hamad Med Corp, Doha, Qatar)
Scand J Urol Nephrol 30:515–516, 1996   11–12

Background.—Priapism has been associated with several drugs given perorally. The current case report is the first to describe the association of priapism and peroral papaverine.

Case Report.—Man, 44, was admitted because of a painful erection that had persisted for more than 7 hours. He had taken 2 papaverine hydrochloride tablets, 150 mg each, for abdominal colic, after which he had sexual intercourse without detumescence. The patient was a heavy smoker with a history of chronic bronchitis and diabetes mellitus. Conservative treatment did not resolve the priapism. The corpora cavernosa were aspirated and irrigated with normal saline solution through a needle in each corpus. About 100 mL of dark red blood was aspirated. Although detumescence occurred during aspiration, the erection recurred afterward. The corpora cavernosa were irrigated with phenylephrine, which immediately resulted in sustained detumescence. The patient was monitored for 48 hours and discharged with the instruction to avoid sexual excitement for 3 weeks. Normal erection and normal coitus occurred after 1 month.

Conclusions.—In this patient, priapism occurred after the oral intake of papaverine hydrochloride, 300 mg. Researchers may want to investigate the potential of oral papaverine in the treatment of impotence.

▶ Intracavernosal injection of papaverine in the treatment of impotence is known to carry a risk of priapism, but this seems to be the first case of this adverse event after oral papaverine.

L. Lasagna, M.D.

12 Infectious Diseases

Programmatic Role of the Infectious Diseases Physician in Controlling Antimicrobial Costs in the Hospital
John JF Jr, Fishman NO (Univ of Medicine and Dentistry of New Jersey, New Brunswick; Univ of Pennsylvania, Philadelphia)
Clin Infect Dis 24:471–485, 1997   12–1

Introduction.—Numerous studies indicate that up to 50% of antimicrobial usage in U.S. hospitals is inappropriate. Because these agents account for up to 30% of hospital drug budgets, a reduction in unnecessary usage could yield significant savings. Infectious diseases physicians are using a variety of strategies to control antimicrobial costs.

Methods.—References for review were obtained from a search of the heading of antimicrobial and antibiotic costs in the 1966–1995 MEDLINE and other databases, personal reference libraries, and articles from relevant journals not appearing in on-line searches. Articles were reviewed for characteristics of the antimicrobial control programs, specific antimicro-

---

TABLE 2.—Strategies to Control Hospital Antibiotic Costs

A. Education* of prescribers
   1. Direct interaction
   2. Peer feedback from performance evaluation
     a. Verbal
     b. Written
B. Antimicrobial formulary restriction
C. Pharmacy justification
   1. Without consultation with infectious diseases physician
     a. Antibiotic order form
     b. Stop orders
   2. With consultation with infectious diseases physician
     a. Direct interaction
     b. Simple chart entry
D. Formulary substitution or switch
E. Computer surveillance
F. Clinical microbiology laboratory item costing
G. Purchase plans
H. Multidisciplinary approach

---

*Considered as education when there is human interaction over choice of the antimicrobial and the recommended change is not necessarily mandatory.
(Courtesy of John JF Jr, Fishman NO: Programmatic role of the infectious diseases physician in controlling antimicrobial costs in the hospital. *Clin Infect Dis* 24:471–485, 1997, by permission of The University of Chicago. All rights reserved.)

TABLE 4.—Steps for Infectious Diseases Physicians to Apply for
Establishment of an Antimicrobial Program

1. Develop knowledge about the local antimicrobial budget and patterns of usage.
2. Collect the necessary data to publish a quarterly antimicrobial susceptibility
   report including the prices of all formulary antimicrobials.
3. Gather baseline usage and cost data and attempt to compare them to those of
   equivalent institutions [60].
4. Outline a structure for participation in the AMP team and estimate the annual
   costs for funding, including salary for the IDP.
5. Meet with administrators of hospitals and managed care companies to discuss
   implementation [79].
6. Focus on the most frequently used and most costly agents on the formulary.
7. Publish a manual, *Guidelines for Antimicrobial Use*, and provide appropriate
   educational or multimedia formats for educating the prescribing staff.
8. Ensure a fail-safe mechanism to resolve disagreements with the prescribing staff.
9. Develop innovative educational methods including computerized interplay to
   explain the use of new antimicrobials, antivirals, and antiinfectious biologics.
10. Reevaluate the AMP annually with quality assurance personnel and review the
    cost-effectiveness with the chief of staff, the president of the hospital, and the
    Vice President for Clinical Affairs.

Abbreviations: AMP, antimicrobial management program; *IDP,* infectious diseases physician.
(Courtesy of John JF Jr, Fishman NO: Programmatic role of the infectious diseases physician in
controlling antimicrobial costs in the hospital. *Clin Infect Dis* 24:471–485, 1997, by permission of
The University of Chicago. All rights reserved.)

bials under investigation, and economic impact of the control programs.
Programs were divided into 1 of 8 types (Table 2).

Specific Strategies.—Because physicians have significant deficiencies in
their knowledge of appropriate prescription of antimicrobials, education
with continuous reinforcement can be an effective strategy. The most
direct method of influencing antimicrobial usage and costs is control of the
hospital formulary. Various restriction and approval mechanisms, although onerous to prescribing physicians, are among the more effective
means of controlling the antimicrobial budget. Formulary substitution or
"switch" policies appear less dictatorial than restrictions but may not be as
strictly enforced. The computer may prove to be the ultimate method for
antibiotic surveillance and education. Many control programs use a multidisciplinary approach with input from various hospital services: infectious diseases, clinical pharmacy, infection control, nursing, and administration.

Discussion.—Infectious diseases physicians have been crucial to the
success of cost-effective antimicrobial control strategies, but multidisciplinary antimicrobial management offers the best potential for sustained
cost savings. With the recommendations (Table 4) provided here, infectious diseases physicians can address cost containment issues, mobilize
their colleagues, and present a comprehensive program to the administration.

► Intelligent prescribing of antibiotics can produce miracles; inappropriate
prescribing wastes money and can harm patients. This thoughtful and sophisticated article on cost control deserves to be read in its original length.

L. Lasagna, M.D.

Oral Administration of Antibiotics: A Rational Alternative to the Parenteral Route

MacGregor RR, Graziani AL (Univ of Pennsylvania, Philadelphia)
Clin Infect Dis 24:457–467, 1997   12–2

Introduction.—The preference for intravenous (IV) antibiotics has recently been reconsidered because of new highly effective oral agents. Data supporting the safety and efficacy of oral antibiotic administration as an alternative to IV therapy were reviewed.

Benefits and Disadvantages of Oral Antibiotics.—When they are effective, oral antibiotics can reduce costs and risks associated with use of IV antibiotics. Patient inconvenience is also decreased with the use of oral antibiotics. Disadvantages include: some organisms are not responsive to oral antibiotic therapy, third-party payers who insist that patients on oral antibiotics do not require hospitalization, and potential legal liability stemming from the impression that oral treatment is not the "standard of care."

Attempts at Changing Medical Culture.—Several infectious disease and pharmacy groups have worked to encourage physicians to use oral instead of IV antibiotics when possible. Programs that seem to be influencing antibiotic administration route choices are those that show physicians within their own institutions that patients can be treated effectively with oral antibiotics and at a significant cost savings and reduction in risks.

Conclusion.—Appropriate use of oral instead of parenteral administration of antibiotics is gaining acceptance within physician groups. The Infectious Disease Society of America and individual infectious disease specialists need to lead efforts to educate colleagues and the public that oral treatment is appropriate and aggressive treatment for sick and even hospitalized patients.

▶ There are advantages and disadvantages to IV antibiotics, and this article reminds us that with sophisticated judgments, oral antibiotics can work just as well, with cost savings and risk reduction.

L. Lasagna, M.D.

Early Switch From Intravenous to Oral Antibiotics in Hospitalized Patients With Infections: A 6-Month Prospective Study

Ahkee S, Smith S, Newman D, et al (Univ of Louisville, KY)
Pharmacotherapy 17:569–575, 1997   12–3

Background.—A short course of IV antibiotics with an early switch to oral treatment may be as effective as a prolonged course of IV antibiotics in some hospitalized patients with infection. This study determined what percentage of hospitalized patients given IV antibiotics would be candidates for early switch to oral therapy and the clinical outcomes of patients after the switch.

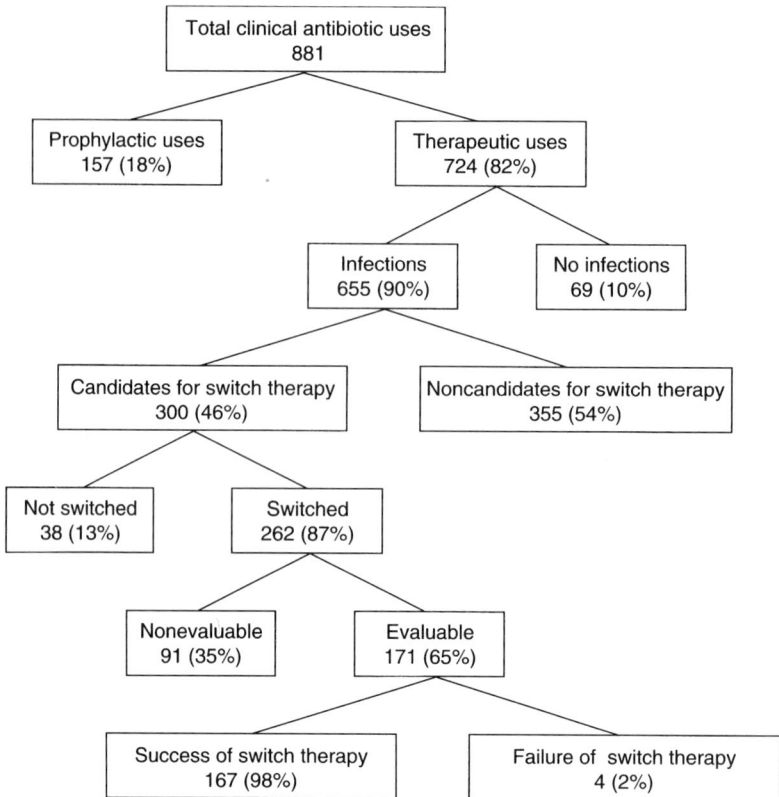

FIGURE 1.—Clinical uses of IV antibiotics and outcomes of switch therapy. (Courtesy of Ahkee S, Smith S, Newman D, et al: Early switch from intravenous to oral antibiotics in hospitalized patients with infections: A 6-month prospective study. *Pharmacotherapy* 17:569–575, 1997.)

Methods and Findings.—All patients at 1 center in whom IV antibiotics were prescribed for infection treatment from October 1, 1993, to March 31, 1994, were screened prospectively to identify candidates for switch therapy. Three hundred of the 655 patients (46%) were considered candidates for a switch. The switch was made in 262 of these patients (40% of the total group). The switch was associated with clinical cure in 98% of the 171 evaluable patients. Thus, the failure rate of this strategy was only 2% (Fig 1).

Conclusions.—The duration of IV antibiotic treatment can be minimized with early switch to oral therapy in hospitalized patients with infections. Patient outcomes after the switch are good.

▶ Hospitalized patients whose infections seem to be showing a good clinical response to IV antibiotics can often be switched to oral antibiotics with cost savings and increased ease of medication.

L. Lasagna, M.D.

Vitamin C, the Placebo Effect, and the Common Cold: A Case Study of How Preconceptions Influence the Analysis of Results

Hemilä H (Univ of Helsinki)
J Clin Epidemiol 49:1079–1084, 1996 12–4

Purpose.—Several placebo-controlled studies have demonstrated that taking supplemental vitamin C can reduce the symptoms of the common cold. Karlowski et al. published an influential study of this issue in 1975. That study used lactose, which tastes different than ascorbic acid, for a placebo. The study found that cold episodes were 17% shorter in participants taking vitamin C, 6 g/day. However, the researchers attributed the difference to a placebo effect. This "placebo explanation" has subsequently been repeated in several reports. The results of the Karlowski study were reinterpreted, focusing on the basis of and the problems with the placebo explanation.

The Placebo Explanation.—In the Karlowski study, most patients were able to correctly identify which prophylactic treatment they were taking. This led Karlowski, et al. to assume that all patients giving a correct answer truly knew whether they were taking placebo or vitamin C, and that none had guessed. They supported this interpretation by subgroup analysis of "blinded" and "unblinded" participants, although the selection criteria for these groups were not made explicit. However, the placebo explanation does not hold for several reasons. First, patients taking therapeutic vitamin C had a greater benefit than those taking placebo, even though there was no statistically valid evidence that any participants knew which therapeutic tablet they were taking. Realizing that one had received the active treatment cannot simply be assumed to cause a decrease in symptoms. The placebo explanation is not consistent with the results of the study. Also, for unexplained reasons, nearly half of all episodes studied were in neither the "blinded" nor the "unblinded" group. No explanation was given for this missing group. The results of subsequent studies using more appropriate placebos also refute the placebo explanation. Rejection of the placebo explanation permits comparison of therapeutic vs. regular supplementation and analysis of dose dependency.

Conclusions.—In contrast to the original investigators' conclusions, taking therapeutic vitamin C supplementation during a cold seems to be as effective as regular supplementation. There is also evidence of linear dose dependency, at least up to a dose of 6 g/day. Thus, taking large doses of vitamin C during a cold may do much to relieve the symptoms. Preconceived notions appear to be responsible for the misinterpretation of previous studies of vitamin C and the common cold.

▶ This article is a delightful rejection of the notion that vitamin C's effects on the symptoms of the common cold are simply placebo phenomena. The article was followed in the same issue by a vigorous dissent from Tom Chalmers,[1] but I am persuaded by Hemilä's analysis.

L. Lasagna, M.D.

Reference

1. Chalmers TC: Dissent to the preceding article by H. Hemilä. *J Clin Epidemiol* 49:1085, 1996.

Comparison of Once-daily Versus Pharmacokinetic Dosing of Aminoglycosides in Elderly Patients

Koo J, Tight R, Rajkumar V, et al (Univ of North Dakota, Fargo)
Am J Med 101:177–183, 1996   12–5

Introduction.—Despite the risk of nephrotoxicity and ototoxicity, aminoglycosides are commonly used to treat severe gram-negative infections. Interest has risen in simplifying therapy and limiting toxicities of aminoglycosides by recommending once-daily dosing rather than twice- or thrice-daily dosing. Currently, the pharmacokinetic dosing method is the most widely recommended because of the substantial inter- and intra-patient variations that occur in the distribution volume and the elimination rate constant of aminoglycosides. A once-daily dosing (4 mg/kg IV) method was compared with a pharmacokinetic dosing method using an initial dose of 2 mg/kg IV every 12 hours.

Methods.—Ninety-six patients, mostly males with a mean age of 69 years, who had a suspected or confirmed infection for which an aminoglycoside was indicated, were randomly assigned to either the once-daily dosing group receiving 4 mg/kg or the pharmacokinetic dosing group receiving an initial dose of 2 mg/kg every 12 hours. To maintain a serum trough concentration of less than 1.5 mg/L regardless of the peak concentration, the dosing interval was extended by 12 to 24 hours in the once-daily dosing group. To achieve a serum peak concentration of 6 to 10 mg/L and a trough concentration of less than 1.5 mg/L, dosing in the other group was adjusted based on the individual pharmacokinetic data.

Results.—With regard to clinical and bacteriologic efficacy, there was no significant difference between the 2 groups. In the once-daily dosing group, the incidence of nephrotoxicity was 24%, and in the pharmacokinetic dosing group, it was 14%; this was statistically significant. In the once-daily dosing group, a correlation was found between a high serum peak concentration and the incidence of nephrotoxicity. In the once-daily dosing group, nephrotoxicity developed in 6 of 10 patients (60%) with an initial serum peak concentration of greater than 12.0 mg/L, whereas 2 of 24 patients (8.3%) with an initial peak concentration of less than 12 mg/L had nephrotoxicity. Nephrotoxicity was not correlated with serum peak concentrations in the pharmacokinetic dosing group.

Conclusions.—There appears to be equal efficacy and toxicity among the groups receiving once-daily dosing and pharmacokinetic dosing of aminoglycosides. The risk of nephrotoxicity, however, may be increased in the elderly population receiving once-daily aminoglycoside dosing resulting in high serum peak concentrations. High doses of aminoglycosides that can lead to initial serum peak concentrations of greater than 12 mg/L may be hazardous to elderly patients, but a prospective study would be necessary to confirm this.

▶ If we want to use aminoglycosides most effectively and most safely, we need to know whether such measurements as age, peak concentration, and trough concentration are closely related to efficacy and toxicity. We also cannot assume that all aminoglycosides are alike. The studies done to date are not in total agreement, for all sorts of reasons (e.g., different drugs, patients of different ages, dose). Nevertheless, it seems to me that a high serum trough concentration (greater than 2 mg/L) probably is related to nephrotoxicity and should be avoided. The present study also suggests that high serum peak concentrations (greater than 12 mg/L) are associated with nephrotoxicity (at least in the elderly) and should be avoided. The authors concluded that once-daily dosing was no different than pharmacokinetic dosing, but I disagree. Nephrotoxicity was seen in 24% of the once-daily dosing group versus 14% of the pharmacokinetic dosing group. That may only come to a *P* value of 0.13, but who says that such a *P* value is totally dismissable?

L. Lasagna, M.D.

A Prospective Randomized Study of Inpatient IV Antibiotics for Community-acquired Pneumonia: The Optimum Duration of Therapy
Siegel RE, Halpern NA, Almenoff PL, et al (Bronx Veterans Affairs Med Ctr, New York; Castle Point Veterans Affairs Med Ctr, New York)
Chest 110:965–971, 1996   12–6

Background.—Few protocols describe the optimal duration of IV and oral antibiotic treatment in patients with community-acquired pneumonia (CAP). Prolonged IV therapy before the switch to oral medication may extend the length of hospitalization and increase costs. The efficacy of a shortened course of IV antibiotic therapy before changing to oral antibiotics was investigated.

Methods.—Seventy-two men and 1 woman in a veterans' hospital were included. Seventy-five CAP episodes occurred. By random assignment, the patients received 2 days of IV and 8 days of oral antibiotic therapy (group 1), 5 days of IV and 5 days of oral therapy (group 2), or 10 days of IV therapy (group 3). The antibiotics given were cefuroxime, 750 mg every 8 hours, for the IV course and cefuroxime axetil, 500 mg every 12 hours, for the oral therapy.

Findings.—The 3 groups did not differ in clinical course, cure rates, or resolution of chest radiograph abnormalities. The length of hospital stay differed among groups—a mean of 6 days in group 1, 8 days in group 2, and 11 days in group 3.

Conclusion.—Adults hospitalized for CAP who are not severely ill may be treated effectively with an abbreviated, 2-day course of IV antibiotic therapy, and then oral therapy. Longer IV courses increase the length of hospitalization and costs without improving the therapeutic cure rate.

▶ This was one of those studies that was set up to check on the money to be saved by specific methodologies of treating patients. It turns out that the patient group with the shortest stay was the one in which patients received 2 days of IV and 8 days of oral therapy. The IV therapy is so much more expensive that the mixture of IV and oral therapy would be of great cost savings to the Veterans Administration. The best news is that the outcome was not sacrificed.

M. Weintraub, M.D.

Ambulatory Patients With Community-acquired Pneumonia: The Frequency of Atypical Agents and Clinical Course
Marrie TJ, Peeling RW, Fine MJ, et al (Dalhousie Univ, Halifax, NS, Canada; Lab Centre for Disease Control, Winnipeg, Man, Canada; Univ of Pittsburgh, Pa; et al)
Am J Med 101:508–515, 1996   12–7

Background.—Although community-acquired pneumonia (CAP) is a common illness, knowledge about its clinical manifestations and outcomes is incomplete. The causes of CAP in patients treated in an ambulatory setting were determined using serologic methods, and initial symptoms, radiographic manifestations, and clinical outcomes of CAP with atypical and undetermined causes were documented.

Methods.—One hundred forty-nine adults (mean age, 41 years) were included in the prospective cohort study. All had acute onset of 1 or more symptoms suggesting pneumonia and radiographic evidence of pneumonia. Sixty-four percent were women.

Findings.—Etiology was established in 49.7% of the patients. Causative agents included *Mycoplasma pneumoniae* in 22.8%, *Chlamydia pneumonia* in 10.7%, *M. pneumoniae* and *C. pneumoniae* in 3.4%, *Coxiella burnetii* in 2.7%, influenza A virus in 2.7%, and other agents in 7.4%. Patients with known and unknown etiologies had similar symptom severity, although a greater proportion of patients with pneumonia of known causes reported sweats, chills, and headaches at the initial assessment. Patients with undetermined causes were more likely to have multilobar pneumonia. Those with atypical pneumonia and those with pneumonia of undetermined causes experienced severe deterioration of physical functioning with a marked but incomplete recovery at 30 days. Patients with atypical pneumonia had better physical function and general mental health scores at this time.

Conclusions.—Nearly half of the patients with ambulatory CAP have illness caused by atypical agents. Patients with atypical pneumonia cannot be distinguished from those with undetermined etiologies by clinical features at baseline. Outcomes are essentially similar in these 2 patient groups.

▶ Ambulatory patients with pneumonia tend to be young and have a good prognosis. Physicians seem in general not to pin down the microbiological culprit with precision, but about half the cases are the result of infection with an "atypical" agent. Most of these patients seem to respond well to either a macrolide or tetracycline (as recommended by the American Thoracic Society), but other antibiotics probably work as well.

L. Lasagna, M.D.

The Changing Epidemiology of Acquired Drug-resistant Tuberculosis in San Francisco, USA
Bradford WZ, Martin JN, Reingold AL, et al (San Francisco Gen Hosp; Univ of California, San Francisco; Frances J Curry Natl Tuberculosis Ctr, San Francisco)
Lancet 348:928–931, 1996   12–8

Introduction.—In the past few years, tuberculosis caused by drug-resistant *Mycobacterium tuberculosis* has emerged as a serious threat to global public health. To design effective tuberculosis control programs and to determine optimum treatment regimens and management schemes for individual patients, a refined understanding of the factors that contribute to drug resistance is important. Lapses in basic control strategies have largely been the cause of drug-resistant tuberculosis. Secular trends were reviewed to identify causal risk factors for acquired drug resistance.

Methods.—Of 3,168 patients with tuberculosis reported in San Francisco between January 1, 1985 and December 31, 1994, 14 met the definition for acquired drug resistance. The definition applied to patients with initially fully susceptible isolates from whom subsequent isolates showed any level of resistance to isoniazid, rifampicin, or ethambutol hydrochloride. Information about HIV status was obtained, as well as co-existing diseases, alcohol misuse, other substance misuse, medications taken at the same time as antituberculous treatment, and the presence of gastrointestinal symptoms. Univariate and multivariate analyses were conducted to study the variables.

Results.—Acquired drug resistance was independently associated with non-compliance with therapy, gastrointestinal symptoms, and AIDS. Acquired drug resistance developed between 1990 and 1994 in 1 of every 16 patients with tuberculosis and AIDS who had either gastrointestinal symptoms or non-compliance. Patients with acquired drug resistance were more likely to be white and unemployed than were control subjects. Variables that were not associated with acquired drug resistance were history of tuberculosis, history of antituberculous treatment, cavitary disease, and initial 4-drug regimen.

Conclusions.—The increasing prevalence of HIV and *M. tuberculosis* co-infection seems to lie behind the substantial increase in acquired drug resistance in San Francisco. Acquired drug resistance is fostered by the interface of the HIV and tuberculosis epidemics. In communities with high rates of HIV infection, traditional tuberculosis control measures may not be sufficient and alternative measures may be necessary. Susceptibility tests should be repeated sooner rather than later. There are grave implications for the global control of tuberculosis because the AIDS epidemic has fostered the emergence of drug resistance in individual patients and AIDS facilitates the rapid dissemination of these resistant bacteria to other patients.

▶ Drug-resistant *M. tuberculosis* is a global problem today, posing serious management problems, costs, morbidity, and mortality. As the authors suggest, a high index of suspicion for acquired drug resistance is amply warranted for all HIV-infected patients with tuberculosis. Increasing trouble with this type of co-infection seems inevitable.

L. Lasagna, M.D.

Rifampin Preventive Therapy for Tuberculosis Infection: Experience With 157 Adolescents
Villarino ME, Ridzon R, Weismuller PC, et al (Ctrs For Disease Control and Prevention, Atlanta, Ga; Orange County Health Care Agency, Calif)
Am J Respir Crit Care Med 155:1735–1738, 1997   12–9

Background.—Rifampin has been recommended for prevention of active disease in persons infected with *Mycobacterium tuberculosis* resistant to isoniazid. However, the adverse effects and acceptability of rifampin have not been well documented.

Methods.—One hundred fifty-seven high school students exposed to and probably infected with *M. tuberculosis* strains resistant to isoniazid were prospectively followed up. All received preventive treatment with rifampin, 10 mg/kg of body weight (maximum, 600 mg) daily, for 24 weeks.

Findings.—Forty-one patients (26%) reported 1 or more adverse effects while taking rifampin. Treatment was temporarily interrupted in 18 of these patients because of adverse effects, and treatment was discontinued in 2. Increases in alanine aminotransferase levels were greater than 2 times the normal upper limit in 4 patients (2.5%); in 1 of these, treatment was discontinued. Six patients (3.8%) stopped taking rifampin without consulting their physicians. During the 2 years of follow-up, none of the students had active disease. Without preventive treatment, 7 cases of tuberculosis would have been expected in that time. Thus, rifampin had an estimated protective effect of 56%.

Conclusions.—Rifampin appears to effectively prevent active tuberculosis. In this large group of high school students, the treatment was well tolerated and accepted.

▶ Isoniazid is an excellent drug for tuberculosis, but resistance to the drug is not that uncommon. Rifampin is an effective and well-tolerated alternative.

L. Lasagna, M.D.

Antimicrobial Prophylaxis Prior to Shock Wave Lithotripsy in Patients With Sterile Urine Before Treatment: A Meta-analysis and Cost-effectiveness Analysis
Pearle MS, Roehrborn CG (Univ of Texas, Dallas)
Urology 49:679–686, 1997   12–10

Objective.—Urosepsis is a rare but serious complication of shock wave lithotripsy (SWL) for renal and ureteral calculi. Preoperative antimicrobial agents are routinely given before SWL in high-risk patients. However, there is controversy as to whether antimicrobial prophylaxis should be given in low-risk patients with sterile preoperative urine. Using published data, the efficacy and cost-effectiveness of antimicrobial prophylaxis before SWL in patients with a sterile pretreatment urine culture were analyzed.

Methods.—Fourteen studies of antimicrobial prophylaxis for SWL were identified by literature search: 8 prospective, randomized, controlled trials (RCTs) comparing active treatment with placebo or no treatment (including 885 subjects) and 6 non-RCT clinical series (including 597 subjects). The RCTs were subjected to meta-analysis, with the main outcome of diagnosed urinary tract infection (UTI) after SWL. Two strategies were compared in cost analysis: a prophylactic strategy in which every patient received prophylaxis and treatment was given for UTIs developing after SWL and a treatment-only strategy in which post-SWL UTIs were treated by various antimicrobial combinations. The meta-analysis was used to determine the median probability of post-SWL UTIs.

Results.—In the reported studies, post-SWL UTIs occurred in 0% to 28% of control patients and 0% to 8% of patients receiving prophylaxis. Bayesian analysis was performed to combine the placebo and no-drug treatment arms of 6 non-RCTs. This produced a median 6% probability of post-SWL UTI, compared with a 2% median probability in the drug treatment arms. The relative risk of post-SWL UTIs for patients receiving prophylaxis was 0.45 (95% confidence interval 0.22 to 0.93). There were some cost variations depending on the antimicrobial regimens used. However, prophylaxis added little to the overall cost of SWL and was cost-beneficial when the costs of serious UTIs requiring inpatient care were considered.

Conclusions.—Giving prophylactic antibiotics before SWL to patients with sterile pretreatment urine reduces the rate of post-SWL UTIs. Prophylaxis is a cost-effective strategy when the costs of inpatient treatment for episodes of sepsis and acute pyelonephritis are accounted for. This cost-effectiveness is based on prophylaxis in the form of sulfamethoxazole/ trimethoprim or Cipro.

▶ Whew! Now here is something we can grab onto and have some justification for our use of prophylactic treatment with antibiotics. The only bad news is that the data result from a meta-analysis.

M. Weintraub, M.D.

Prospective, Randomized, Controlled Study Comparing Two Dosing Regimens of Gentamicin/Oral Ciprofloxacin Switch Therapy for Acute Pyelonephritis
Bailey RR, Begg EJ, Smith AH, et al (Christchurch Hosp, New Zealand)
Clin Nephrol 46:183–186, 1996   12–11

Background.—Many clinicians prefer aminoglycosides for severe gram-negative infections. Recent evidence indicates that aminoglycosides may be as effective, but less nephrotoxic and ototoxic, if given in a single dose, rather than divided doses. A very large IV dose of aminoglycoside followed by a different oral antibiotic may also be effective, as well as a simple and economical therapy.

Methods.—There were 41 evaluable patients with acute pyelonephritis who were hospitalized for antibiotic therapy. Thirty-eight patients were women; the mean patient age was 32 years. Patients were randomly assigned to either a large single dose of gentamicin, 10 mg/kg administered IV, or multiple doses of gentamicin, with an initial dose of 2.5 mg/kg IV, then computer-determined doses using target peak concentrations of 8 mg/L and trough concentrations of 1.5 mg/L. Patients were changed to oral ciprofloxacin either 4 hours after administration of gentamicin or after clinical improvement with the multiple dose regimen. The treatment time was 5 days.

Results.—The single large IV dose of gentamicin was given to 16 patients; 13 were clinically cured, 3 had clinical improvement, and 15 were cured bacteriologically. The multiple dose regimen was given to 25 patients; 24 were clinically cured, 1 had clinical improvement, and 23 were cured bacteriologically. High-tone audiometry was performed before treatment or immediately after the start of treatment and when treatment ended. Ototoxicity was defined as at least 10 dB loss in at least 2 frequencies in both ears. It occurred in 3 of 18 patients given the single large dose and in 7 of 23 patients given the multiple dose regimen. Other side effects and toxicities were mild and were similar in both groups. The single dose of gentamicin was substantially cheaper than the multiple dose protocol.

Discussion.—In these patients with severe acute pyelonephritis, a single large dose of IV gentamicin had similar efficacy and toxicity, compared with a multiple dose regimen, but it was cheaper and more convenient. A single IV dose of gentamicin is more efficient and more comfortable for the patient than prolonged IV dosing.

▶ Studies nowadays are being done for a variety of reasons. This one had an economic reason. The investigators showed substantial cost savings in the case of the single, large IV dose followed by oral ciprofloxacin vs. the continued standard gentamicin therapy. The second reason is found in the comparative toxicity study. Ototoxicity was less in the switch group than in the standard therapy group. Of course, in the United States, we would also be interested in the length of hospitalization, as all these patients were hospitalized. Obviously, hospitalization could have been much shorter in the two-treatment group.

M. Weintraub, M.D.

How Many Antibiotics Are Necessary to Treat Abdominal Trauma Victims?

Sims EH, Thadepalli H, Ganesan K, et al (Drew Univ, Los Angeles; King-Drew Med Ctr, Los Angeles)
Am Surg 63:525–535, 1997   12–12

Introduction.—Although patients undergoing surgery for penetrating abdominal trauma are often given 2 or 3 antibiotics to prevent sepsis, several reports suggest that a single antibiotic is effective. A prospective study evaluated the efficacy of a single antibiotic vs. double-antibiotic and triple-antibiotic regimens in cases of abdominal trauma.

Methods.—Antibiotics used in the randomized, examiner-blinded study were cefoperazone, a third-generation cephalosporin; ceftriaxone plus metronidazole; and the combination of metronidazole, gentamicin, and ampicillin. Patients were given IV antibiotics as soon as the decision was made to explore the abdomen. The duration of therapy was determined by the nature of the injury. Cultures for aerobic and anaerobic bacteria were obtained upon opening and closing of the peritoneum. Patients also had sputum and urine cultures taken and were evaluated every day for local and systemic infections. During the 15-month study, 291 patients met the protocol criteria; 101 were randomized to a single antibiotic regimen, 95 to 2 antibiotics, and 95 to 3 antibiotics. The 3 groups had comparable demographic and clinical characteristics. Most patients were young adults who had sustained gunshot wounds (67.4%) or stab wounds (32.6%).

Results.—The 3 antibiotic therapy groups did not differ significantly in median number of febrile days, morbidity, incisional wound infection, intra-abdominal abscess, septicemia, other infections, hospital stay, or mortality rates. Two patients in each group died. Noninfectious complications were more frequent in the triple-antibiotic group, and this difference was statistically significant.

Conclusion.—A single antibiotic, cefoperazone, was adequate to prevent sepsis in patients undergoing exploration for abdominal trauma. Additional antibiotics to cover for enterococcus may not be required.

▶ What a great antibiotic study! It was prospective, it was randomized, and the examiner was blinded. Therefore, the patient care was excellent and the investigation could go forward. Even the fact that the patients received 1 medication, or 2 or 3 was randomized. I almost made a mistake in reading this paper. I thought that the authors had probably followed a group of people in an epidemiologic study, but this really was a clinical trial, and the end result is that somebody will have to justify the use of treatment to cover for enterococcus in abdominal trauma.

M. Weintraub, M.D.

---

p55 Tumor Necrosis Factor Receptor Fusion Protein in the Treatment of Patients With Severe Sepsis and Septic Shock
Abraham E, for the Ro 45–2081 Study Group (Univ of Colorado, Denver; Centre Hospitalier Universitaire Vaudois, Lausanne, Switzerland; Texas Tech Univ, Lubbock; et al)
JAMA 277:1531–1538, 1997   12–13

Background.—Because tumor necrosis factor-α is implicated in systemic manifestations of severe sepsis and septic shock, the p55 tumor necrosis factor receptor fusion protein (p55-IgG) was evaluated for safety and efficacy in the treatment of severe sepsis or septic shock.

Methods.—A randomized, prospective, multicenter, double-blind, placebo-controlled clinical trial enrolled 498 patients with signs of severe sepsis or septic shock. Interventions, assigned randomly, were placebo or single infusion of 0.083, 0.042, or 0.008 mg of p55-IgG per kilogram, all with standard aggressive medical and surgical care. Clinical condition and laboratory values were monitored at baseline (before treatment) and throughout the 28-day protocol. The primary efficacy variable was 28-day mortality from all causes.

Results.—Interim analysis showed no benefit for the 0.008 mg/kg dose of p55-IgG, which was discontinued. A total of 444 patients from the 3 remaining arms of the study were available for the final analysis on day 28. Of those, 197 (44%) were in refractory septic shock at enrollment; the remaining 247 were in the severe sepsis group (including early septic shock). There was a nonsignificant trend toward reduced 28-day mortality from all causes among all patients treated with p55-IgG (5% reduction vs. placebo for 0.042 mg/kg and 15% reduction vs. placebo for 0.083 mg/kg, $P = 0.30$), primarily as a result of decreased mortality among patients with severe sepsis; there was no survival increase among patients with refractory shock. Overall 28-day mortalities among patients with severe sepsis were 23% for the 0.83 mg/kg group, 37% for the 0.042 mg/kg group, and 36% for the placebo group. Reduction in mortality among patients treated for severe sepsis with the 0.083 mg/kg dose of p55-IgG was 36% ($P = 0.07$), greater among patients with baseline hypotension (48%) than among those without (24%). Significantly improved outcome, which included decrease in mortality from that expected and decreased interleukin-6, was demonstrated in the 0.82 mg/kg group of patients with severe sepsis ($P = 0.01$). Serious adverse events were reported in 65% of patients in the placebo group and 56% in the treatment groups. No hypersensitivity was reported.

Discussion.—Treatment of severe sepsis or early septic shock, but not refractory septic shock, was apparently enhanced by the infusion of 0.083 mg of p55-IgG per kilogram. A large confirmatory clinical trial is underway.

▶ This was a dose-ranging study, but it contains some of the features that have always troubled studies with severe sepsis and septic shock. It's just very difficult to show an effect of anything, just trends. Either our drugs aren't very good, or our method of studying them is not very good, or a combination of these 2 things, plus many others that I can't even contemplate. I hope folks keep looking for something that will help in the treatment of septic shock.

M. Weintraub, M.D.

Antimicrobial Resistance in *Neisseria gonorrhoeae* in the United States, 1988–1994: The Emergence of Decreased Susceptibility to the Fluoroquinolones
Fox KK, Knapp JS, Holmes KK, et al (Ctrs for Disease Control and Prevention, Atlanta, Ga; Emory Univ, Atlanta, Ga; Univ of North Carolina, Chapel Hill; et al)
J Infect Dis 175:1396–1403, 1997   12–14

Purpose.—The current primary treatment for gonorrhea—still an important sexually transmitted disease—is the fluoroquinolones. Previous reports from around the world have described gonococcal strains with reduced susceptibility to fluoroquinolones. New Centers for Disease Control and Prevention data describing the emergence of fluoroquinolone resistance in the United States were reported.

Findings.—The findings were based on susceptibility typing of 35,263 isolates from 27 clinics in the Gonococcal Isolate Surveillance Project. The demographic characteristics of the patients examined were compared with those of nationally reported gonorrhea cases. The rate of chromosomally mediated or plasmid-mediated resistance to penicillin or tetracycline was 30.5% in 1994. The rate of penicillin resistance increased from 8.4% in 1988 to 19.5% in 1991, before decreasing to 15.6% in 1994. The rate of tetracycline resistance decreased from 23.4% in 1988 to 17.3% in 1989, then increased to 21.7% in 1994. The percentage of isolates showing decreased susceptibility to ciprofloxacin increased from 0.4% in 1991 to 1.3% in 1994; the figures included 4 ciprofloxacin-resistant isolates. Strains with decreased susceptibility to ciprofloxacin were more likely to have chromosomally mediated resistance to penicillin and tetracycline and had higher minimal inhibitory concentrations of the broad-spectrum cephalosporins than did ciprofloxacin-susceptible strains.

Conclusion.—These data document the emergence of decreased susceptibility to fluoroquinolone of Neisseria gonorrhoeae in the United States. The clinical significance of strains with decreased susceptibility remains to be determined. The development of fluoroquinolone resistance threatens the future value of these drugs for antigonococcal therapy.

▶ This nationwide laboratory and clinical center collaboration is the only way to find out about things like the impact of the development of resistance in gonorrhea infections. The percentage of resistance varied from Anchorage, Alaska (the lowest), to Long Beach, California (one of the highest). Also, the fact that the figures differed between plasmid-mediated and the chromosomally mediated type of resistance prevented easy characterization. There just is no way that the rate of resistance can be predicted from a particular hospital or clinical setting in 1 part of the country. Of course, some might say that the incidence of resistance in the particular area where your patient lives is really the information needed to treat patients appropriately. But given Americans' propensity for traveling around and for not seeking treatment immediately means that we should keep our eyes open for the development of more severe fluoroquinolone resistance.

M. Weintraub, M.D.

Topical Undecylenic Acid for Herpes Simplex Labialis: A Multicenter, Placebo-controlled Trial

Shafran SD, Sacks SL, Aoki FY, et al (Univ of Saskatchewan, Saskatoon, Canada; Univ of Alberta, Edmonton, Canada; Univ of British Columbia, Vancouver, Canada; et al)

J Infect Dis 176:78–83, 1997   12–15

Background.—Undecylenic acid has been shown to be virucidal against both herpes simplex types 1 and 2 in vitro. It decreases lesion size, new lesion formation, and titer of recoverable virus from lesions of experimentally induced herpes simplex type 1 cutaneous lesions in guinea pigs. The potential use of this agent as a topical antiviral agent for orolabial herpes infection was investigated.

Methods.—Five hundred seventy-three patients with recurrent herpes labialis were enrolled in the multicenter, double-blind, placebo-controlled, patient-initiated trial. Fifteen percent undecylenic acid cream was applied 5 or 6 times a day until crusting, then 3 times a day until healing. Patients were evaluated daily until 48 hours after crusting, then every other day until healing.

Findings.—Undecylenic acid significantly decreased the incidence and duration of viral shedding as well as the duration and severity of itching. However, it did not increase abortive episodes or shorten time to healing, crusting, or progression of lesion size. When treatment was begun during the prodrome, time to crusting was decreased and the area under the symptom-time curve for pain and tenderness was reduced. Although active treatment was generally well tolerated, it caused dysgeusia and local irritation.

Conclusions.—Undecylenic acid 15% cream was found to decrease viral shedding in patients with recurrent herpes labialis. However, the associated clinical benefits are minimal and primarily limited to patients beginning treatment during the prodrome.

▶ The outcome of treatment of herpes labialis was better when patients started treatment during the prodrome. That's really almost universally true with all the many therapies that there are for this annoying and often uncomfortable infectious disease. In the study, it would have been interesting to see a no-treatment group as well. It probably would have helped the undecylenic acid group by increasing its comparative effectiveness. Many times, a dermatologic placebo group does fairly well because it contains the excipients and may protect the lesion or contribute to its healing. It's always daunting to see how little difference there may be between active dermatologic therapy and the placebo ointment, cream, or lotion.

M. Weintraub, M.D.

Epidemiological Study of an Outbreak Due to Multidrug-resistant *Enterobacter aerogenes* in a Medical Intensive Care Unit
Arpin C, Coze C, Rogues AM, et al (Université de Bordeaux II, France; Hôpital Pellegrin, Bordeaux, France)
J Clin Microbiol 34:2163–2169, 1996   12–16

Introduction.—*Enterobacter aerogenes* has become an important pathogen in the hospital setting. During a 10-month period in 1993, 63 strains of *E. aerogenes* were collected from a medical ICU, most of them resistant to multiple antibiotics. Antibiotic resistance phenotyping was used to determine whether these strains were epidemiologically related.

Methods.—The 63 isolates were obtained from 41 medical ICU patients. By comparison, only 46 isolates were collected from 32 patients in other parts of the hospital during the same period. Antibiotic resistance phenotyping, a nonmolecular biology-based method, was used to analyze each isolate. A representative sample of 77 isolates was then analyzed by plasmid restriction analysis, ribotyping, and arbitrarily primed polymerase chain reaction (AP-PCR). Twenty-two strains produced extended-spectrum β-lactamases, which were studied by determination of their isoelectric points and by hybridization of plasmid DNA using specific probes.

Results.—Of the 77 isolates, 21 were susceptible and 56 were resistant to aminoglycosides. There were 15 different plasmid profiles, 14 ribotypes, and 15 AP-PCR patterns. Plasmid profiles differed for the resistant isolates. However, their chromosomal pattern was identical on ribotyping and AP-PCR analysis. Most of these epidemiologically related strains were found in the medical ICU. In contrast, the susceptible strains had differing markers and were mainly found in other units.

Conclusions.—This study documents a nosocomial outbreak of *E. aerogenes* in a medical ICU and the spread of a multidrug-resistant epidemic strain throughout the hospital. It is important to identify patients who carry multidrug-resistant bacteria when they are first admitted, as these strains tend to cause nosocomial outbreaks once they are established. In this situation, ribotyping and AP-PCR can be important discriminatory tools.

▶ *Enterobacter* organisms can cause opportunistic infections in debilitated patients, and the prevalence of these species has greatly increased with the clinical use of extended-spectrum cephalosporins. The bowels of colonized or infected patients are thought to be the reservoir for such nosocomial infections. Once established in a hospital unit, these bugs tend to replace more susceptible resident pathogens and cause nosocomial outbreaks, so it is important to detect patients colonized or infected with resistant bacteria when they are newly admitted to hospital.

L. Lasagna, M.D.

Manipulation of a Hospital Antimicrobial Formulary to Control an Outbreak of Vancomycin-resistant Enterococci
Quale J, Landman D, Saurina G, et al (State Univ of New York Health Science Ctr)
Clin Infect Dis 23:1020–1025, 1996   12–17

Purpose.—Outbreaks of vancomycin-resistant enterococci (VRE) may occur despite hospital infection control measures. At the authors' hospital, despite barrier precautions for patients with VRE infection, nearly one half of inpatients were found to have gastrointestinal colonization with these organisms. The successful management of this problem through changes in the hospital formulary and physician prescribing habits is described.

Methods and Findings.—The changes were made after initial infection control measures failed to control the hospital-wide outbreak of VRE. The hospital antibiotic formulary was changed to limit the use of cefotaxime and vancomycin, and third-generation cephalosporins were replaced with β-lactamase inhibitors. Clindamycin use was restricted at the same time because of an outbreak of *Clostridium difficile* colitis. By 6 months, average monthly antibiotic use decreased by 84% for cefotaxime, 55% for

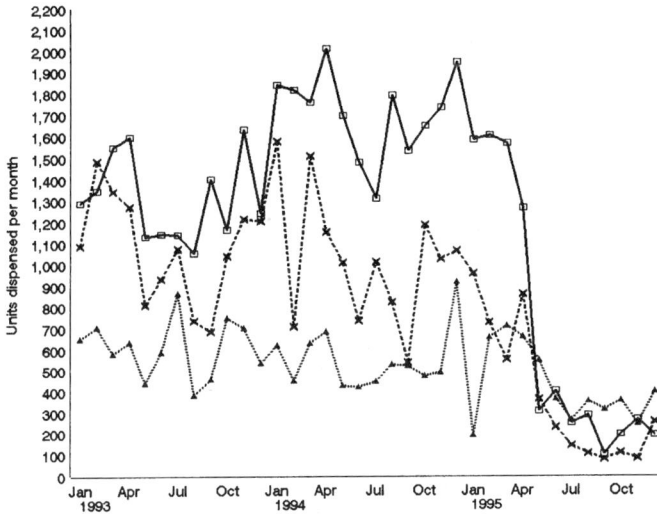

ceftazidine, and 80% for clindamycin (Fig 2). The rate of colonization with VRE decreased from 47% before the intervention to 15% afterward. The number of new patients with positive cultures decreased from 5.4 to 3.3 patients/month. The rate of *C. difficile* diarrhea was significantly reduced at the same time.

Conclusions.—Changes in antibiotic use may reduce outbreaks of VRE in settings where barrier measures have failed. For outbreaks involving multiples strains of VRE, it may be necessary to reduce the use of various broad-spectrum antibiotics, not just vancomycin. Time will tell if the changes made at the authors' hospital lead to sustained reductions in the rate of VRE infection or colonization.

▶ Nosocomial spread of VRE is alarmingly common. Some outbreaks are localized to a single area of a hospital, but others are hospitalwide. Initiation of traditional infection control measures (barrier precautions and surveillance cultures) is not uniformly successful in reducing the spread of VRE.

The hospital described in the preceding abstract had this problem in all of its medical and surgical units despite barrier precautions. The restriction of cefotaxime and vancomycin use and the addition to the formulary of β-lactamase inhibitors to replace third-generation cephalosporins seem to have done the trick. Using gowns and gloves was deemed of minor importance.

L. Lasagna, M.D.

Management of Invasive Candidal Infections: Results of a Prospective, Randomized, Multicenter Study of Fluconazole Versus Amphotericin B and Review of the Literature

Anaissie EJ, Darouiche RO, Abi-Said D, et al (Univ of Texas, Houston; Veterans Affairs Med Ctr, Houston; Methodist Hosp, Houston; et al)

Clin Infect Dis 23:964–972, 1996   12–18

Introduction.—In susceptible patients, hematogenous candidiasis and other invasive organ candidiasis are life-threatening infections. Candidiasis is the 4th most common nosocomial bloodstream infection in the United States, and is associated with a 38% attributed mortality rate and a hospital stay that is prolonged by 30 days. To treat invasive candidiasis, amphotericin B has been used routinely and fluconazole has been used in experimental candidiasis. To compare the activities and toxicities of amphotericin B and fluconazole in the treatment of presumed or proven invasive candidiasis, a prospective, randomized, multicenter study was conducted and a literature review was performed.

Methods.—Treatment with either fluconazole (400 mg daily) or amphotericin B (25 to 50 mg daily; 0.67 mg/kg daily for patients with neutropenia) was given to 164 patients, 60 of whom had neutropenia. At 48 hours, after 4 days, and at the end of therapy, clinical response and survival rates were measured. Disappearance of all clinical and laboratory indicators of infection was defined as a clinical response. For all study reports published from 1980 to 1996, a MEDLINE search was conducted on the use of fluconazole and amphotericin B for treating hematogenous candidiasis.

Results.—There was a similar response rate between fluconazole (66%) and amphotericin B (64%). As related to site of infection, time to defervescence, relapse, pathogen, or survival rate, there were no differences in response between the 2 groups. Adverse effects were more frequent with amphotericin B (35%) than with fluconazole (5%).

Conclusions.—In the treatment of candidal infections, fluconazole is as effective as amphotericin B, and is better tolerated. Fluconazole is the drug of choice for candidal infections caused by fluconazole-susceptible pathogens in hemodynamically stable patients, because of its therapeutic activity and safety profile, and the convenience and lower cost of oral administration. Empiric antifungal therapy is recommended for high-risk patients in view of the high mortality rate associated with hematogenous candidiasis. High-risk patients are those with known risk factors for the disease such as neutropenia of at least 12 weeks' duration or other immunosuppression, those who have no obvious focus of infection, those who remain febrile despite broad-spectrum antibiotic therapy, and those who are colonized by *Candida* species.

▶ Candidiasis is the 4th most common nosocomial bloodstream infection, it significantly prolongs the hospital stay, and it is associated with a 38% attributable mortality rate. Because *Candida* organisms are hard to isolate from blood, antifungal therapy often is given empirically to patients presumed to have invasive candidiasis. In the present study, response rates were similar with fluconazole and amphotericin B, but adverse events were 7 times as common with the latter as with the former. Other studies agree.

L. Lasagna, M.D.

Susceptibility of Vancomycin-resistant Enterococci to Environmental Disinfectants

Anderson RL, Carr JH, Bond WW, et al (US Dept of Health and Human Services, Atlanta, Ga)
Infect Control Hosp Epidemiol 18:195–199, 1997   12–19

Background.—Concern has arisen regarding environmental contamination within hospitals by vancomycin-resistant enterococci (VRE). Susceptibilities of both VRE and vancomycin-sensitive enterococci (VSE) to commercial, hospital-grade disinfectants were tested.

Methods.—A microbial suspension test was used to determine inactivation by various test dilutions of disinfectant solutions of 2 VRE and 2 VSE strains. Four preparations were evaluated: 2 quaternary ammonium germicidal detergents, a phenolic germicidal detergent, and an iodophor detergent-germicide. All were evaluated both at recommended use dilutions and extended dilutions (dilutions greater than recommended). Inocula were exposed to various concentrations of detergents for varying durations, neutralized, and plated. Colonies were counted to produce curves for various disinfectant exposures.

Results.—Both VRE and VSE were killed by 15-second exposure to at-use dilutions of all detergents. Extended dilution curves were similar for VRE and VSE, indicating similar inactivation kinetics. Quaternary ammonium solutions showed greater extended microbicidal activity than did either phenolic or iodophor disinfectants.

Conclusions.—Some concern has been raised that VRE might be more resistant than VSE to germicidal detergents used in hospital disinfection. No such difference was found, and no need is currently seen for the use of germicides with higher potency in the rooms of patients with VRE.

▶ Physicians don't often think enough about the use of environmental disinfectants. Their use is most likely associated with housekeeping functions in hospitals. Still, we have to think about them because, in many cases, machines and eating surfaces, as well as areas all around the patient's room, may be treated with disinfectants, which might have lost their ability to kill VRE. We too often depend on the hospital infection monitoring committee to handle those things, but I think all of us have to participate. Fortunately, both VSE and VRE can still be killed by even greatly diluted environmental disinfectants.

M. Weintraub, M.D.

Parental Attitudes Do Not Explain Underimmunization

Strobino D, Keane V, Holt E, et al (Johns Hopkins School of Hygiene and Public Health, Baltimore, Md; Univ of Maryland, Baltimore)
Pediatrics 98:1076–1083, 1996   12–20

Background.—The reasons for underimmunization are not completely clear. A community-based study of the effect of family knowledge and attitudes on immunization rates was reported.

Methods.—The parents of 557 children younger than 2 years of age in the poorest census tracts of Baltimore were interviewed. Data regarding immunization status were obtained from the children's medical records.

Findings.—Mothers were well informed regarding immunizations and generally had favorable attitudes toward immunizing their children. Immunization status was more strongly associated with the sociodemographic characteristics of the children than the protection motivation theory variables. However, the children of mothers who believed that timing of vaccination did not matter were less likely to be immunized than those of mothers who thought it did matter. Also, children whose parents believed in the safety of multiple immunizations were less likely to be immunized than children whose parents did not believe in this.

Conclusion.—Parental attitudes and beliefs appear to have little effect on the immunization status of their children. African-American children whose mothers are young and who have many siblings, live in poor urban areas, and do not attend the Women, Infants and Children program may be at greatest risk for delayed immunization.

▶ A goal has been set for the year 2000: 90% of children will be immunized with the basic vaccines by the time they are 2 years old. But we are not making great progress toward achieving this goal; we are probably protecting against diphtheria, pertussis, tetanus, polio, mumps, measles, and rubella in only two thirds of our child population, and the figure is less than that for children from poor families. This study suggests that this underimmunization is not just a reflection of uninformed parents or parents with a negative attitude toward vaccines.

L. Lasagna, M.D.

Cost-effectiveness of Incorporating Inactivated Poliovirus Vaccine Into the Routine Childhood Immunization Schedule

Miller MA, Sutter RW, Strebel PM, et al (Ctrs for Disease Control and Prevention, Atlanta, Ga)
JAMA 276:967–971, 1996   12–21

Introduction.—Poliomyelitis vaccination routinely has involved 4 doses of live oral poliovirus vaccine (OPV) since the 1960s. In 1996, the Advisory Committee on Immunization Practices adopted a new recommended schedule of 2 doses of inactivated poliovirus vaccine (IPV) followed by 2 doses of OPV. A cost-benefit and cost-effectiveness analysis was conducted to determine the economic consequences of a greater reliance on IPV.

Methods.—Models were created to simulate the outcomes of 3 poliomyelitis vaccine schedules using estimates of national poliovirus vaccination coverage and national surveillance data for vaccine-associated paralytic poliomyelitis (VAPP). The model used a cohort of children up to 6 years of age who were given 4 doses of OPV, 4 doses of IPV, or 2 doses of IPV followed by 2 doses of OPV. The main outcome measures were annual societal incremental cost relative to the current schedule for the cost-benefit model, and cost per VAPP case prevented for the cost-effectiveness model.

Results.—The estimated cost of 15.4 million doses of OPV administered yearly is $375 million for a schedule of OPV doses only. The additional cost for an IPV-only schedule would be $28.1 million; for a sequential schedule, it would be $14.7 million. The cost per case of VAPP prevented was estimated to be $3 million for children receiving IPV only and $3.1 million for children receiving a sequential schedule. The outcomes were most sensitive to the number of extra visits that would occur to avoid multiple injections.

Conclusions.—At current vaccine prices and current costs of VAPP, the introduction of IPV into the routine vaccination schedule would not be cost-effective. These costs are higher than those of other public health prevention programs, but may be justified because VAPP continues to occur as a result of government-mandated vaccination policies in the United States.

▶ The Salk and Sabin vaccines have essentially eliminated wild poliovirus as a cause of poliomyelitis in the western hemisphere, but a few cases occur each year that are related to the attenuated virus in the oral vaccine. This study shows how much it would cost to use IPV instead of OPV. The latter does provide an important benefit—mucosal immunity to prevent the spread of imported wild poliovirus. The goal now is to repeat the smallpox story (i.e., eliminate poliomyelitis on this planet by the year 2000) so that we could halt all poliovirus vaccination programs.

L. Lasagna, M.D.

Clinical Varicella Following Varicella Vaccination: Don't Be Fooled

Feder HM Jr, LaRussa P, Steinberg S, et al (Univ of Connecticut, Farmington; Columbia Univ, New York)
Pediatrics 99:897–899, 1997   12–22

Background.—Adverse effects are uncommon after administration of varicella vaccine to healthy persons. The development of a high fever and more than 100 varicella lesions 2 weeks after varicella vaccination in a previously healthy boy, 8 years, is described.

Case Report.—Three days after the boy's varicella vaccination, a 10-day-tapered course of oral prednisone (at a maximum dose of 1.7 mg/kg/day) was begun for allergic rhinitis. Nine days after the prednisone was initiated, the boy had fatigue, myalgias, fever, and a vesicular eruption on his face and trunk. No known exposure to varicella had occurred. His pediatrician diagnosed varicella, prescribed oral acyclovir (80 mg/kg/day for 5 days), and, concerned that the prednisone had made the boy susceptible to vaccine-induced disease, referred him for further evaluation at a university health center. Forty-eight hours after the patient was seen at that center, he became afebrile and all the lesions had crusted. The results of a culture done on referral were positive for varicella-zoster virus. Further analysis showed it to be a wild-type varicella-zoster virus.

Conclusions.—Apparent severe reactions to varicella vaccine need to be investigated, so that the safety and efficacy of this vaccine can be better defined. Reports of the possible transmission of vaccine-strain varicella-zoster virus have been filed with the manufacturer, who has established a registry for reports of adverse reactions.

▶ Adverse effects of varicella vaccine in healthy individuals are unusual and usually take the form of varicelliform eruptions. In the case discussed here, high-technology laboratory analysis showed that the villain with regard to the rash and high fever was *not* a vaccine strain, but a wild-strain varicella-zoster virus.

L. Lasagna, M.D.

Epidemiology of Invasive Pneumococcal Disease in Southern California: Implications for the Design and Conduct of a Pneumococcal Conjugate Vaccine Efficacy Trial

Zangwill KM, Vadheim CM, Vannier AM, et al (Harbor UCLA Med Ctr, Torrance, Calif; UCLA Ctr for Vaccine Research, Torrance, Calif; Kaiser Permanente Southern California Region, North Hollywood)
J Infect Dis 174:752–759, 1996   12–23

Background.—A better understanding of the epidemiology of pneumococcal disease will help improve the development and assessment of pneumococcal conjugate vaccine (PCV). The results of an epidemiologic study conducted in a large HMO population were reported.

Methods and Findings.—In a population-based prospective surveillance of invasive pneumococcal disease performed in southern California between 1992 and 1995, 814 patients were identified for an incidence of 12.5 per 100,000 individuals per year. The incidence per 100,000 among individuals aged 2 years or younger, 5 years or younger, and 65 years or older was 145, 72, and 32, respectively (Table 1). In more than 95% of the

TABLE 1.—Invasive Pneumococcal Disease: Clinical Presentation by Age

Clinical Presentation†	Incidence* (No. of Cases) in Age Group				Mortality* in Age Group	
	All Ages	≤2 yr	3–64 yr	≥65 yr	≤2 yr	≥65 yr
Bacteremia	13 (796)	143 (249)	6 (368)	31 (179)	1.7	5
Pneumonia	6 (385)	17 (29)	4 (209)	26 (147)	0	4
Meningitis	0.8 (53)	10 (18)	<1 (30)	<1 (5)	0	<1
Otitis media	0.9 (55)	20 (34)	<1 (20)	<1 (1)	<1	0
Arthritis	<1 (20)	5 (8)	<1 (7)	<1 (5)	0	0
Cellulitis	<1 (22)	8 (14)	<1 (6)	<1 (2)	0	0
Osteomyelitis	<1 (5)	2 (3)	<1 (2)	0 (0)	0	0
Other	<1 (10)	<1 (1)	<1 (7)	<1 (2)	0	0
Total	13 (814)	145 (253)	7 (375)	32 (184)	1.7	5

*Per 100,000 population per year.
†Several patients had more than 1 clinical diagnosis.
(Courtesy of Zangwill KM, Vadheim CM, Vannier AM, et al: Epidemiology of invasive pneumococcal disease in southern California: Implications for the design and conduct of a pneumococcal conjugate vaccine efficacy trial. *J Infect Dis* 174:752–759, 1996. Published by The University of Chicago. Copyright 1996 by The University of Chicago. All rights reserved.)

patients, bacteremia was involved. The incidence of meningitis was 0.8 per 100,000. Seventy-nine percent of the isolates were obtained in the outpatient setting in children aged 2 years and younger as compared with 16% of the isolates in those aged 15 years and older. Eighty percent of the isolates were serotypes included in heptavalent PCVs under investigation. The greatest risk of having an isolate resistant to penicillin occurred in children aged 2 years or younger. High-level resistance among resistant isolates rose from 4% to 21% during a 3-year period.

Conclusions.—A PCV efficacy trial should target children 2 years old or younger and assess protection against invasive disease. Enhanced surveillance for invasive pneumococcal disease in the outpatient setting would markedly facilitate such a study.

► *Streptococcus pneumoniae* remains an important cause of serious infection, but it is potentially vaccine-preventable. Deaths in the United States from such infections are said to total 40,000 annually. Meanwhile, resistance of this microorganism to penicillin is increasing. Up until now, pneumococcal vaccines have not been immunogenic in children under 2 years of age, but the success with *Haemophilus influenzae* conjugate vaccines in young children has raised hopes that the newer vaccines now being studied will allow successful vaccination in infants.

L. Lasagna, M.D.

Framing Effects on Expectations, Decisions, and Side Effects Experienced: The Case of Influenza Immunization

O'Connor AM, Pennie RA, Dales RE (Univ of Ottawa, Ont, Canada; McMaster Univ, Hamilton, Ont, Canada)

J Clin Epidemiol 49:1271–1276, 1996   12–24

Background.—Explanations of the risks and benefits associated with vaccinations may be framed positively—in terms of the percentage of patients who remain free of disease and adverse vaccine effects—or negatively—in terms of the percentage who acquire the disease or have adverse effects. The influences of positive or negative "frames" on patient expectations, decisions, decisional conflict, and reported side effects were investigated.

Methods and Findings.—Two hundred ninety-two previously immunized patients with chronic respiratory or cardiac disease were randomly assigned to receive risk-benefit information framed positively or negatively. Immunization rates and decisional conflict scores were similar in the 2 groups. Patients receiving a positively framed explanation had more realistic expectations of adverse vaccine effects, fewer systemic side effects, and less work absenteeism.

Conclusions.—Contrary to expectation, the way in which benefit-risk information was framed apparently did not influence these patients' decisions, possibly because of the patients' awareness of their higher risk of influenza complications and greater desire to follow recommendations. The common practice of describing the probabilities of adverse effects with negative frames may need to be reassessed, because it appears to have a negative effect on self-reported adverse effects and work absenteeism.

▶ Several studies have reported that framing information negatively affects at least hypothetic treatment decisions. In the choice between surgery and radiation therapy, for example postoperative mortality risk discourages more people from surgery when it is described as 10% mortality rather than 90% survival. Similarly, chemotherapy treatments are interpreted as less desirable when benefit is described as lessening mortality rather than increasing survival.

This study attempted to discover whether real life decisions (not hypothetic choices) would be affected by framing. In fact, decisions seemed not to be affected differentially, but negative framing did increase self-reported side effects and work absenteeism. It is not possible to state whether there were actually more side effects or patients were simply more *aware* of them. In any case, however, the increased absenteeism looks as if it could be decreased by positive framing.

L. Lasagna, M.D.

Influenza Vaccination of Health Care Workers in Long-term–care Hospitals Reduces the Mortality of Elderly Patients
Potter J, Stott DJ, Roberts MA, et al (Univ of Glasgow, Scotland; Greater Glasgow Health Board, Scotland; Western Infirmary Glasgow, Scotland)
J Infect Dis 175:1–6, 1997   12–25

Objective.—Because of the health risks to elderly patients caused by influenza, the Centers for Disease Control recommend vaccination. Vaccination of health care workers (HCWs) caring for the elderly has been suggested as a means of reducing the transmission to patients. Results of a study assessing whether vaccination of HCWs caring for long-term-care elderly patients reduces the incidence of influenza, lower respiratory tract infection, and death were evaluated.

Methods.—On October 31, 1994, the vaccination status of 1,059 patients (302 men), aged 55–119 years, in 12 geriatric long-term-care hospitals in Glasgow was assessed. Six hospitals had an "opt-out" policy where patients were vaccinated unless they refused or had a contraindication, and 6 hospitals had an "opt-in" policy where patients were vaccinated only if relatives requested it. Staff vaccination status was also recorded. Four groups resulted: staff and patients unvaccinated (S0P0), staff vaccinated and patients not vaccinated (SVP0), staff unvaccinated and patients vaccinated (S0PV), and staff and patients vaccinated (SVPV). Vaccination began in October 1994, and patients were monitored for symptoms and signs through the end of March 1995. Deaths were recorded.

Results.—There was a significant reduction in mortality from 17% in the S0PV and S0P0 groups to 10% in the SVPV and SVP0 groups. There was no significant difference in mortality between hospitals that offered or did not offer vaccination to patients. There was a significant difference in the prevalence of influenza-like illnesses in patients in sites that vaccinated HCWs.

Conclusion.—Whereas influenza vaccination of HCWs reduced mortality in long-term-care elderly patients, vaccination of the patients themselves did not decrease mortality.

▶ Perhaps presenting results, such as shown in this study, to HCWs will improve their percentage of immunization. Perhaps not.

M. Weintraub, M.D.

New and Improved Vaccines: Promising Weapons Against Varicella, Hepatitis A, and Typhoid Fever
Conrad DA, Jenson HB (Univ of Texas, San Antonio)
Postgrad Med 100:113–118, 121–127, 1996   12–26

Objective.—Four new vaccines have recently been approved for use in the United States: the live-virus varicella vaccine, 2 inactivated-virus vaccines against hepatitis A virus, and a purified polysaccharide typhoid vaccine. These diverse preparations raise some complex issues related to their use. The 4 new vaccines are reviewed, with focus on their most appropriate use.

Varicella Virus Vaccine.—The main benefit of the varicella vaccine is not to prevent chickenpox per se but to avoid its serious complications. The vaccine is indicated for all children aged 12 months through 12 years. It may also be given to certain high-risk groups. There are concerns about waning immunity, but these are insufficient to withhold vaccination. The cost of universal vaccination is justifiable from a medical and financial standpoint.

Hepatitis A Virus Vaccine.—Two inactivated vaccines against hepatitis A virus have been developed: Havrix and Vaqta. They are nearly 100% effective in producing immunity to hepatitis A virus and in preventing the associated disease. The vaccines are recommended for use in high-risk groups, including certain racial groups and children in communities with high rates of hepatitis A. The main indication is travel to countries endemic for this disease, including Mexico and all other developing countries. The vaccines may be given with immune serum globulin in patients requiring both immediate and short-term protection.

Typhoid Fever Vaccines.—Typhoid fever is still an important problem in some parts of the world. The new parenteral purified polysaccharide vaccine is 1 of 3 licensed vaccines. All 3 vaccines are of demonstrated efficacy, although recipients should still practice enteric precautions. The new parenteral vaccine is indicated for high-risk children older than 2 years of age. It replaces the older parenteral heat-phenol inactivated vaccine, which is the only typhoid vaccine approved for children aged 6 months to 2 years.

Discussion.—These 4 diverse new vaccines are important additions to our immunization options. Immunization recommendations will probably change quickly in the future. Universal varicella vaccination is recommended, and universal vaccination for hepatitis A virus may be recommended soon. Typhoid vaccination will probably continue to be recommended for patients in contact with the causative organism or those traveling to endemic areas.

▶ Vaccines still represent the only way to eliminate an infectious disease. Of these 4 new Food and Drug Administration–approved vaccines, the one against chickenpox is perhaps the most important. Although varicella-zoster virus infection in mostly self-limited, about 10,000 persons are hospitalized each year in the United States for complications; approximately 100 of these die. Furthermore, 1%–2% of persons who have had this infection have a reactivation of the virus to cause herpes zoster, an unpleasant disease in the aged, with possible post-herpetic neuralgia.

Although the varicella vaccine is recommended for all children, the hepatitis A virus and typhoid vaccines are recommended only for high-risk groups.

L. Lasagna, M.D.

13 Neoplastic Diseases

Why Has Induction Chemotherapy for Advanced Head and Neck Cancer Become a United States Community Standard of Practice?

Harari PM (Univ of Wisconsin, Madison)

J Clin Oncol 15:2050–2055, 1997

13–1

Background.—The use of induction chemotherapy for advanced head and neck cancer has become common in the United States, despite the failure of clinical trials for 2 decades to demonstrate a clear benefit in locoregional tumor control or overall survival. Some of the factors that may have contributed to this were studied.

Methods.—A total of 300 community cancer specialists were mailed a questionnaire to elicit data on their treatment approaches for patients with locoregionally advanced, nonmetastatic head and neck cancer. The response rate was 73%.

Findings.—The most common treatment approach, used by 61% of the respondents, was sequential chemoradiation. Specifically, these physicians used induction chemotherapy with fluorouracil (5-FU) and cisplatin followed by radiation therapy. Only 4% of respondents gave induction chemotherapy in controlled clinical trials. The main reasons cited for using induction chemotherapy were the desire to improve locoregional tumor control (67%), to improve overall survival (56%), to maintain a spirit of multidisciplinary care (34%), to improve quality of life (29%), and to reduce distant metastases (26%).

Conclusions.—Despite the lack of clear evidence that induction chemotherapy improves locoregional control or overall survival in patients with advanced head and neck cancer, this treatment has become common among U.S. community cancer specialists. Furthermore, more than half the physicians responding to the current survey specifically identified improved locoregional control and overall survival as primary objectives for using induction chemotherapy in such patients.

▶ The value of chemotherapy for squamous cell cancers of the head and neck is a contentious area, with a lot of disagreement about how to interpret the published literature. One important question is whether chemotherapy is best given before, during, or after radiation.

This review of published trials and meta-analysis over the last quarter century concludes that there is no evidence of benefit for these patients when treated with 5–FU and cisplatin induction chemotherapy. So why is such use common practice?

L. Lasagna, M.D.

Survival of Patients With Limited-stage Small Cell Lung Cancer Treated With Individualized Chemotherapy Selected by In Vitro Drug Sensitivity Testing
Cortazar P, Gazdar AF, Woods E, et al (Natl Cancer Inst, Bethesda, Md; Natl Naval Med Ctr, Bethesda, Md)
Clin Cancer Res 3:741–747, 1997   13–2

Background.—To improve the therapeutic benefit of chemotherapy, various types of in vitro drug sensitivity testing have been developed for identifying drugs likely to kill tumor cells in a given patient. Only a few prospective studies have chosen chemotherapy regimens from assay results. There may be greater benefit from drug sensitivity testing in cases of more sensitive cancers. Patients with limited-stage small-cell lung cancer are twice as likely as patients with extensive-stage disease to have a complete response to chemotherapy. The value of determining individualized chemotherapy protocols by in vitro drug sensitivity testing for limited-stage small-cell lung cancer was evaluated, as well as patient response and survival.

Methods.—There were 54 patients with limited-stage small-cell lung cancer who had not had previous treatment. Fresh tumor specimens were obtained. The in vitro sensitivity of tumor cells to different drugs was determined by differential staining cytotoxicity assays. An in vitro best regimen was determined from these results. This regimen was a combination of 3 of 7 active drugs with proven efficacy in small-cell lung cancer.

Results.—Initial treatment was 4 cycles of etoposide/cisplatin and concurrent radiation therapy. Patients were then treated with 4 cycles of individualized chemotherapy based on results of drug sensitivity testing when available, or 4 cycles of vincristine, doxorubicin, and cyclophosphamide. Biopsy to obtain specimens for drug sensitivity testing was done in 18 patients. The median time from diagnosis to start of treatment was 22 days for the 18 patients who had biopsy, and 21 days for patients who did not have biopsy. The median time from thoracic biopsy to start of chemotherapy was 4 days. In vitro drug sensitivity testing was done in 10 patients, and in vitro best regimen was administered to 8 patients. The median survival was 38.5 months in these 8 patients and 19 months for the 46 patients treated with empiric chemotherapy (Fig 2).

Discussion.—Determining individualized chemotherapy regimens is time consuming but feasible and safe in patients with small-cell lung cancer. In these patients, individualized chemotherapy was associated with longer survival, but because of the study design, other factors could have been involved.

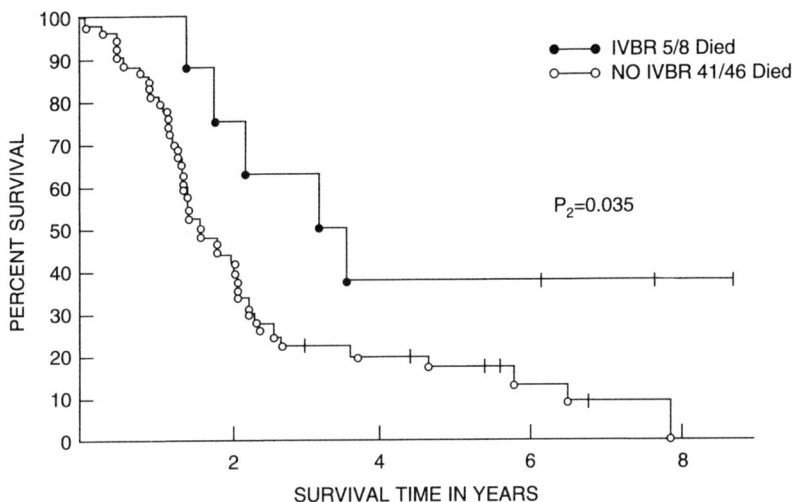

FIGURE 2.—Actuarial survival of patients who were treated with their in vitro best regimen (IVBR) (*solid circles*) compared with survival of patients treated with empiric chemotherapy (*open circles*). Tick marks represent patients still alive. (Courtesy of Cortazar P, Gazdar AF, Woods E, et al: Survival of patients with limited-stage small cell lung cancer treated with individualized chemotherapy selected by in vitro drug sensitivity testing. *Clin Cancer Res* 3:741–747, 1997.)

▶ Periodically, somebody tries to use some in vitro drug sensitivity testing to individualize chemotherapy for patients with cancer. Such an approach is eminently reasonable, and this study provides some hope for its clinical utility.

L. Lasagna, M.D.

Comparison of Melphalan and Prednisone With Vincristine, Carmustine, Melphalan, Cyclophosphamide, and Prednisone in the Treatment of Multiple Myeloma: Results of Eastern Cooperative Oncology Group Study E2479
Oken MM, Harrington DP, Abramson N, et al (Univ of Minnesota, Minneapolis; Harvard School of Public Health, Boston; Baptist Regional Cancer Inst, Jacksonville, Fla; et al)
Cancer 79:1561–1567, 1997   13–3

Background.—A regimen of melphalan and prednisone (MP) is standard treatment for multiple myeloma. Because cure is rarely achieved with the available treatments for myeloma, current treatment goals are long-term survival, relief from symptoms, and ability to function. A response rate of 78% and a median survival of 38 months have been reported in patients with myeloma after treatment with vincristine, carmustine, melphalan, cyclophosphamide and prednisone (VBMCP).

Methods.—There were 479 patients with multiple myeloma randomly assigned to treatment with MP for 4-week cycles or VBMCP for 5-week cycles. After 1 year, patients received maintenance therapy with MP for 6-week cycles, or VBMCP for 8-week cycles until relapse. Patients who did not respond to MP were eligible for crossover to the VBMCP regimen.

Results.—An objective response was seen in 51% of patients given MP and 72% of patients given VBMCP. Patients given VBMCP also had a longer response. Overall survival was similar in both groups. The 5-year survival rate was 26% in patients given VBMCP and 19% in patients given MP. Patients given VBMCP had more nausea, peripheral nerve toxicity, alopecia, and neutropenia. The infection rate was similar in both groups. Both regimens were well tolerated, except that a higher risk of death was seen with VBMCP in elderly patients who were confined to bed. The rate of late secondary myelodysplastic syndrome and acute leukemia was similar in both groups. In patients who did not respond to MP, crossover to VBMCP was minimally effective, with an objective response rate of 20% and median survival of 11 months after crossover.

Discussion.—In these patients, VBMCP produced superior and longer responses compared with the responses seen with MP. Survival associated with these 2 regimens was similar. It may be advantageous to base new treatment regimens on VBMCP rather than MP. Promising results have been seen with alternating courses of interferon and VBMCP.

▶ For many years, the standard therapy for multiple myeloma has been MP. The 5–drug regimen evaluated in this paper seems to be superior with regard to objective responses and duration thereof, but average survival time does not seem to be improved. Disappointing.

L. Lasagna, M.D.

Treatment of Metastatic Melanoma With Combined Chemotherapy Containing Cisplatin, Vinblastine and Dacarbazine (CVD) and Biotherapy Using Interleukin-2 and Interferon-α

Legha SS, Ring S, Bedikian A, et al (Univ of Texas M.D. Anderson Cancer Ctr, Houston)
Ann Oncol 7:827–835, 1996   13–4

Introduction.—The usual treatment for metastatic melanoma has been chemotherapy and/or biological agents used separately. The efficacy of combined chemotherapy using cisplatin, vinblastine, DTIC (CVD) and biological therapy using interleukin-2 (IL-2) and interferon-α (INF-α) was evaluated in patients with advanced inoperable metastatic melanoma and no prior chemotherapy or biotherapy treatment.

Methods.—Patients were randomly assigned to a CVD or biotherapy regimen. The CVD regimen was cisplatin 20 mg/m²/day × 4, vinblastine 1.6 mg/m²/day × 5, and DTIC 800 mg/m²/day × 1, repeated at 21-day intervals. The biotherapy regimen was IL-2, 9 × 10⁶ IU/m²/day × 4 days and INF-α 5 × 10⁶ U/m²/day subcutaneously × 5 days. The CVD and biotherapy regimens were integrated in an alternating manner at 6-week intervals in 40 patients and sequentially in 62 patients.

Results.—In the alternating biochemotherapy program, there were 2 complete responses (CRs) and 11 partial responses (PRs). The overall response rate was 33% in 39 evaluable patients. In the sequential biochemotherapy group, there were 14 CRs and 23 PRs. The overall response rate was 60%. The CVD/Bio sequence resulted in a 69% response rate, compared with a response rate of 50% for the Bio/CVD sequence. The duration of PRs was a median of 8 months. The duration of CRs was 3+ years, with 10 of 16 patients disease free for periods of 3+ to 6+ years at final evaluation. The median survival was 13 and 9 months, respectively, in patients receiving sequential biochemotherapy and CVD. Biochemotherapy was associated with severe toxicity that included intense myelosuppression, infections, IL-2–induced constitutional toxicity, and hypotension. The IL-2–induced toxicities were usually managed during hospitalization, but 15% of patients required transfer to the ICU for treatment of complications associated with treatment.

Conclusions.—The sequential combination of CVD and IL-2 plus INF-α seemed to create an increase in the number of durable responses in patients with advanced malignant melanoma. Toxicity was severe but considered manageable. An increase in survival was observed with the biochemotherapy regimen that was not detected with the CVD regimen.

▶ The toxicity of this treatment combination is relatively great and seems, at least to me, really serious. The constitutional toxicity category, which consists of fever and fatigue often with chills and muscle pain, sometimes labeled a "flu-like syndrome," occurred at level 2 in 92% of the people in this study. It makes you want to be certain that continuous therapy with these drugs (as well as many others) that causes such a high symptom level, produces a real benefit in terms of the length and quality of life.

M. Weintraub, M.D.

Clinical and Immunomodulatory Effects of Repetitive 2–Day Cycles of High-dose Continuous Infusion IL-2
Englehardt M, Wirth K, Mertelsmann R, et al (Univ of Freiburg, Germany; Goedecke/Parke Davis, Freiburg, Germany)
Eur J Cancer 33:1050–1054, 1997   13–5

Introduction.—Malignant melanoma (MM) and renal cell carcinoma (RCC) are two chemotherapy-resistant tumors with a particularly dismal prognosis. High-dose interleukin-2 (HD IL-2) offers promising antitumor activity, but the optimal schedule balancing efficacy and toxicity remains to be defined. The efficacy of a treatment schedule consisting of 5 repetitive cycles of high-dose recombinant (rh) IL-2 (24×10^6 U/m^2/day) administered weekly on 2 consecutive days by continuous intravenous infusion was reported.

Methods.—Of 19 patients treated with HD IL-2, 17 had metastatic RCC and 2 had stage IV MM. Treatment was administered as described and patients were followed up for toxicity. Response rate was evaluated at 4 and 8 weeks after IL-2 therapy. A second IL-2 cycle was recommended for patients with complete or partial response or stable disease after 8 weeks rest.

Results.—Eight of 17 patients with RCC responded to HD IL-2: 2 had a complete response, 3 had a partial response, 1 had a minor response, and 2 had stable disease (median response duration, 11.5+ months). The remaining 9 patients with RCC and both patients with MM had disease progression. Toxicity was generally well tolerated with the HD IL-2 regimen. Interleukin-2 therapy induced a noticeable increase in lymphocytes and proinflammatory cytokines IL-9, IL-5, γ-interferon, tumor necrosis factor-α (TNF-α), and TNF-β that peaked in cycle 3. The serum levels of these cytokines, natural killer (NK) cells, T cells, and eosinophils decreased with subsequent therapy, and serum IL-10 levels progressively increased. Progressive increases in IL-10 were observed, with maximum levels achieved after the fifth week of therapy. Absolute numbers of activated T cells and NK cells remained at increased levels for at least 4 weeks after treatment cessation, compared with baseline levels.

Conclusions.—This regimen was well-tolerated. It is suggested that further protocols include 3 weekly 2-day cycles, separated by a 4-week treatment-free interval before continuing therapy.

▶ It seems to me that many of these cancer chemotherapeutic interventions, and rheumatoid arthritis treatments, and perhaps even the drugs for amyotrophic lateral sclerosis should be individualized for the patient. We may not know what the best therapy is and we have no clue from the groups of patients. If we only had markers that could be measured to help individualize the therapy, the outcome would be better. Still, giving 2-day cycles of IL-2, which reduces the adverse effects, can be very helpful. Now, we either ought to have a better methodology for determining the therapy in groups of patients, or measure it in individual patients.

M. Weintraub, M.D.

Double-blind, Multicenter, Randomized Trial to Compare the Effect of Two Doses of Adrenocorticotropic Hormone Versus Placebo in Controlling Delayed Emesis After High-dose Cisplatin in Adult Patients With Cancer
Passalacqua R, Cocconi G, Caminiti C, et al (Inst of Pharmacology, Milan, Italy)
J Clin Oncol 15:2467–2473, 1997   13–6

Background.—Adrenocorticotropic hormone (ACTH) effectively prevents acute cisplatin-induced vomiting. Two different doses of the depot formulation of ACTH were compared in a double-blind, placebo-controlled, randomized trial.

Methods.—One hundred fifty-two patients were given cisplatin, 60 to 120 mg/m², on day 1, and a combination of dexamethasone, 20 mg, plus ondansetron or metoclopramide to prevent acute emesis. Twenty-four hours after cisplatin administration, the patients randomly received placebo or ACTH, 1 mg intramuscularly or 2 mg intramuscularly plus another dose of 1 mg on day 4.

Findings.—All but 2 patients were evaluable. During the 5 days of the study, delayed vomiting was less frequent in patients given ACTH, 2 mg plus 1 mg, than in patients given ACTH, 1 mg, or placebo (28%, 38%, and 65%, respectively). The differences were most pronounced on days 2 and 3. No significant differences were seen among the 3 groups on days 4, 5, and 6. Severity of delayed emesis, expressed as the mean number of emetic episodes per day, was 0.48 in the 2-mg ACTH group, 0.70 in the 1-mg ACTH group, and 0.80 in the placebo group. Adrenal cortisol secretion increased rapidly after ACTH injection, but was suppressed for about 44 hours in the placebo group. In all groups, toxicity was mild and transient.

Conclusions.—A 2-mg dose of ACTH given 24 hours after cisplatin administration is superior to a 1-mg dose. Further research is needed to verify whether ACTH activity is mediated only by adrenal corticosteroids.

▶ The advent of 5-HT$_3$ receptor antagonists has been a wonderful addition to the pharmacopeia of antiemetic agents when one is trying to control acute vomiting after cisplatin. These drugs are not helpful when the patient has delayed emesis (1 to 5 days after such treatment), perhaps because different pathogenetic mechanisms are involved.

Adrenocorticotropic hormone seems to be reasonably effective in this situation in a dose-related fashion. Whether corticosteroids would work as well or better is not known.

L. Lasagna, M.D.

14 Neurologic Diseases

Families Are Content to Discontinue Antiepileptic Drugs at Different Risks Than Their Physicians
Gordon K, MacSween J, Dooley J, et al (Dalhousie Univ, Halifax, Nova Scotia, Canada)
Epilepsia 37:557–562, 1996   14–1

Objective.—Although it is common practice to recommend discontinuation of antiepileptic drugs in children after a sufficient seizure-free period, some families accept the decision more readily than others. The factors influencing families' and physicians' treatment decisions were explored to determine the frequency of disagreement between the two.

Methods.—Between October 1991 and August 1992, the families of 76 children, aged 1 to 21 years, attending a pediatric epilepsy clinic and having been seizure free for at least 3 months, completed a survey about opinions of acceptable risk of seizure recurrence after discontinuing medication and factors that might be useful in predicting their responses. Their physicians filled out a survey that included acceptable risk of seizure recurrence, a prediction of the families' decision, and predictive factors including a subjective assessment of family anxiety. Survey results for the 2 groups were compared statistically.

Results.- The 1-year seizure-free rate is 30% to 40%. Although 31 families were unwilling to discontinue medication with a recurrence risk of 25%, 15 families were willing to discontinue treatment when their recurrence risk was more than 75%. Risk-averse behavior increased with increasing frequency of previous seizures ($\geq$ 1/week, < 1/week, and > 2/year, and $\leq$ 2/yr), multiple vs. single seizure types, and when the child had repeated grades in school. Whereas families and physicians accepted similar risks (35% and 40%, respectively), there was no correlation between their answers ($r^2=-0.07$). None of the responding physicians was able to predict the families' risk responses ($r^2=0.09$).

Conclusion.—Whereas the 1-year seizure-free rate of 30% to 40% was unacceptable to approximately half the families, 20% of families would accept a risk higher than 75%. Physicians were not able to predict the degree of risk a family would be willing to accept. Possibly, if these

215

differences are discussed at the time of drug discontinuation, physicians may be better able to deal with family anxiety.

▶ Actually, I love the premise of this article. One of the questions the authors asked was the families' strategy for playing lotteries. Some years ago, some colleagues of mine and I were trying to figure out how to tell whether a physician was a "thought leader" when it came to using new medications. One day, we were sitting around and trying to devise a questionnaire and we came up with the idea that their lottery playing strategies would be an acceptable way of actually telling which physicians would use new medications very rapidly after they were introduced. This study examines a different risk assessment, the families' acceptance of how they play the lottery, whether they want the computer to pick the numbers, or whether they actually pick the numbers. By the way, in our never-published study, one of the big determinants of whether physicians were willing to take risks in prescribing a new drug was what kind of hobbies they had. Those folks who were less risk averse in their hobbies tended to use the new medication.

M. Weintraub, M.D.

Continuous Midazolam Infusion as Treatment of Status Epilepticus
Koul RL, Aithala GR, Chacko A, et al (Sultan Qaboos Univ, Sultanate of Oman)
Arch Dis Child 76:445–448, 1997   14–2

Objective.—Status epilepticus occurs more commonly in children and carries a death rate of from 3% to 20%. Because of its anticonvulsant activity, wide safety margin, and broad therapeutic index, midazolam was tested for 2 years as a treatment for status epilepticus in children.

Methods.—Twenty children (15 boys), aged 2 months to 13 years, admitted between November 1993 and November 1995 received an IV infusion of 0.15 mg/kg midazolam as a bolus followed by a constant infusion beginning at 1 µ/kg/min and increasing up to 5 µ/kg/min in 1-µ increments every 15 minutes until seizures were controlled. Vital signs were monitored and any adverse events were noted. Blood samples were drawn on admission and at 24 hours.

Results.—Eleven children had a history of seizures and were already taking antiepileptic medication; 8 children had idiopathic epilepsy. Eight children received only midazolam. Midazolam completely arrested seizures in all children except 1 with Batten's disease. On average, seizure control in refractory status epilepticus was achieved in 64.6 minutes and in established status epilepticus in 34.3 minutes. The time from the start of infusion to complete cessation of seizures averaged 54 minutes at an average infusion rate of 2 µ/kg/min. Although no child experienced hypotension or change in heart rate, 2 children required oxygen by mask for a transient fall in oxygen saturation. Both had received phenobarbital before transferring to the treating hospital. Children regained consciousness an average of 5.1 hours after the infusion was discontinued. No adverse reactions were noted after recovery.

Conclusion.—Infusion of midazolam is a safe and effective treatment for both refractory and established status epilepticus in children.

▶ Status epilepticus demands prompt treatment, as prolonged seizure activity can produce irreversible cerebral damage. Midazolam infusion is an excellent therapeutic choice for status patients. It is safe and effective and has a short duration of action. These authors suggest that it is the drug of choice.

L. Lasagna, M.D.

Sudden Unexplained Death in Epilepsy: Observations From a Large Clinical Development Program
Leestma JE, Annegers JF, Brodie MJ, et al (Chicago Inst of Neurosurgery and Neuroresearch; Univ of Texas, Houston; Univ of Glasgow, Scotland; et al)
Epilepsia 38:47–55, 1997   14–3

Objective.—The cause of sudden unexplained death in epilepsy (SUDEP) is unknown; therefore SUDEP rates are difficult to determine. The rate of SUDEP in the patient population participating in the worldwide lamotrigine (LTG) clinical development database was determined. Seven cases are discussed.

Methods.—A panel of 6 epilepsy experts reviewed 45 SUDEP case summaries from the LTG clinical studies involving 4,700 patients. The experts classified each death as definitely or highly probably SUDEP, possibly SUDEP, non-SUDEP, or insufficient data to classify.

Results.—Eighteen deaths were classified as SUDEP, 6 as non-SUDEP, 20 deaths as other, and 1 as indeterminate because of insufficient information. The overall rate of definite or probable SUDEP per 1,000 patient-years of LTG exposure was 2.78. The overall rate of definite or probable and possible SUDEP per 1,000 patient-years of LTG exposure was 3.48.

Conclusion.—Because the rate of SUDEP per 1,000 patient-years of LTG exposure is comparable to that expected for these severely epileptic patients, it appears that the SUDEP rate is related to the population rather than to the drug.

▶ The value in this particular study is that it presents a baseline for all future studies for sudden unexplained and unexpected death in patients with epilepsy. In many ways, this knowledge will allow for the development of new antiepileptic drugs in add-on studies that maintain the effect, even partially, of 1 of the medications.

M. Weintraub, M.D.

Anticonvulsants and Congenital Malformations

Jick SS, Terris BZ (Boston Univ)
Pharmacotherapy 17:561–564, 1997   14–4

Background.—Previous research has shown that congenital anomalies are more prevalent in the infants of epileptic mothers given anticonvulsants than in those of nonepileptic mothers. The prevalence of major congenital disorders among the children of epileptic women given anticonvulsant agents in the first trimester of pregnancy was further investigated.

Methods and Findings.—Data were obtained from the General Practice Research Database on women delivering live-born infants between 1988 and 1993. The analysis included 297 women treated for epilepsy and 594 nonepileptic women matched by age at delivery, date of baby's birth, and general practice. Major anomalies were documented in 10 infants of the epileptic women and in 6 infants of the nonepileptic, untreated women. Thus, the prevalences were 3.4% and 1%, respectively, yielding a relative risk of 3.3. There was a greater than expected number of clefts and cardiac defects in the babies of treated epileptic mothers.

Conclusions.—Epileptic women given anticonvulsant agents in the first trimester of pregnancy are at increased risk of giving birth to infants with major congenital anomalies. The percentage of all anomalies was higher in exposed than in unexposed infants.

▶ An important study. The prevalence of congenital anomalies has long been thought to be higher in babies born of anticonvulsant-treated epileptic mothers than in infants of nonepileptic mothers. What has not been clear is whether the increased risk is the consequence of the drugs, the epilepsy, or both.

This study helps nail down the villains, i.e., the anticonvulsants, although there is still the nagging possibility that the treated epileptic mothers are different from the untreated epileptic mothers in ways that might complicate nondrug factors.

L. Lasagna, M.D.

CAST: Randomised Placebo-controlled Trial of Early Aspirin Use in 20000 Patients With Acute Ischaemic Stroke

Chen Z-M, for the CAST Collaborative Group (Radcliffe Infirmary, Oxford, England)
Lancet 349:1641–1649, 1997   14–5

Background.—In China, about 15 million people are expected to die of stroke during the current decade, and many others are expected to have stroke-related disabilities. Aspirin is effective in treating acute myocardial infarction, and long-term, low-dose aspirin therapy is effective in preventing serious vascular events among survivors of stroke and myocardial infarction. There is little evidence for the benefits and risks of early aspirin therapy during the acute phase of ischemic stroke.

Methods.—The Chinese Acute Stroke Trial, a randomized, placebo-controlled trial, enrolled 21,106 patients with acute ischemic stroke a mean of 25 hours after onset of symptoms. The mean age of patients was about 63. Before random assignment, 87% of patients underwent a CT scan. Treatment was continued in the hospital for as long as 4 weeks. Main outcome measures were death from any cause and death or dependence at discharge; analyses were according to intention to treat.

Results.—During the treatment period, a significant 14% decrease in mortality rate was observed. In the group treated with aspirin, there were significantly fewer cases of recurrent ischemic stroke but somewhat more cases of hemorrhagic stroke. In the group treated with aspirin, there was a 12% reduction in risk of death or nonfatal stroke at 4 weeks; this resulted in an absolute difference of 6.8 fewer cases per 1,000 patients. At discharge, 3,153 patients given aspirin and 3,266 patients given placebo were dead or dependent.

Discussion.—The results of this trial were to be reported with results of the concurrent International Stroke Trial of 20,000 patients with acute stroke from other countries. The results of the Chinese Acute Stroke Trial and the International Stroke Trial show small but definite benefits of early in-hospital aspirin treatment for patients with acute ischemic stroke. About 9 fewer deaths or nonfatal strokes occurred per 1,000 patients, and 13 fewer patients per 1,000 patients were dead or dependent after several weeks or months of follow-up.

▶ In this study, aspirin use was associated with 1.6% recurrent ischemic strokes versus 2.1% in the control group, but with slightly more hemorrhagic strokes (1.1% vs 0.9%). At discharge, 30.5% of the aspirin group were dead or dependent, versus 31.6% of the control group. Microstatistics?

L. Lasagna, M.D.

Lubeluzole in Acute Ischemic Stroke: A Double-blind, Placebo-controlled Phase II Trial
Diener HC, for the Lubeluzole International Study Group (Neurologische Universitätsklinik, Essen, Germany; Neurologische Universitätsklinik, Heidelberg, Germany; Neurologische Universitätsklinik, Mannheim, Germany, et al)
Stroke 27:76–81, 1996   14–6

Introduction.—Animal experiments showed improved neurologic outcome and reduced infarct volume when lubeluzole was administered up to 6 hours after induction of thrombotic cerebral infarcts. A randomized trial evaluated the safety and efficacy of this new compound in patients with acute ischemic stroke.

Methods.—The multicenter, double-blind study randomized 232 patients, 69 to placebo, 83 to 10 mg/d lubeluzole, and 80 to 20 mg/d lubeluzole. Treatment continued for 5 days after an initial loading dose. Recruitment was halted when the higher dose lubeluzole group was found to have increased 28-day mortality (31%) compared with placebo (19%) and 10 mg/d (10%) groups. The final study group consisted of 193 patients with acute ischemic stroke in the carotid artery territory (the target population).

Results.—At the final follow-up of 28 days, mortality rates were 18% for placebo, 6% for lubeluzole 10 mg/d, and 35% for lubeluzole 20 mg/d. The 3 groups were comparable at baseline, except that European Stroke Scale and National Institutes of Health scores were significantly worse for the lubeluzole 20 mg/d group, and significantly more patients in this group had severe stroke. Multivariate logistic regression analysis revealed significantly lowered mortality in the 10 mg/d treatment group, but more patients in this group had mild stroke. The rates of adverse events were similar (84% to 89%) in the 3 groups.

Conclusion.—Lubeluzole (7.5 mg over 1 hour, then 10 mg/d IV) safely reduced mortality in patients with acute ischemic stroke and resulted in a trend toward a better functional outcome.

▶ Although this trial was stopped early because of a significant difference in patient mortality within the 3 treatment groups, the high dose produced greater mortality than the placebo. This result has been seen in a number of different studies, for example, studies on cardiovascular agents. Something needs to be done about getting an accurate feeling for the higher doses of this medication. Perhaps 15 mg of the medication should be tried in another study. The authors note that clinical trials with a larger number of patients are ongoing to confirm an efficacious result and the dose where this result occurs. Certainly, we don't have any medications for ischemic stroke, so the results of other studies will be very important.

M. Weintraub, M.D.

European Stroke Prevention Study 2: Dipyridamole and Acetylsalicylic Acid in the Secondary Prevention of Stroke
Diener HC, Cunha L, Forbes C, et al (Univ of Essen, Germany; Hospitais da Universidade de Coimbra, Portugal; Ninewells Hosp, Dundee, Scotland; et al)
J Neurol Sci 143:1–13, 1996   14–7

Background.—The European Stroke Prevention Study, first published in 1987, showed that combined treatment with dipyridamole and acetylsalicylic acid (ASA) reduced secondary stroke by 38%, compared with placebo, in patients with prior stroke or transient ischemic attack (TIA). This was a markedly greater reduction than that achieved with ASA alone.

The second European Stroke Prevention Study determined the efficacy of dipyridamole and ASA alone for preventing secondary stroke, whether combined treatment is better than each agent alone, and whether low-dose ASA (50 mg daily) eliminates the propensity to induce bleeding.

Methods.—Data were obtained from 6,602 patients. The primary end points were stroke, death, and the combination of stroke and death. Secondary end points were TIA and other vascular events. Treatment and follow-up was continued for 2 years.

Findings.—In a factorial analysis, ASA and dipyridamole alone significantly reduced the risk of stroke and stroke and death combined. Compared with placebo, stroke risk was reduced by 18% with ASA alone, 16% with dipyridamole alone, and 37% with combined treatment. The risk of stroke or death was decreased by 13%, 15%, and 24% with ASA alone, dipyridamole alone, and combined treatment, respectively. Treatment did not significantly affect death rate alone. Dipyridamole and ASA also significantly prevented TIA. Compared with placebo, combined treatment reduced the risk by 36%. The most common adverse event was headache, occurring more often in patients receiving dipyridamole. Patients receiving ASA had significantly more common instances of all-site and GI bleeding.

Conclusions.—The efficacy of ASA, 25 mg twice daily, and modified-release dipyridamole, 200 mg twice daily, is equal in the secondary prevention of ischemic stroke and TIA. When prescribed together, the protective effects are additive. Combined treatment is significantly more effective than either agent used alone. Low-dose ASA does not eliminate the propensity for induced bleeding.

▶ In many studies looking at the prevention of specific problems such as secondary myocardial infarction or stroke, the difference in the combined end points, which, in this case is stroke or death, often is not significant. There may not be a significant difference for death alone, as in this study. Sometimes it's because the trial hasn't been carried out long enough. At least, that's what some investigators say. It could be that adverse effects of the medications will shift the balance for total death to another cause, even though they are helpful in the main cause of death under study. Most often, however, I believe it's a combination of many factors. If you don't die from a heart attack or a stroke, two of the biggest killers, you may die of cancer, accident, or some organ failure. That's why we have to be so careful in applying these results from studies that are quite well done, as in this case, but do not give significant results for total death. If you believe that it's because the studies weren't carried out long enough or for another good reason and that the treatment hasn't caused the patient a more painful or debilitating type of death, then we should go ahead and prescribe this therapy.

M. Weintraub, M.D.

Stroke, Statins, and Cholesterol: A Meta-analysis of Randomized, Placebo-controlled, Double-blind Trials With HMG-CoA Reductase Inhibitors

Blauw GJ, Lagaay AM, Smelt AHM, et al (Leiden Univ, The Netherlands)
Stroke 28:946–950, 1997   14–8

Objective.—The 3-hydroxy-3-methylglutaryl–coenzyme A (HMG-CoA) reductase inhibitors, or "statins," have proved effective in the prevention of coronary heart disease. However, their effects on stroke and other manifestations of atherosclerotic disease are unclear. To answer this question, the investigators combined all data on stroke occurrence from published randomized, placebo-controlled, double-blind trials of HMG-CoA reductase inhibitor treatment.

Methods.—Thirteen trials published between 1980 and 1996 met criteria for inclusion in the analysis. Design aspects considered included placebo control, monotherapy, and double-blinding. When there were incomplete data on the type of stroke or the rates of clinical events or adverse effects, the study authors were contacted. For each study, the number of strokes occurring in patents receiving active statin treatment was compared with the number of strokes expected.

Results.—In 20,438 study participants, there were 462 evaluable strokes. One hundred eighty-one strokes occurred in patients receiving HMG-CoA reductase inhibitor treatment and 261 in patients receiving placebo. Twelve of the 13 trials showed a smaller than expected number of strokes with statin treatment. The overall odds ratio of stroke with HMG-CoA reductase inhibitor treatment was 0.69, with a 95% confidence interval of 0.57 to 0.83.

Conclusion.—Meta-analysis of randomized trial data suggests that treatment with HMG-CoA reductase inhibitor reduces the risk of stroke in middle-aged patients. The 31% reduction shown in this study is comparable with the effects of statins in preventing coronary heart disease. The findings underscore the need to test the ability of statins to prevent stroke in the elderly.

▶ The statins unquestionably can prevent some coronary artery disease, but their effect on stroke is not clear. This meta-analysis suggests a beneficial effect with regard to stroke prevention in middle-aged patients. As the authors point out, we need data on the elderly, in whom most strokes occur. To confuse matters, hypercholesterolemia is not an independent risk factor for cardiovascular disease beyond the age of 70 years.

L. Lasagna, M.D.

Piracetam as an Adjuvant to Language Therapy for Aphasia: A Randomized Double-blind Placebo-controlled Pilot Study
Huber W, Willmes K, Poeck K, et al (Westfälische Technische Hochschule, Aachen, Germany; UCB Pharmaceutical Sector, Braine-l'Alleud, Belgium)
Arch Phys Med Rehabil 78:245–250, 1997   14–9

Introduction.—Aphasia develops in approximately 20% of stroke patients and can cause long-lasting disability. A pilot study was conducted to evaluate whether piracetam (4.8 g/day) had a positive adjuvant effect on patients with aphasia who were receiving language therapy.

Methods.—The double-blind study enrolled 66 consecutive patients admitted to an aphasia ward for intensive language therapy. Thirty-two were randomized to piracetam and 34 to placebo. The 2 groups were well matched in prognostic factors and in type and severity of aphasia. All patients took part in intensive language therapy for 6 weeks and were evaluated at baseline and after treatment using the Aachen Aphasia Test (AAT).

Results.—Fifty patients (24 men and 26 women) were evaluable for efficacy, 24 in the piracetam group and 26 in the placebo group. The mean scores for all AAT subtests were higher with piracetam, although only "written language" test results were significant in univariate analysis. The weighted average of all subtests reflecting overall severity of aphasia was significantly better on piracetam than on placebo. No statistically significant differences were present between the groups for any of the 6 scales of spontaneous speech, although improvement in syntactic structure in patients on piracetam approached significance.

Conclusion.—Preliminary results suggest that piracetam may hasten recovery in aphasic patients receiving speech therapy. The drug's action may be attributed to its neuroprotective qualities of enhanced cell metabolism and neurotransmission.

▶ Unfortunately, piracetam, which has been around for a long time, did not improve language learning by a statistically significant amount. There was, however, a trend in favor of the medication. This has been true of other studies of piracetam in other cognitive dysfunctions, such as learning and memory. The individual patient scores are illustrated in the study by Huber et al. Language therapy is considered the best treatment for aphasic patients. Perhaps the patients who improved the most should be investigated to see if there is any difference between the patients who improved and those who did not. The other approach, in a setting like this with so much interpatient difference at the start, is to use some sort of stratification procedure. Conversely, you can make the groups more homogenous at the beginning by making the diagnoses more similar or by limiting the scores to a certain type.

M. Weintraub, M.D.

Sumatriptan Nonresponders: A Survey in 366 Migraine Patients

Visser WH, de Vriend RHM, Jaspers NHWM, et al (Univ Hosp, Leiden, The Netherlands)

Headache 36:471–475, 1996   14–10

Background.—Sumatriptan is very effective in the acute treatment of migraine in most patients, especially after subcutaneous administration. The clinical characteristics of responders and nonresponders were compared to determine risk factors for nonresponse to this treatment.

Methods and Findings.—A questionnaire about the use of sumatriptan was mailed to 869 patients with migraine. The response rate was 85%. In patients taking sumatriptan subcutaneously, nonresponders tended to have a higher body mass index, to have migraine onset at an earlier age, and to treat their migraine attacks earlier. In patients taking the drug orally, nonresponders tended to have attacks associated with more severe vomiting and photophobia, to want to sleep or rest more often, and to experience initial worsening of the headache more frequently after taking the drug. None of these differences were statistically significant. Within-patient comparisons indicated no differences between attacks with and without response.

Conclusions.—Few, if any, clinically relevant risk factors for nonresponse to sumatriptan were found. Administering the drug too early was the strongest indicator.

▶ The authors tried to carry out an interesting exercise. They tried to look at who didn't respond to sumatriptan and figure out if there were any differences. At least at the present state of knowledge of migraine headaches, no differences could be ascertained. They did figure out that the patients who were nonresponders treated their headaches too early, but even that was not statistically significant by their criteria. Still, I believe that we should always be looking for responders and nonresponders to all treatments. It's the only way that we are going to have any hint as to who will respond. We shouldn't withhold therapy, but we should remember to keep something in reserve, such as another analgesic or some other anti-hypertensive agent, when we are faced with a nonresponder. Also, we have to remember the role of compliance and the role of pharmacokinetics in deciding who is really a nonresponder.

M. Weintraub, M.D.

Ocular Myasthenia Gravis: Response to Long Term Immunosuppressive Treatment

Sommer N, Sigg B, Melms A, et al (Eberhard-Karls-Univ Tübingen, Germany)

J Neurol Neurosurg Psychiatry 62:156–162, 1997   14–11

Background.—Myasthenia gravis is an autoimmune disease that sometimes manifests as a relatively mild ocular disease. The best method for treating ocular myasthenia gravis has not been determined. Results of the current therapies used to treat this condition were examined retrospectively.

Methods.—Of 178 patients with myasthenia gravis, 78 had ocular myasthenia gravis based on eye muscle weakness not attributable to other causes. In these 78 patients, myasthenia gravis had been diagnosed quite late, a mean (±SD) of 39.8 ± 93.5 months after symptoms developed. The mean disease duration was 8 years (range, 6 months to 58 years). The disease had been treated with immunosuppressants, corticosteroids, or thymectomy.

Findings.—Generalized muscle weakness developed secondarily in 24 of 78 patients (31%) within 3–132 months after ocular symptoms became apparent. Treatments led to remission in 29 patients, improvement in 18, and no change in 7; no patient experienced a worsening of ocular symptoms. Pyridostigmine was given to 60 of 78 patients for an average of 45 months, and in 14 patients this was the sole treatment. Of those 14, 7 had considerable improvement, 6 had mild improvement, and 1 had no effect. Patients treated with the immunosuppressive drugs prednisolone (45 patients) or azathioprine or a combination (27 patients) were less likely to progress to generalized myasthenia gravis (only 12% did so, compared to 18 of 28 patients [64%] who did not receive immunosuppressants). Thymectomy was performed in 12 patients an average of 50 months after symptom onset, and all but 1 were also treated with immunosuppressants. Of those 12, 6 achieved remission, 4 showed improved ocular muscle strength, and 2 subsequently had generalized disease.

Conclusions.—Overall, the prognosis for ocular myasthenia gravis is good. Treatment generally confines the disease to the eye muscles and achieves remission or improvement. In particular, early immunosuppressive treatment was associated with superior results. Thymectomy also provided a good outcome, but its results were not superior to those of medical management alone. On the basis of these results, in the majority of patients a combination of short-term pyridostigmine and long-term azathioprine should achieve disease remission.

▶ This may be good news! It appears that immunosuppressive therapy (corticosteroids and/or azathioprine) prevents progression of ocular disease to a more generalized myasthenia gravis.

M. Weintraub, M.D.

Therapy of Myasthenic Crisis
Berrouschot J, Baumann I, Kalischewski P, et al (Univ of Leipzig, Germany)
Crit Care Med 25:1228–1235, 1997   14–12

Purpose.—The term "myasthenic crisis" refers to acute respiratory failure requiring mechanical ventilation. It is a life-threatening but rare condition, with few valid data about its causes, frequency, duration, and course. Three treatments for myasthenic crisis—continuous intravenous infusion of pyridostigmine, pyridostigmine plus prednisolone, and plasma exchange—were compared retrospectively.

Methods.—The population for the study was 235 patients with myasthenia gravis treated at a specialist medical center. Forty-four of these patients had a total of 63 myasthenic crises, for an average annual incidence of 2.5%. Treatment for the myasthenic crises was pyridostigmine in 24 cases, pyridostigmine plus prednisolone in 18, and plasma exchange in 21. The 3 treatments were compared for duration of ventilation and patient outcome.

Results.—The 3 groups had similar clinical characteristics. The treatments did not differ significantly in terms of duration of mechanical ventilation, complications, and outcome at discharge from the intensive care unit and 3 months' follow-up. Of 11 patients with severe cardiac arrhythmia, 6 died.

Conclusions.—The 3 treatment regimens for myasthenic crisis give similar results. Each is effective and should be used according to the circumstances. The key to treatment is early intubation and mechanical ventilation. Cardiac monitoring is essential, with a temporary pacemaker as indicated.

▶ Respiratory failure of sufficient severity to require mechanical ventilation is the most dangerous complication of myasthenia gravis. Such crises occur—rarely, to be sure—even in patients treated vigorously with early thymectomy and immunosuppression.

There is no standard therapy for myasthenic crisis, and the present study suggests that with the 3 therapeutic regimens compared by these authors the end results were not significantly different. All seemed to help, but careful cardiac monitoring and a temporary pacemaker in some patients must not be ignored.

L. Lasagna, M.D.

A Meta-analysis of Trials on Aldose Reductase Inhibitors in Diabetic Peripheral Neuropathy

Nicolucci A, and the Italian Study Group for the Implementation of the St Vincent Declaration (Univ of Perugia, Italy; Istituto Mario Negri, Milano, Italy)
Diabet Med 13:1017–1026, 1996   14–13

Introduction.—One of the most common and disabling long-term sequelae of diabetes mellitus is peripheral neuropathy. The prevalence of this condition is as high as 50%. Typical symptoms are loss of sensation in the feet, deformation, development of ulcers, and gangrene, which can result in amputation. The polyol pathway hypothesis proposes that high tissue glucose levels lead to an accumulation of sorbitol and fructose within the nerves, which are associated with decreased sodium-potassium adenosine triphosphatase activity, myoinositol depletion, and axoglial dysfunction in peripheral nerves. In diabetic animals, these abnormalities may be prevented with inhibitors of aldose reductase, the first end rate-limiting enzyme of the polyol pathway that catalyzes the reduction of glucose to sorbitol. For the prevention and treatment of diabetic neuropathy, aldose reductase inhibitors have been proposed and are increasingly used in many countries. Existing evidence on the effectiveness of aldose reductase inhibitors was reviewed in a meta-analysis.

Methods.—The meta-analysis included 13 randomized clinical trials, published between 1981 and 1993, that compared aldose reductase inhibitors with placebo. In all of these trials nerve conduction velocity was the end point. Treatment effect on nerve conduction velocity was evaluated

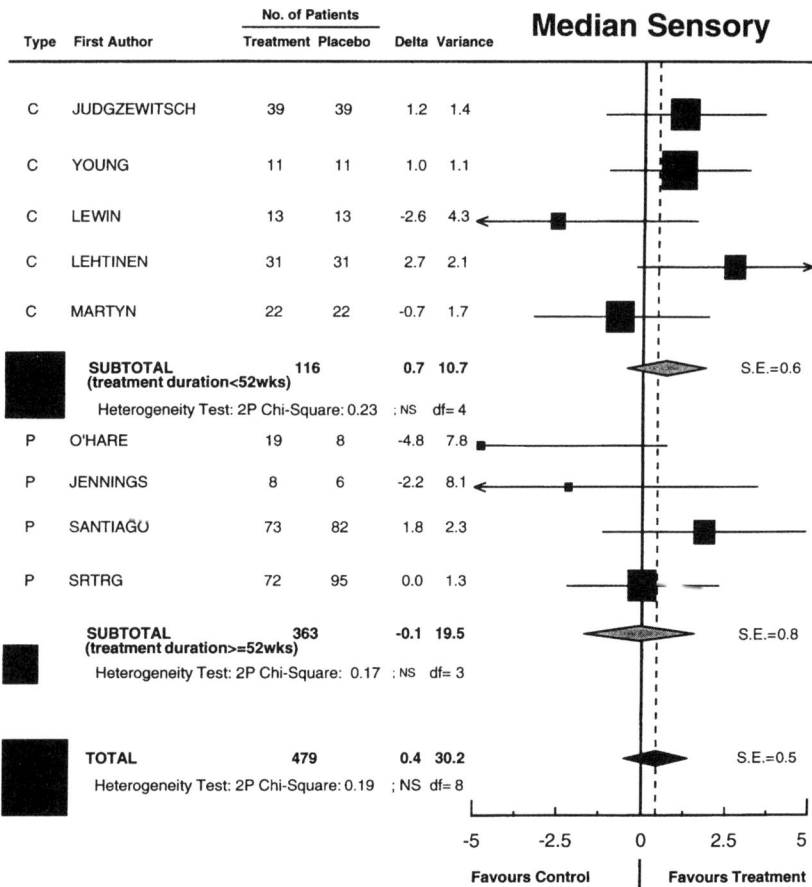

FIGURE 3.—Effect of aldose reductase inhibitors as compared with placebo on median sensory nerve conduction velocity (ms^{-1}): overall results and subgroup analysis by treatment duration (< 1 year compared with ≥ 1 year). *Abbreviations: df*, degrees of freedom; *NS*, not significant; SE, standard error. (Courtesy of Nicolucci A, and the Italian Study Group for the Implementation of the St Vincent Declaration: A meta-analysis of trials on aldose reductase inhibitors in diabetic peripheral neuropathy. *Diabet Med* 13:1017–1026, 1996. Reprinted by permission of John Wiley & Sons, Ltd.)

by using 4 different nerves: sural sensory, peroneal motor, median sensory, and median motor.

Results.—The treated group had a statistically significant reduction in decline of median motor nerve conduction velocity when compared with the control group (mean, 0.91 ms^{-1}, 95% confidence interval, 0.41–1.42 ms^{-1}). For patients treated with aldose reductase inhibitors, no clear benefit was seen in peroneal motor, median sensory, or sural sensory nerve results. For peroneal motor nerve conduction velocity, a significant effect was seen when the analysis was limited to trials in which treatment lasted at least 1 year (Fig 3). For median motor nerve conduction velocity, statistical significance was borderline when the analysis was limited to trials with at least 1 year of treatment.

Conclusion.—No clear conclusion can yet be drawn about the efficacy of aldose reductase inhibitors in treating peripheral diabetic neuropathy. However, the results of 1-year treatment on motor nerve conduction velocity seem encouraging.

▶ As shown by the figure, there really is no hope for aldose reductase inhibitors, even according to a meta-analysis. The authors discuss the many factors for bias and failure to include all of the studies that are present in systematic overviews of data. Even if a treatment effect was missed, it would have to be relatively small and therefore probably not of clinical benefit. The one problem is the kind of patients that participated in these studies. They really may have been too sick and therefore could not respond to the treatment at all. However, using less sick patients means that one would have to wait a very long time to see an effect and be burdened with the problem of patients' not developing diabetic neuropathy at all. The problem is very difficult and, in fact, may currently be insurmountable. However, with the continued development of measures for diabetic neuropathy, one can hope that simple, very reproducible, early measures will be developed so that the studies can be done and the questions answered once and for all.

M. Weintraub, M.D.

Differential Effects of Transdermal Nicotine on Microstructured Analyses of Tics in Tourette's Syndrome: An Open Study
Dursun SM, Reveley MA (Univ of Leicester, England)
Psychol Med 27:483–487, 1997   14–14

Introduction.—Tourette's syndrome (TS), the most severe form of tic disorder, is both socially and functionally disabling, and drug therapy has often been unsatisfactory. An open study examined whether transdermal nicotine patch (TNP) application can improve tics in patients in whom haloperidol treatment failed.

Methods.—Study participants were 5 male non-smokers with TS; 4 had not responded to haloperidol and 1 had never been medicated. All were free of other significant diseases and had no history of epilepsy, drug addiction, or alcoholism. Patients were videotaped before and after TNP application and assessed for tics with the Yale Global Tic Severity Scale (YGTSS). All tics were counted under 3 conditions of 5 minutes each: sitting quietly, reading aloud, and performing written calculations.

Results.—Application of TNP (10 mg) significantly reduced the YGTSS by an average of 50%, compared with baseline, for up to 4 weeks. At each of the 3 assessment periods (24 hours, 4 weeks, and 16 weeks after TNP), different tics (head-shake, eye-blink, vocalization, facial grimace, and other body tics) showed different levels of reduction.

Conclusion.—Overall, total tic counts significantly decreased for up to 4 weeks (but not 16 weeks) after TNP application. The varied effect on individual tics suggests a differential role for nicotine receptors involved in the generation of TS. Further study is needed to clarify the effects of TNP on individual tics and to establish dose-response parameters.

▶ Of course, this observation needs a double-blind study, but it's very interesting and may be helpful for people who get little benefit from current therapies for Tourette's syndrome.

M. Weintraub, M.D.

A Double-blind Controlled Study of Gabapentin and Baclofen as Treatment for Acquired Nystagmus
Averbuch-Heller L, Tusa RJ, Fuhry L, et al (Case Western Reserve Univ, Cleveland, Ohio; Bascom Palmer Eye Inst, Miami, Fla; Ludwig-Maximilians Univ, Munich; et al)
Ann Neurol 41:818–825, 1997   14–15

Introduction.—The symptoms of acquired nystagmus may be alleviated if the ocular oscillations are reduced or abolished, but few reliable clinical therapies are available. A double-blind, crossover trial compared gabapentin to baclofen as therapy for acquired nystagmus.

Methods.—Fifteen patients had acquired pendular nystagmus (APN) and 6 had jerk nystagmus that was either downbeat or torsional downbeat. Several had tried a variety of other medications with only minor or temporary relief. Treatment consisted of gabapentin (up to 900 mg/day) and baclofen (up to 30 mg/day). Experimental studies suggest that γ-aminobutyric acid (GABA) plays an important role in the mechanism by which gaze is held steady during visual fixation, and both gabapentin and baclofen involve GABAergic mechanisms. Visual acuity and nystagmus were measured before and at the end of 2 weeks for each agent.

Results.—Twenty patients completed both 2-week test periods. The 2 patient groups differed in their responses to each agent. Only gabapentin significantly improved visual acuity in patients with APN; median eye speed was significantly reduced in all 3 planes with gabapentin, but baclofen affected only the vertical plane. Eight patients with APN elected to continue gabapentin treatment. With both therapies, patients with down-beat or torsional downbeat nystagmus had less consistent changes in median slow-phase eye speed. Only 1 of 6 patients had consistent reduction in median eye speed, and the 2 drugs were similarly effective in this case.

Conclusion.—Gabapentin proved to be an effective therapy for most patients with APN. Visual acuity was improved and all components of the nystagmus were reduced. Ataxia may be worsened, however, and care should be taken to avoid falls. Both gabapentin and baclofen may benefit some patients with downbeat nystagmus.

▶ This study demonstrates quite well that crossover trials are not as good as they are believed to be by many nonclinical trialists. There really are too many questions. For example, the results at the end of the washout period (1–2 weeks) would be really crucial to make sure that the drug did not produce long-standing control of nystagmus. Given the side effects of the gabapentin, a perhaps better approach would be to stop the dose escalation at a time when the patients' nystagmus was almost controlled.

Too often, others say, American physicians try for perfection in their therapeutic interventions. I am not sure that is true, but I do believe that we attempt to look for complete responses, perhaps more than European or Japanese physicians do.

M. Weintraub, M.D.

Hiccups Associated With Lateral Medullary Syndrome: A Case Report
Nickerson RB, Atchison JW, Van Hoose JD, et al (Univ of Kentucky, Lexington)
Am J Phys Med Rehabil 76:144–146, 1997   14–16

Introduction.—Hiccups (singultus) are usually a temporary annoyance that resolves spontaneously or with home remedies. Persistent hiccups that are chronic (lasting more than 48 hours) or intractable (lasting more than 1 month) have been associated with various diseases, alcohol ingestion, drug use, and ischemic events. In the case presented here, hiccups that persisted after a lateral medullary cerebrovascular accident were treated successfully with baclofen.

> *Case Report.*—Man, 69, had a history of multiple transient ischemic attacks. When seen at the emergency room with a 2-day history of nausea and vomiting, he had experienced loss of pain and temperature on the left side of the face and the right side of the trunk. Also evident were left-sided ataxia, nystagmus, diplopia, and hiccups. He received a diagnosis of a left lateral medullary syndrome in the vascular distribution of the posterior inferior cerebellar artery. Systemic anticoagulation was started, and the patient was subsequently transferred to a rehabilitation facility.

Hiccups continued to be his most troublesome symptom. A search of the literature led to selection of baclofen (5 mg by mouth 3 times per day) to treat hiccups. The hiccups and nausea resolved within 48 hours and baclofen was tapered off after 1 week. Hiccups and nausea were still absent at 8-week follow-up.

Discussion.—Hiccups appear to be common among patients with a lateral medullary syndrome. As in other cases of chronic and intractable hiccups, simple remedies and physical maneuvers are ineffective. Baclofen was successful in treating persistent hiccups after prochlorperazine, promethazine, and chlorpromazine failed.

▶ Why do we always have to have a special word like "singultus" for diseases like hiccups? Actually, I think hiccups seems not be important enough to be treated and reported. Thus, the use of singultus. The patient described in this article had very severe hiccups that interfered with sleep and activities of daily living, including eating. Using the baclofen was a clever idea. We should congratulate the investigators on doing a good job.

M. Weintraub, M.D.

15 Obstetrics and Gynecology

Little Knowledge and Limited Practice: Emergency Contraceptive Pills, the Public, and the Obstetrician-Gynecologist
Delbanco SF, Mauldon J, Smith MD (Henry J Kaiser Family Found, Menlo Park, Calif; Univ of California, Berkley; California HealthCare Found, Woodland Hills)
Obstet Gynecol 89:1006–1011, 1997   15–1

Background.—Lack of public knowledge about emergency contraception may partly explain its limited use. Americans' knowledge of and attitudes toward emergency contraceptive pills were assessed, along with obstetrician-gynecologists' knowledge, attitudes, and practices.

Methods and Findings.—A random sample of a national cross-section of 1,000 women and 1,002 men and a nationally representative sample of 307 obstetrician-gynecologists were surveyed. Only 36% of the laypersons knew that "anything could be done" to prevent pregnancy within a few days after unprotected sex. Fifty-five percent said that they had heard of emergency contraceptive pills. Only 1% had ever used them. Ninety-nine percent of the physicians said that they were familiar with emergency contraceptive pills. Seventy-seven percent said that they were "very familiar" with such contraception; most of these considered it to be extremely safe and effective. Overall, 70% of the physicians said they had prescribed emergency contraception, though infrequently. Seventy-seven percent of those who reported prescribing emergency contraceptive pills had done so 5 or fewer times.

Conclusions.—Americans have limited knowledge about the availability and use of emergency contraceptive pills. The practice of prescribing such pills is also limited. Health care providers can improve knowledge and availability of emergency contraceptive pills.

▶ Although unplanned pregnancy is obviously a greater risk among women who do not use any contraceptive method, 1.7 million pregnancies (almost half the total number of unwanted pregnancies) occur in women who are said to be using some method, which has seemingly failed for one reason or another. It has long been known that high doses of oral contraceptives administered within 72 hours of unprotected intercourse and followed by a second dose 12 hours later reduce the risk of pregnancy by about 75%. This study suggests that this information is not sufficiently appreciated by either the public or the obstetric-gynecologic physician community.

L. Lasagna, M.D.

Emergency Contraception: A Survey of Women's Knowledge and Attitudes
Smith BH, Gurney EM, Aboulela L, et al (Univ of Aberdeen, Scotland; Aberdeen Maternity Hosp, Scotland)
Br J Obstet Gynaecol 103:1109–1116, 1996   15–2

Background.—In the United Kingdom, increasing knowledge and availability of emergency contraception has been recommended to reduce the number of unwanted pregnancies. Women's knowledge of and attitudes about emergency contraception were surveyed.

Methods and Findings.—A survey was mailed to a stratified random sample of 2,000 Grampian women, aged 18–47 years, identified through the Community Health Index. Ninety-four percent of the women were aware of emergency contraception and could identify an appropriate source. Only 39% knew the correct timing for its use. These percentages were generally greater among younger, single women. The most common source of information was the popular media. General practitioners and family planning clinics were rarely cited as information sources. Seventy-one percent of the women, primarily older ones, felt that increased advertising was desirable. Only 36% (primarily younger, single women) thought that over-the-counter availability was desirable.

Conclusions.—Knowledge of the correct timing for emergency contraceptive use and its use in relation to intrauterine contraceptive methods is still deficient. Health professionals appear to be underutilized sources of information on such contraception.

▶ In this British study, 36% of the women felt that the emergency contraception pills should be available over-the-counter. These pills are not now available in the United States or in the United Kingdom over-the-counter. Although 94% of the women knew of the existence of emergency contraception, only a third knew how and when to use it. Certainly, more instruction is needed on the use of the pill by the average woman.

M. Weintraub, M.D.

Postcoital Contraception: Who Uses the 'Morning After Pill?'
Pyett PM (La Trobe Univ, Melbourne)
Aust N Z J Obstet Gynaecol 36:347–350, 1996   15–3

Introduction.—The "morning after pill" is the common term for post-coital contraception. It is widely assumed that this intervention is effective only within 24 hours of sexual encounter, but it is actually effective within 72 hours. Providers of family planning services are concerned about the number of women using this emergency measure. Unprotected sex leaves a woman open to the risk for acquiring a sexually transmitted disease. The sociodemographic characteristics of women coming to family planning clinics for postcoital contraception were examined to determine why they engage in unprotected heterosexual intercourse.

Methods.—During a 3-month period, 206 women who requested post-coital contraception completed a self-administered questionnaire. The mean age was 23 years (range, 14 to 43 years). More than a quarter of the women had used postcoital contraception more than twice before and more than half had used it once previously. There were 79% single women, 16% married women, and 5% separated women. Most (79%) had postsecondary education, and 38% of those 20 years and older had completed a university course.

Results.—The most commonly used form of contraception was condoms (60%), but only 34% reported that condoms were their only usual form of contraception. For 45% of the women surveyed, the oral contraceptive pill was the usual form of contraception. Three quarters of the women had sex with their regular partner, and 24% had sex with a casual partner. Three fourths of the women were at home or at their sexual partner's home before the sexual encounter. Only 11% were at a nightclub (most of these women were younger than 20 years of age). Nonuse of condoms (34%), condom breakage (31%), and missing an oral contraceptive pill (20%) were the main reasons given for needing postcoital contraception

Conclusion.—Women who use postcoital contraception do not appear to represent women in the general population. Those who use this method regularly are not taking adequate precautions to ensure prevention of sexually transmitted disease.

▶ In the United States, the use of postcoital contraception with double-the-dose (or even higher) contraceptives has recently been promulgated. Unfortunately, this means that the women will have to have access to the pills. They'll also need a good relationship with a physician and they'll need a pharmacy that can provide them with the medication.

M. Weintraub, M.D.

Oral Contraceptive Failure Rates and Oral Antibiotics
Helms SE, Bredle DL, Zajic J, et al (Northeastern Ohio Univs, Cleveland)
J Am Acad Dermatol 36:705–710, 1997   15–4

Background.—Anecdotal evidence suggests that some antibiotics may reduce the efficacy of oral contraceptives (OCs). The effect of tetracyclines, penicillins, and cephalosporins (commonly used in dermatologic practices) on OC failure rates was studied.

Methods.—The records of 356 patients seen at 3 dermatologic practices were reviewed. All had a history of combined oral antibiotic and OC use. Two hundred sixty-three of these women sometimes used OCs alone, thus providing control data. Control data only were obtained for another 162 patients.

Findings.—Five pregnancies occurred in 311 woman-years of combined antibiotic and OC use, for a 1.6% per year failure rate. In the control group, this rate was 0.96% per year. This difference was statistically nonsignificant. All the groups in the current study had failure rates of less than 3% per year, which is typically reported with OC use in the United States.

Conclusions.—The antibiotics studied apparently do not increase the risk of pregnancy in OC users. Regardless of antibiotic use, the OC failure rate is at least 1% per year. Patients and physicians need to appreciate this and the fact that predicting OC failure in individuals is not yet possible.

▶ The literature on the possible interference of oral antibiotics with the efficacy of OCs is not persuasive. This retrospective survey suggests that antibiotics do not increase the failure rate of OCs but reminds us that OCs have a failure rate of 1% per annum anyway.

L. Lasagna, M.D.

Evidence-guided Prescribing of Combined Oral Contraceptives: Consensus Statement
Hannaford PC, and the participants at an International Workshop (Manchester Research Unit, England)
Contraception 54:125–129, 1996   15–5

Background.—When combined oral contraceptives (COCs) are prescribed, the provision of safe and effective contraception must be balanced against interventions that might unnecessarily restrict the availability of birth control pills. The screening procedure to follow when prescribing COCs has been debated. If women who use COCs are to be screened differently from nonusers, evidence of differing disease risk should be clear. A consensus statement, based on review of the available evidence, was prepared regarding the value of screening procedures in premenopausal women.

Recommendations.—An expert panel identified only 2 prerequisites for safe prescription of COCs: a careful personal and family medical history must be taken (with emphasis on cardiovascular risk factors), and blood pressure must be measured accurately. A small minority of women will require further evaluation if they have a relevant personal or family history or if they have high blood pressure. The risk for serious disease associated with COC use is very small for most women.

Discussion.—The risks and benefits of oral contraceptive use must be weighed against those of other contraceptive methods and of unintended pregnancy. Health care providers involved in contraceptive services play a key role in informing women of the benefits and risks of COC use.

▶ The fact that oral contraceptives are imperfect (what isn't?) has led to their underuse. This sensible consensus statement advises that a few simple things (personal and family history; blood pressure measurement) suffice to predict excellent contraception with minimal risk. Unintended pregnancy and abortion also involve risks.

L. Lasagna, M.D.

A Comparison of "U" and Standard Techniques for Norplant Removal
Rosenberg MJ, Alvarez F, Barone MA, et al (Health Decisions Inc, Chapel Hill, NC; Biomedical Research, Profamilia, Santo Domingo, Dominican Republic; AVSC Internatl, New York)
Obstet Gynecol 89:168–173, 1997   15–6

Background.—Many women with Norplant contraceptive implants ask for early removal. Several methods for Norplant removal have been reported. The "U" technique was compared with the manufacturer-recommended technique for removal in a randomized study.

Methods.—Two hundred Norplant removals were performed by 21 physicians, 18 of whom were not experienced at such removals. The "U" technique requires an incision between and parallel to the third and fourth implants. The implants are removed by using a modified vasectomy clamp and pulling perpendicular to the implant axis.

Findings.—The "U" technique was significantly less time-consuming than the standard method for inexperienced physicians. Although it was also less time-consuming for experienced physicians, it was not significantly so after adjustment for other factors. Experienced and inexperienced physicians broke implants more often when using the standard method, although the difference was only significant for inexperienced physicians. Tissue damage and patient reports of pain during and after removal did not differ.

Conclusions.—The "U" technique appears to be an improvement over the standard method of Norplant removal, especially for personnel who are not highly experienced in Norplant removal. In general, the new technique required less time and resulted in fewer broken implants.

▶ Norplant's long-acting contraceptive effect is achieved via the subdermal implantation of 6 levonorgestrel-containing units. While it seems to work for 5 years, many women decide to have the implants removed earlier, a feat that is not always easy to carry out (e.g., envelope of fibrous tissue, too deep a placement, or an implant not in the recommended fan-shaped pattern) and make failure a threat.

This article suggests a good way to remove the Norplant.

L. Lasagna, M.D.

Safety of First Trimester Exposure to Histamine H₂ Blockers: A Prospective Cohort Study

Magee LA, Inocencion G, Kamboj L, et al (Hosp for Sick Children, Toronto)
Dig Dis Sci 41:1145–1149, 1996   15–7

Background.—Pregnant women commonly have gastroesophageal reflux. H₂-receptor antagonists are effective in the treatment of this condition. The possible teratogenic effects of H₂ blockers were assessed.

Methods.—One hundred seventy-eight women who contacted a Canadian teratology information service about gestational H₂-blocker use were included in the prospective study. One hundred seventy-eight women matched for maternal age, smoking, and heavy alcohol consumption comprised a control group.

Findings.—The incidence of major malformations was not increased after first-trimester exposure to H₂ blockers. Major malformations occurred in 2.1% and 3.5% of the infants in the H₂-blocker and control groups, respectively. The 2 groups did not differ in any other aspect of pregnancy outcome or neonatal health.

Conclusion.—The use of H₂ blockers for gastroesophageal reflux in the first trimester of pregnancy appears to be safe. However, a small teratogenic risk cannot be ruled out. Continuing surveillance of pregnancy outcomes in women taking H₂ blockers is needed.

▶ Heartburn is a serious problem in pregnancy. Fortunately, the drugs used to treat it are generally without adverse effects. This study was done by Motherisk, which collects information regarding standardized data forms and conducts follow-ups by telephone. Such systems are relatively small but provide excellent data and complement programs like the record-linkage studies (done in Canada and in various states of the United States) and postmarketing studies done by manufacturers. Both of these studies may have larger patient populations but cannot get the kind of information that a study like this one provides. In some ways, this is almost like a concentration-controlled study. In this case, the group of interest for comparison is one that took a high dose of alcohol. The study is set up as a prospective cohort study, which is a really good study design.

M. Weintraub, M.D.

Dose Ranging Study of the Oxytocin Antagonist Atosiban in the Treatment of Preterm Labor

Goodwin TM, and the Atosiban Study Group (Women's Hosp, Los Angeles)
Obstet Gynecol 88:331–336, 1996   15–8

Background.—Atosiban, a competitive oxytocin inhibitor, reportedly decreases preterm uterine activity in women when given in a continuous infusion at a rate of 300 µg/min. The minimal effective dose of atosiban in the initial treatment of uterine activity in preterm labor was established.

Methods.—Three hundred two patients were enrolled in this double-blind, parallel group, multicenter trial. The patients received either 6.5 mg bolus plus 300 µg/min, placebo bolus plus 300 µg/minute, 2 mg bolus plus 100 µg/min, 0.6 mg plus 30 µg/min, or IV ritodrine.

Findings.—The lowest atosiban dose was significantly less effective than ritodrine in stopping contractions and in achieving 4 or fewer contractions per hour in the last hour of treatment. The other atosiban regimens were comparable to ritodrine, except for the drug discontinuation rate because of adverse events, which was higher for ritodrine. Atosiban was discontinued in 1 of 244 patients and ritodrine in 15 of 58 patients. High-dose atosiban given in a bolus resulted in a significantly higher percentage of patients whose contractions stopped in the first 2 hours of treatment, compared with patients not receiving a bolus.

Conclusion.—Bolus infusion enhanced the effect of atosiban on uterine activity in preterm labor, making it comparable to that of ritodrine. In addition, atosiban was associated with fewer adverse effects than ritodrine.

▶ In this study of the effect of a whole series of doses of atosiban on preterm labor, the comparative agent was ritodrine, a commonly used drug with perhaps no great efficacy and a good deal of toxicity. Therefore, the effect of the new drug should be greeted with some enthusiasm, albeit quiet and watchful. The authors claim that future therapy in preterm labor will involve dividing patients into treatment groups according to the mechanism precipitating labor and then choosing therapies appropriately. That will be an effective strategy—if we have the treatments.

M. Weintraub, M.D.

Taxol as Second-line Treatment in Patients With Advanced Ovarian Cancer After Platinum-based First-line Chemotherapy

Mayerhofer K, Kucera E, Zeisler H, et al (Univ Hosp of Vienna)
Gynecol Oncol 64:109–113, 1997   15–9

Introduction.—Most patients with advanced ovarian cancer respond initially to surgery followed by platinum-based chemotherapy, but fewer than 25% will be alive 5 years later. Salvage therapy after recurrence typically yields low response rates. A retrospective study of patients treated with paclitaxel (Taxol) investigated the response, toxicity, and survival when this agent was administered as second-line therapy.

Methods.—Twenty-eight patients received Taxol between April 1993 and January 1995. All had previously been treated with cisplatin, or carboplatin, or both. Taxol was given at a dose of 175 mg/m^2, infused over 3 hours, every 21 days. The dose was reduced for severe toxicity and increased for patients with significant clinical response and low toxicity. One hundred forty-five courses of Taxol were infused. Premedication consisted of dexamethasone, diphenhydramine, and ranitidine.

Results.—There were 3 complete and 4 partial remissions, for an overall response rate of 25%; the median survival was 15 months. The response rate was lower (15%, with 3 partial remissions) in patients resistant to platinum-based therapy. Leukopenia was the most common severe toxicity (grade 3 in 10% of courses), and some patients experienced neurologic toxicity.

Discussion.—A prospective randomized trial showed Taxol to have significant activity in ovarian cancer, but only a few platinum-resistant patients in this study showed any response. The response rate was significantly higher among patients considered sensitive to platinum-based therapy.

▶ These data are not what I would have guessed. Taxol is thought to be the most effective treatment for advanced ovarian cancer, but here it yielded little benefit to platinum-resistant patients.

L. Lasagna, M.D.

16 Pain

Summary of the Mayday Fund Survey: Public Attitudes About Pain and Analgesics
Bostrom M (Trahan, Burden and Charles Inc, Baltimore, Md)
J Pain Symptom Manage 13:166–168, 1997   16–1

Background.—Previous research on pain has not tried to understand the human aspect of pain or the emotions associated with it. The Mayday Fund Survey sought to understand people's underlying assumptions about pain and its treatment.

Methods and Findings.—Telephone interviews were conducted in an unbiased sample of 1,004 adults in the United States. Forty-six respondents reported having severe pain at some time in their lives. Seventy-seven percent had experienced childbirth; 63%, surgical pain; 49%, chronic backaches; 41%, migraine headaches; 45%, a broken bone; and 34%, arthritis. Twenty-four percent had had pain severe enough to interfere with daily activities a couple times each month. Eighty-eight percent of the respondents agreed that it was more important to treat the cause of pain than the pain itself, being more concerned with the meaning of the pain than with alleviating it. Most respondents preferred to bear pain for a while, 66% saying that the last time they had fairly serious pain, they withstood it. Only 30% had acted quickly to relieve such pain. Seventy-one percent said they generally avoid calling a physician when in pain. The respondents tended to avoid taking pain medication because of fears of becoming addicted or too dependent on drugs. Eighty-two percent felt that it was easy to become too reliant on pain medication. To avoid taking medications to alleviate pain, the respondents reported seeking alternatives. Interestingly, blue collar workers and lower income respondents were more likely to avoid medication than were professional and higher income respondents.

Conclusions.—These survey respondents indicated that they would rather bear pain than take action to relieve it, primarily because they fear becoming addicted or dependent on medication. Alternatives to drugs, such as relaxation and exercise, were seen as effective pain relievers.

Public Attitudes About Pain and Analgesics: Clinical Implications

Fins JJ (Cornell Univ, New York; Hastings Ctr, Briarcliff Manor, NY)
J Pain Symptom Manage 13:169–171, 1997   16–2

Background.—In addition to assessing the prevalence of pain in daily American life, the Mayday Fund Survey investigated the experience of pain in individuals who had not entered the health care system for evaluation and treatment. The clinical implications of the general public's attitudes toward pain and analgesics were discussed.

Methods and Findings.—The findings of the Mayday Fund Survey indicate that Americans experience pain frequently and that when they do, they tend to be stoic about it. Generally, Americans hope that their pain will pass quickly and is not symptomatic of a serious underlying illness. The implicit message is that response to pain is motivated more by the fear of suffering than by the pain itself. *Suffering* has been defined as the meaning that people attach to the pain experienced. Experiencing pain makes people try to understand what the pain portends for their future health and happiness. Until people know whether the pain will pass quickly, if it means more severe distress, or if it is life threatening, they will suffer profoundly. When a patient understands that the pain can be attended to and, more important, what it represents, the patient will feel relief even before the physical source of pain is treated.

The decision to seek medical attention for pain, then, is determined by a balance between pain and suffering. Medical care will be sought when the pain overwhelms the potential suffering associated with the visit to the physician, which involves a loss of personal control. The issue of loss of control may partly explain the profound fear of addiction reported by the respondents in the Mayday Fund Survey.

Conclusions.—Physicians need to be sensitive to the difference between pain and suffering. Paradoxically, the general public will tolerate pain to avoid suffering. Physicians must understand and address the suffering and anxiety of patients in pain to provide effective treatment.

▶ Many people who teach professionals about the treatment of pain have a feeling of being Sisyphus and rolling the rock up the mountain. Of course, if you turn your back, the stone begins to roll down, necessitating your repeating the process over and over again. Fortunately, the Agency for Health Care Policy and Research came out with their pain treatment guidelines. The use of narcotic analgesics in the appropriate patient was discussed and lauded. Unfortunately, we also have to deal with the patient who may reject pain medication for a variety of reasons. However, as we learn more about the benefits of the patients themselves controlling their medications and of pain-relieving procedures not related to medications, we can mix the factors to help them feel and function better and cease suffering. Of course, we always have to teach about who gets addicted and that very few patients who need narcotic analgesics will ever develop addiction.

M. Weintraub, M.D.

Assessment of Knowledge About Cancer Pain Management by Physicians in Training
Mortimer JE, Bartlett NL (Washington Univ, St Louis)
J Pain Symptom Manage 14:21–28, 1997   16–3

Objective.—Studies have shown that blame for inadequate pain management in cancer patients lies with physicians, patients, and patients' families. Part of the responsibility lies with inadequate training. Results of a questionnaire to assess trainees' objective knowledge of cancer pain management are discussed.

Methods.—Of the 187 internal medicine housestaff, radiation oncology residents, and hematology-oncology fellows at 2 tertiary care hospitals associated with Washington University Medical Center, 81 (43%) completed questionnaires addressing palliative therapy of a hypothetical patient with metastatic lung cancer and included questions on opioid selection, conversion of parenteral morphine to oral, management of opioid toxicities, opioid addition in cancer patients, and efficacy and time course of radiation therapy in treating cancer pain.

Results.—Median time since completion of medical school was 2 years. Whereas 18 correct answers were considered reasonable, the average number of correct answers was 12. Most physicians in training were unaware of World Health Organization guidelines on stepwise progression of analgesic medications. Approximately 75% of physicians in training, when asked to convert a parenteral dose of morphine to an equivalent dose of a controlled-release preparation, calculated a dose one third of the correct dose. Only 2% knew that resolution of pain from radiation therapy may occur after 12 weeks.

Conclusion.—Despite the fact that cancer pain relief has been addressed in lay and medical literature, the majority of physicians in training were deficient in their knowledge of cancer pain management, opioid bioequivalency and pharmacology, and pain management benefits of radiation therapy.

Cancer Pain Emergencies: A Protocol for Management
Hagen NA, Elwood T, Ernst S (Univ of Calgary, Alberta, Canada)
J Pain Symptom Manage 14:45–50, 1997   16–4

Objective.—Established algorithms can be used to manage severe, chronic cancer pain. A treatment protocol is presented to provide rapid and effective relief for severe sustained episodes of excruciating pain (pain emergencies). The clinical course and outcomes of treatment were determined for 9 consecutive patients with metastatic cancer who received treatment for a pain emergency in a prospective pilot study.

Methods.—A pain emergency was defined as a subjective pain intensity score of 8 or higher on a scale of 0 to 10. Nine patients aged 31 to 70 were evaluated during 10 pain emergencies, and pain was assessed. Morphine sulfate 10 to 20 mg IV or an equianalgesic dose of an alternative opioid was infused over a period of 15 minutes. Thirty minutes after evaluation, the patients' vital signs were reassessed and the effective bolus dose was repeated as needed and increased as needed after 12 to 24 hours of stable analgesia or, if necessary, the bolus size was doubled every 30 minutes and infused for 15 minutes. Dose was titrated upward until analgesia was achieved or toxicity developed.

Results.—Pain escalation time ranged from 6 hours to 21 days. All patients had satisfactory pain relief within an average of 89 minutes. No significant toxicity was observed.

Conclusion.—Doubling the intravenous bolus dose of opioid until pain was relieved was an effective, rapid, and safe way of managing intractable pain emergencies in cancer patients.

▶ Unfortunately, young doctors (and some older ones, as well) still don't know much about the treatment of patients with pain as part of their cancer syndrome. Abstract 16–3 describes some of the problems and recommends a potential solution, which is the dissemination of the Agency for Health Care Policy and Research guidelines and local ones as well.

Abstract 16–4 looked at the rapid increasing intravenous opioid dose, which included a doubling every 30 minutes until analgesia was achieved. The authors do recommend validation of the protocol before acceptance by hospital pharmacy and therapeutics committees.

M. Weintraub, M.D.

Self-administration of Over-the-Counter Medication for Pain Among Adolescents
Chambers CT, Reid GJ, McGrath PJ, et al (Dalhousie Univ, Halifax, Nova Scotia)
Arch Pediatr Adolesc Med 151:449–455, 1997   16–5

Objective.—The age at which children begin to self-medicate with over-the-counter (OTC) products is not known. Because numerous studies have suggested that there is a high prevalence of OTC medication use among children and adolescents, the self-administration of medications by adolescents for various types of pain was examined in a community-based survey.

Methods.—A total of 651 students in the seventh, eighth, and ninth grades at 3 junior high schools in Halifax, Nova Scotia, were surveyed (with parental consent) regarding the self-administration of pain medications for pain of the head; stomach; ear and throat; and muscle, joint, and back, as well as menstrual cramps. Demographic information and the frequency and intensity of pain characteristics were also collected.

Results.—Within the previous 3 months, 90.9% of the subjects reported head pain; 80.4%, stomach pain; 83.8%, muscle, joint, or back pain; 76.9%, ear and throat pain; and 58.6%, menstrual pain. Approximately

45% to 65% of children reported 1 to 6 instances of pain in the previous 3 months. Frequencies of medication use were 95.9% for head pain; 90.4% for stomach pain; 58.7% for ear or throat pain; 88.2% for muscle, joint, or back pain; and 88.5% for menstrual pain. Acetaminophen was the most commonly used OTC medication for all types of pain and was taken by 67.8% to 89.2% of children. Children obtained medications from parents 68.5% to 82.3% of the time or from home medicine cabinets 42.9% to 60.9% of the time. Information sources regarding medications were parents (70.4% to 82.1%), bottle or package (35.7% to 40.7%), doctors and nurses (14.8% and 26.5%), and peers (14.0% for medications in general and 18.5% for menstrual pain). Girls had higher-intensity head pain than boys. The degree of self-medication increased with grade. Boys had more stomach pain than girls in seventh grade, but by ninth grade, the situation was reversed. Ninth graders had more ear and throat pain and more muscle, joint, and back pain than seventh graders. Ninth grade girls had more menstrual pain than seventh grade girls. The tendency to self-medicate increased significantly with pain frequency and intensity for all pain except muscle, joint, and back. Self-medication began for most children at age 11.5.

Conclusion.—Although this study is retrospective and is based on self-reporting, it does show that self-administration of OTC drugs among adolescents is common and widespread. How self-medication decisions are made is unclear as is the degree of inappropriate self-medication. Better access to quality information about medications and legislation restricting access of adolescents to OTC medications may be worth considering.

▶ Self-administration of OTC medications is common among adolescents, with both good and bad results.

L. Lasagna, M.D.

EMLA Cream as a Topical Anesthetic Before Office Phlebotomy in Children
Young SS, Schwartz R, Sheridan MJ (Utah Valley Family Practice Residency, Provo; Vienna Pediatric Associates Ltd, Va; Inst of Research and Education, Falls Church, Va)
South Med J 89:1184–1187, 1996   16–6

Background.—For children, venipuncture can be one of the most distressing events in a medical encounter, needlessly eroding the doctor-patient relationship. A mixture of 2.5% lidocaine and 2.5% prilocaine—EMLA cream—can produce dermal anesthesia through intact skin. The value of EMLA cream in reducing distress among children undergoing venipuncture as outpatients was investigated.

Methods and Findings.—Sixty children and adolescents aged 6 months to 18 years were included in the randomized, double-blind, placebo-controlled study. One hour before phlebotomy, EMLA cream or placebo was applied. When compared with placebo, the use of EMLA cream resulted in significant decrease in patient distress, increased ease of the procedure, and less change in heart rate. The EMLA cream also reduced pain. The 2 groups had comparable levels of anticipatory anxiety. Parents and observers rated the efficacy of EMLA cream better than that of placebo.

Conclusions.—The use of EMLA cream is safe and effective in reducing pain and distress among children undergoing venipuncture. Further study of the use of EMLA cream in conjunction with similar medical and surgical procedures is warranted.

▶ Children often hate even the sight of needles after having sustained pain or discomfort in an earlier experience. The advent of EMLA cream, which produces dermal anesthesia through intact skin, is a step forward. This study shows a beneficial effect on everything except anticipatory anxiety.

L. Lasagna, M.D.

Effect of Racemic Mixture and the (S+)-Isomer of Ketamine on Temporal and Spatial Summation of Pain

Arendt-Nielsen L, Nielson J, Petersen-Felix S, et al (Aalborg Univ, Denmark; Inselspital Bern, Switzerland)

Br J Anaesth 77:625–631, 1996   16–7

Background.—Few NMDA antagonists are available for use in humans, and the existing agents have severe psychomimetic effects. Ketamine is available commercially. The analgesic efficacy of racemic mixture and the stereoisomer (S+)-isomer of ketamine on temporal and spatial summation of pain was reported.

Methods.—Twelve healthy subjects participated in the double-blind, 3-way crossover, placebo-controlled study. Pain evoked by small and large area pressure stimuli, pain detection threshold and pain ratings to small and large area of heat stimuli, pain detection threshold and pain rating to heat stimuli of brief and long duration, summation pain threshold and pain ratings to repeated heat and electrical stimuli, adverse effects, and reaction times were assessed. Ketamine (racemic) and ketamine (S+) were assessed at plasma levels of 350 and 180 ng mL^{-1}, respectively.

Findings.—Ketamine (racemic) prolonged reaction time more than ketamine (S+). Both agents affected pain resulting from repeated stimuli or stimuli of long duration equally or more than a single stimulus of short duration. In addition, both agents affected pain evoked from large areas equally or more than pain from small areas. The (S+)-isomer was about twice as potent as the racemic mixture in inhibiting central summation.

Conclusions.—Ketamine (racemic) and ketamine (S+) both had a general analgesic effect and an effect on repeated stimuli, on long duration stimuli, and on stimuli covering large areas. The doses tested had the same number of adverse effects, which were minimal.

▶ This is one case where the (S+)-isomer appeared to have the activity of twice as much of the racemic mixture. This supports the evidence of other studies which show that the (S+)-isomer was greater in potency than the (R−)-isomer for the management of postoperative pain. It doesn't work out exactly this way every time. For example, with some drugs there is a conversion back to the racemate version, all or in part, once the drug enters the body so that you may find only a third or less difference in the amount of the 2 isomers in the body. Also, sometimes the 2 isomers have similar effects on 1 receptor although one has more of an effect on another receptor. Thus, the racemate is just as easy to give. Years ago, when it was so much more difficult to make 1 isomer, we had to make do with the racemate. Now for ketamine, the isomers are so different in their effects and we can more easily manufacture them. We should choose the one that is more active and has less side effects.

M. Weintraub, M.D.

Extradural Morphine Gives Better Pain Relief Than Patient-controlled I.V. Morphine After Hysterectomy

Eriksson-Mjöberg M, Svensson J-O, Almkvist O, et al (Karolinska Inst, Huddinge, Sweden)
Br J Anaesth 78:10–16, 1997   16–8

Introduction.—Comparisons of single doses of extradural morphine and IV morphine by patient-controlled analgesia (PCA) have yielded contradictory results. The effects of PCA administration of IV morphine and extradural morphine were compared during the first 18 hours after hysterectomy.

Methods.—Patients were randomized to receive either extradural morphine, 0.06 mg/kg, by completion of surgery and 6 hours postoperatively or IV infusion of morphine, 0.2 mg/kg, after surgery. Both groups received PCA with morphine, 0.04 mg/kg. A visual analogue scale (VAS) was used to monitor pain relief, and patients were assessed for side effects and cognitive function for 18 hours after surgery. Serum morphine concentrations were evaluated.

Results.—The mean PCA morphine consumption was 2.4 mg/h and 1 mg/h, respectively, for the IV and extradural groups. The IV group had significantly higher VAS scores, compared with the extradural group. Patients with IV morphine experienced itching, tiredness, blurred vision, and vertigo that correlated with cumulative consumption, compared with tiredness only for patients in the extradural group. Patients in both groups experienced decreased ability to perform tests of cognitive function, despite markedly lower plasma morphine concentrations for patients in the extradural group.

Conclusion.—Patients in the IV morphine group had unlimited access to morphine but had higher VAS pain scores than patients receiving extradural morphine. The quality of pain relief afforded by extradural morphine in patients undergoing hysterectomy was superior to that of IV morphine.

▶ The literature on comparisons of patient-controlled IV morphine and extradural morphine is contradictory and inconsistent in its conclusions. In this study, the extradural route was clearly the winner, and the authors speculate that the explanation lies in the lower effectiveness of IV morphine in treating visceral pain, hysterectomy being a cause of both somatic (cutaneous and muscular) and visceral pain.

L. Lasagna, M.D.

Monitoring of Opioid Therapy in Advanced Cancer Pain Patients
Mercadante S, Dardanoni G, Salvaggio L, et al (Pain Relief and Palliative Care SAMOT, Palermo, Italy; Buccheri La Ferla Fatebenefratelli Hosp Palermo, Italy; Ingrassia Hosp, Palermo, Italy)
J Pain Symptom Manage 13:204–212, 1997   16–9

Background.—No parameters for monitoring opioid treatment for pain in cancer patients have been available to date. Factors that may be associated with response to opioids in this population were evaluated.

Methods.—Three hundred twenty-five consecutive patients with advanced cancer were scheduled for the prospective longitudinal survey. After exclusions, the study population included 67 patients. All had advanced cancer and pain requiring opioid treatment for more than 6 weeks before they died.

Findings.—Advanced age, being female, and previous chemotherapy all decreased the opioid escalation index (OEI). A higher OEI was associated with head and neck cancer. An increased OEI was also correlated with the presence of confusion, which in turn was correlated with neuropathic pain. However, neuropathic pain alone did not affect the score. Sex-specific cancer affected the sex differences reported for the length of the stable dose period. Twenty-eight patients had a good response; 33, partial response; and 6 patients, no response. Psychological factors were correlated with poor pain relief, probably because of decreased compliance with therapy.

Conclusions.—The indices used in the current study may be useful as audit tools and in clinical research. Additional surveys are needed to validate these indices.

▶ Intelligent prescribing of opioids to patients with advanced cancer can achieve good pain control in at least half of this population. This study is a nice attempt to determine what factors seem important in determining response to these analgesics.

Increases in dosage can be caused by increased severity of disease, pharmacologic tolerance, or both.

L. Lasagna, M.D.

Day-to-Day Titration to Initiate Transdermal Fentanyl in Patients With Cancer Pain: Short- and Long-term Experiences in a Prospective Study of 39 Patients
Korte W, de Stoutz N, Morant R (Kantonsspital, St Gallen, Switzerland)
J Pain Symptom Manage 11:139–146, 1996   16–10

Background.—Transdermal fentanyl is used to treat patients with chronic pain. Plasma levels stabilize within about 72 hours. Steady state plasma concentrations have been reported with additional doses of transdermal fentanyl at 72-hour intervals. If shorter intervals are used, accumulation may be a concern. Experience with converting patients to transdermal fentanyl from other opioids with the recommended dosages has been unsatisfactory. Because some studies have indicated that a relative steady state occurs 15 to 20 hours after application of transdermal fentanyl, early titration at 24-hour intervals should be possible.

Methods.—In a prospective study, increased initial doses and day-to-day titration of transdermal fentanyl were studied in 39 patients with uncontrolled cancer pain. There were 16 men and 23 women; the mean age was 62 years. Morphine was available for breakthrough pain.

Results.—After 24 hours, patients reported significant reduction in pain. Within 48 hours, satisfactory analgesia was obtained and maintained throughout the study. During weeks 1 to 4, significant increases in transdermal fentanyl were needed to control pain. Almost half of the patients needed 1 or more early dose increases. Side effects in 1 patient resulted partially from the specific properties of transdermal fentanyl. In general, side effects were less common than with morphine.

Discussion.—Dose-finding in patients who are to be given transdermal fentanyl can be effective and safe by day-to-day titration. Patients should be monitored carefully, and rescue medication for breakthrough pain should always be available. The initial doses recommended by the manufacturer are too low; 150% of the recommended dose was appropriate. Transdermal fentanyl caused less constipation than expected.

▶ I have believed for many years that an analgesic regimen should start with higher doses and then taper down to standard doses. In a sense, this is the so-called "sponge" theory of disease treatment. At a time when pain levels are very high, adverse effects are not likely to occur from high doses of analgesics. Pain control is much more rapid when performed in this way, and the total analgesic used over the first few days or over a course of analgesic therapy will be much less.

M. Weintraub, M.D.

Intravenous Methadone for Cancer Pain Unrelieved by Morphine and Hydromorphone: Clinical Observations
Manfredi PL, Borsook D, Chandler SW, et al (Massachusetts Gen Hosp, Boston; Univ of Texas, Houston)
Pain 70:99–101, 1997   16–11

Background.—Methadone is very effective as a second-line opioid in the treatment of pain from cancer. However, the starting doses shown on the opioid conversion charts may overestimate the IV dose needed. Four patients with cancer-related pain treated with continuous IV morphine and hydromorphone were reported.

      Case Reports.—The patients were 2 women and 2 men, aged 44 to 54. In all patients, persistent pain and opioid side effects limited increases in opioid dose. Thus, the patients were switched to IV methadone. The starting dose in each patient was about 3% of the calculated equivalent dose of hydromorphone according to the available conversion charts. Excellent pain relief was achieved with these low doses in all 4 patients. No significant side effects occurred.

Conclusions.—These 4 patients had excellent relief of cancer pain without significant side effects with an IV methadone dose that, according to the conversion charts, was only about 3% of the calculated equivalent dose of hydromorphone. Clinicians should use such low doses when converting from continuous IV hydromorphone to continuous IV methadone.

▶ The intelligent prescribing of oral opioids can control most patients with cancer pain. In the remainder, intravenous medication is required. These case reports remind us that IV methadone is a fine drug and more potent than is suggested by current opioid conversion charts.

L. Lasagna, M.D.

Patient Controlled Oral Analgesia With Morphine
Striebel HW, Römer M, Kopf A, et al (Free Univ, Berlin, Germany)
Can J Anaesth 43:749–753, 1996   16–12

Objective.—Intravenous patient-controlled analgesia is widely used for severe postoperative pain. For many patients who can drink and eat on the evening after surgery, some form of demand-adapted oral opioid titration is desirable. A new device for patient-controlled oral analgesia (PCORA) was evaluated for use in postoperative pain management.

      Methods.—The PCORA system was developed by modifying a Baxter IV patient-controlled analgesia system, with a maximum bolus volume of

0.5 mL and a flow rate for filling bolus volume of 0.5 mL·hr^{-1}. The PCORA system was compared with customarily prescribed pain therapy (CPPT) in 20 patients having orthopedic surgery. The patients were randomly assigned to 300 minutes of PCORA or CPPT, followed by 300 minutes of the other method. The maximum PCORA dose was 15 mg of morphine per hour. Pain and side effects were evaluated every 30 minutes.

Results.—The bolus volume delivered by the PCORA system was 89% accurate compared with the manufacturer's specifications. Pain intensity decreased over time with PCORA, but not with physician- or nurse-administered CPPT. No significant difference in the mean morphine requirement was seen between groups. The patients had no problems using the PCORA system.

Conclusions.—The PCORA system offers an effective, noninvasive method of postoperative pain management. It is reliable and easy to use, and patients like it better than CPPT. The authors call for further studies to compare oral and IV patient-controlled analgesia.

▶ This device is a modification of the Baxter PCA-on-demand system. It was set to deliver a maximum of 15 mg of morphine per hour. The results are another plus for patient-controlled analgesia.

L. Lasagna, M.D.

Antiemetic Efficacy of Ondansetron With Patient-controlled Analgesia
Davies PRF, Warwick P, O'Connor M (Princess Margaret Hosp, Swindon, England)
Anaesthesia 51:880–882, 1996   16–13

Objective.—The most frequent complication of postoperative patient-controlled analgesia (PCA) is nausea and vomiting (PONV). Previous studies have suggested that ondansetron can reduce nausea and vomiting after chemotherapy and surgery. The effects of ondansetron on PONV in patients receiving PCA were assessed in a double-blind, randomized, placebo-controlled trial.

Methods.—The study included 66 patients who were scheduled for total abdominal hysterectomy. All received the same regimen of anesthesia and PCA. Patients assigned to group 1 also received ondansetron, 4 mg, given at induction of anesthesia and again 8 hours later. Patients in group 2 received a saline placebo. The antiemetic efficacy of ondansetron during PCA was assessed.

Results.—There was no difference in pain scores, nausea scores, number of episodes of vomiting, use of rescue antiemetics, or recollection of nausea and vomiting. In the first 24 postoperative hours, 70% of patients in the placebo group and 85% of those in the ondansetron group had nausea or vomiting.

Conclusions.—At the dose studied, ondansetron does not reduce PONV in patients receiving PCA after total abdominal hysterectomy. In this study,

PONV was actually more common in women receiving ondansetron than in those receiving placebo.

▶ The commonest complication of PCA is postoperative nausea and vomiting. Sad to say, in the present study, the antiemetic ondansetron failed to prevent nausea and vomiting in most patients who had undergone total abdominal hysterectomy and in fact results were worse than with placebo. Would higher doses have worked better?

L. Lasagna, M.D.

Effect of Intramuscular Intraoperative Pain Medication on Narcotic Usage After Laparoscopic Cholecystectomy
Lane GE, Lathrop JC, Boysen DA, et al (Saginaw Cooperative Hosps Inc, Mich; Michigan State Univ, Saginaw)
Am Surg 62:907–910, 1996   16–14

Introduction.—Pain control in the early postoperative period can be a significant problem in patients undergoing outpatient surgery. Injection of local anesthetic into the wound can reduce postoperative pain but is not always effective. For patients undergoing laparoscopic cholecystectomy, some long-acting injectable medication without side effects would be desirable. The effects of intraoperative ketorolac tromethamine injection on postoperative pain relief in patients undergoing elective laparoscopic cholecystectomy were evaluated.

Methods.—The randomized, double-blind clinical trial included 125 patients undergoing laparoscopic cholecystectomy. They were assigned to receive placebo; 100 mg of intramuscular meperidine intraoperatively, before or after the procedure; or 60 mg of intramuscular ketorolac tromethamine intraoperatively, before or after the procedure. The groups were compared for postoperative pain ratings and narcotic use.

Results.—All 4 active treatment groups used less pain medication in the recovery room than did the control group. The pain-free interval was longer in patients receiving preprocedural ketorolac than in those receiving meperidine or placebo. Postoperative narcotic use was significantly reduced in both ketorolac groups. Pain ratings showed less postoperative pain in the ketorolac groups than in the control group but no significant difference between the meperidine groups and the control group.

Conclusions.—Intraoperative ketorolac injection can reduce postoperative pain for patients undergoing laparoscopic cholecystectomy. Postoperative use of narcotics is reduced for patients receiving ketorolac. Giving this long-acting nonsteroidal anti-inflammatory drug during surgery may ease the transition to oral pain medication after surgery.

▶ In the typical hospital, pain is most often encountered after surgery. It is often treated poorly by an every-4-hour approach, which ignores the greater need for patient analgesia in the immediate postoperative period. Inadequate dosing often reflects the unfounded fears of doctors and nurses regarding opioid-induced respiratory depression and addiction.

Laparoscopic surgery is on the rise; for patients having such surgery, patient-controlled analgesia and epidural catheters are not the answer. A long-acting analgesic makes sense in this venue, and the present study describes some promising results from the use of intraoperative analgesia, especially with ketorolac.

L. Lasagna, M.D.

A Double-blind Comparison of Codeine and Morphine for Postoperative Analgesia Following Intracranial Surgery
Goldsack C, Scuplak SM, Smith M (Natl Hosp for Neurology and Neurosurgery, Queen Square, London; Great Ormond Street Hosp, London)
Anaesthesia 51:1029–1032, 1996   16–15

Background.—Codeine phosphate is preferred to stronger opioid analgesics after intracranial neurosurgery. The efficacy and safety of codeine phosphate and morphine sulphate were compared for postoperative craniotomy analgesia.

Methods.—Forty patients undergoing intracranial neurosurgery were enrolled in the double-blind comparison. Eighteen patients were given codeine phosphate, 60 mg, for postoperative analgesia, and 18 patients received morphine sulfate, 10 mg. Both agents were administered by intramuscular injection. Four patients needed no analgesia.

Findings.—Both agents provided analgesia within 20 minutes of injection. However, morphine was more effective than codeine after 60 minutes, and fewer doses of morphine than of codeine were needed. Nine patients asked for 1 dose of morphine, and 9 asked for 2 doses. By contrast, 7 patients required 3 doses of codeine and 1 patient required 4 doses. There were no instances of respiratory depression, sedation, pupillary constriction, or unwanted cardiovascular effects in either group.

Conclusions.—Morphine, with a more persistent action than codeine, appears to be a safe alternative to codeine for analgesia after neurosurgery. Further research is needed to determine the efficacy of morphine given intravenously after neurosurgery.

▶ Codeine has been the preferred medication after intracranial surgery for a lot of reasons. One of the most important is a feeling that morphine would raise intracranial pressure and might do damage to these patients who have just undergone intracranial surgery. This was not shown in this particular study. In fact, the morphine worked for a longer time and didn't cause respiratory depression or signs of increased intracranial pressure.

M. Weintraub, M.D.

Preoperative Local Infiltration With Ropivacaine for Postoperative Pain Relief After Inguinal Hernia Repair: A Randomised Controlled Trial

Johansson B, Hallerbäck B, Stubberöd A, et al (Norra Älvsborgs Länssjukhus, Trollhättan, Sweden; Värnamo Sjukhus, Sweden; Diakonhjemmets Sykehus, Oslo, Norway; et al)

Eur J Surg 163:371–378, 1997   16–16

Objective.—Whereas infiltration of a surgical wound with local anesthesia reduces postoperative pain, studies of the effect of preoperative infiltration of local anesthetics are inconsistent. One study found long-term pain relief from preoperative infiltration of local anesthetic, after hernia repair, whereas another study of pain relief after cholecystectomy showed no long-term effect from preincisional local anesthetic. The effects of preoperative local infiltration with ropivacaine in 2 doses on postoperative pain after inguinal hernia repair were evaluated immediately postoperatively and during the first postoperative week. Also evaluated were patients' perceptions of well-being and ability to function in daily activities during the week after surgery.

Methods.—In a multicenter, parallel, randomized, double-blind, placebo-controlled study, 131 men, aged 18 to 70 years, received preoperative local infiltration in the surgical wound area with 200 mg 0.5% ropivacaine, 100 mg 0.25% ropivacaine, or saline. Postoperative pain at rest and during mobilization was evaluated 3, 6, 10, and 24 hours and 7 days after infiltration on a visual analogue scale from 0 (no pain) to 100 (worst pain). An electronic pressure transducer was used to determine the pain threshold and maximum pain tolerance to wound pressure. Quality of life was assessed by the Psychological General Well-Being Index and the Minor Symptoms Evaluation Profile. Adverse events were recorded. The difference between groups was analyzed statistically.

Results.—Five patients were withdrawn from the study. Wound pain at rest was significantly lower in the ropivacaine groups than in the placebo group 3 hours after infiltration. Wound pain during mobilization, maximum pain threshold, and pressure causing maximum pain tolerance were significantly lower in the 200 mg ropivacaine group than in the 100 mg ropivacaine and placebo groups. Time until first request for analgesics after infiltration was significantly shorter for the saline group than for the ropivacaine groups. Significantly more patients in the saline group than in the ropivacaine groups requested analgesics. Results of well-being and quality of life assessments were similar among the 3 groups. Treatments were generally well tolerated and adverse events reported were not judged to be related to treatment.

Conclusion.—Preoperative infiltration of local anesthetics resulted in significant pain relief for 3 to 6 hours after inguinal hernia surgery. The treatment was generally well-tolerated.

▶ One theory supporting the use of local anesthetics preoperatively is that the patients, having never had painful stimuli, will recover more easily and more quickly from the operation. Unfortunately, that did not happen in this study. The theory is more theoretical than actual. However, it would be very important if this could be shown to occur.

One interesting thing about this paper is that it was in the *European Journal of Surgery* and contained abstracts in French, German, and Russian as well as English. Together with interpretation of the graphs, that would make this paper very easy to understand if one were a speaker of only 1 of those languages.

M. Weintraub, M.D.

A Double-blind Randomised Comparison of the Effects of Epidural Clonidine, Lignocaine and the Combination of Clonidine and Lignocaine in Patients With Chronic Pain
Glynn C, O'Sullivan K (Univ of Oxford, England; Adelaide Hosp, Dublin)
Pain 64:337–343, 1995   16–17

Objective.—Few controlled studies have investigated the analgesic effects of epidural clonidine in the treatment of chronic pain. When epidural clonidine and local anesthetics are given in combination, it is not clear whether the analgesic effect is due to clonidine, the local anesthetic, or both. The effect of epidural clonidine, lignocaine, and clonidine plus lignocaine were compared in a randomized, double-blind, crossover study in patients with chronic pain who had obtained relief from the combination.

Methods.—Either 150 μg clonidine, 40 mg lignocaine, or the combination were administered to 20 patients (9 men), aged 23 to 78, with chronic lower back or leg pain (n=9), neuropathic pain (n=9), pelvic pain (n=1), and Wegner's granulomatosis (n=1). Pain intensity was recorded every 10 minutes for 30 minutes and then every 30 minutes for 2 hours. Patients were crossed over to the other 2 arms of the study in 24 hours or when the pain returned to its original intensity.

Results.—The 17 patients who completed all 3 arms of the study reported their best pain relief. Twelve patients preferred the combination, 4 preferred clonidine, none preferred lignocaine, and 1 had no relief from any of the injections. Summed pain intensity difference analysis showed a significant difference between the combination and lignocaine only, whereas total pain score (TOTPAR) analysis revealed no significant differences between any of the injections. Clonidine produced a motor blockade in 3 patients and a sensory blockade in 3. Lignocaine produced a sensory blockade in 6 patients, and a motor blockade in 3. The combination produced a neurological blockade in 17 patients, a sensory blockade in 6, and a motor blockade in 11. Neurological blockage and analgesia were not related. Six clonidine patients and 1 lignocaine patient had side effects.

Conclusion.—The combination of clonidine and lignocaine was most effective in treating patients with chronic lower body pain.

▶ This study used a sophisticated technique called enrichment. The patients had already responded to clonidine and lidocaine. That may be the reason why no patient in the study reported that lidocaine was, by itself, the superior analgesic. The vast majority picked out the lidocane plus clonidine, even though clonidine itself was rated poorly and chosen as the best analgesic by only 4 of the 17 patients. The question we have to answer and deal with is what is the meaning of co-analgesia and supra-additive in this setting? Perhaps these patients were the most sensitive to this particular combination of analgesic drugs, or maybe it is really that the combination is the most effective treatment. There are newer statistical techniques for testing potentiation and supra-additivity of drugs. They may be the answer to help us understand the effect of clonidine in this combination.

M. Weintraub, M.D.

Erythromelalgia Pain Managed With Gabapentin
McGraw T, Kosek P (Oregon Health Sciences Univ, Portland)
Anesthesiology 86:988–990, 1997   16–18

Objective.—Two cases of erythromelalgia, episodic burning pain, erythema, and elevated temperature of the hands and/or feet, controlled with the anticonvulsant gabapentin, are presented.

> *Case 1.*—A man, 42, with severe pain and swelling in his legs and feet of 3 months' duration, had been diagnosed with multiple sclerosis 9 months earlier. His legs were erythematous, warm, edematous, and tender with easily palpable pulses. His pain was unrelieved even by intravenous morphine. Oral gabapentin (100 mg 3 times daily) relieved his pain within 30 minutes. His dosage was increased to 300 mg 3 times daily, and his edema largely resolved. He has been pain-free for 4 months.
> *Case 2.*—A child, 9, was evaluated for unrelieved, severe foot and hand pain of 1 month's duration and no history of trauma. Lumbar epidural bupivacaine relieved the foot pain, but the loss of sensation distressed the patient. Gabapentin, 100 mg 3 times daily, increased to 300 mg 3 times daily relieved her pain completely within 1 month. After 4 months she was weaned from her medications and has remained pain-free for months.

Conclusion.—Gabapentin relieved the pain of erythromelalgia in 2 patients. The treatment was safe and well tolerated.

▶ Reading the details of the 2 cases is really very instructive. It's possible that these patients would have improved without the gabapentin. However, erythromelalgia is really a very difficult to treat disease in which the hands or feet, or both, have severe burning type of pain, they are red, and they have higher temperature. The tricyclic antidepressants have been tried, I believe, with little success. However, they seem to be better than nothing and can be used in combination with aspirin, which may help as well. The patients get serious emersion problems from keeping their feet or hands or both in ice water. It is certainly worth a try of gabapentin for a couple of weeks to see if it will work.

M. Weintraub, M.D.

A Non-selective (Amitriptyline), But Not a Selective (Citalopram), Serotonin Reuptake Inhibitor Is Effective in the Prophylactic Treatment of Chronic Tension-type Headache
Bendtsen L, Jensen R, Olesen J (Univ of Copenhagen, Glostrup, Denmark)
J Neurol Neurosurg Psychiatry 61:285–290, 1996   16–19

Background.—Although tension-type headache is the most common type of headache and has important socioeconomic impact, little is known about its pathophysiology and treatment. Amitriptyline is a tricyclic antidepressant and is the only established prophylaxis for tension-type headache. Studies of this treatment have reported inconsistent results. There is little scientific evidence for the widespread use of amitriptyline for chronic tension-type headache. Citalopram is a selective serotonin reuptake inhibitor with antidepressant properties similar to those of tricyclic drugs. Citalopram may be effective treatment for chronic tension-type headache. The effectiveness of amitriptyline and citalopram for chronic tension-type headache was studied in a double-blind, placebo-controlled, 3-way crossover trial.

Methods.—There were 40 patients with chronic tension-type headache who were randomly assigned to one of 6 treatment sequences with amitriptyline, citalopram, and placebo. The treatment periods were 8 weeks and the study period was 32 weeks.

Results.—Of the 40 patients, 34 completed the trial. Compared to placebo, amitriptyline reduced areas under the headache curve by 30%. Citalopram had no significant effect. Amitriptyline significantly reduced the duration of headache, headache frequency, and use of analgesics. Amitriptyline did not reduce headache intensity.

Discussion.—In this group of treatment-resistant patients with chronic tension-type headache, amitriptyline had a significant effect, though it did not eliminate the headache. Mechanisms other than inhibition of serotonin reuptake are involved in the analgesic effect of tricyclic drugs.

▶ Tension-type headache is very common and has significant socioeconomic impact. Data to support the prophylactic use of amitriptyline in such patients have not been easy to come by. The present positive study is a welcome addition. Amitriptyline's efficacy as an analgesic here and in patients with postherpetic neuralgia, and the drug's superiority over specific serotonin reuptake inhibitors strengthens the belief that amitriptyline analgesia is independent of antidepressant activity. It also reminds us that "dirty" drugs (i.e., those that affect multiple receptors) may at times be better than "clean" ones.

L. Lasagna, M.D.

Nonprescription Ibuprofen and Acetaminophen in the Treatment of Tension-type Headache
Schachtel BP, Furey SA, Thoden WR (McGill Univ, Montreal; Whitehall-Robins Healthcare, Madison, NJ)
J Clin Pharmacol 36:1120–1125, 1996   16–20

Objective.—There are no studies directly comparing acetaminophen and ibuprofen in the treatment of tension-type headache. The efficacy of 400 mg ibuprofen and 1,000 mg of acetaminophen on tension-type headache was compared in a single-center, randomized, placebo-controlled trial.

Methods.—Either acetaminophen (n=151), ibuprofen (n=153), or placebo (n=151) was administered to 455 patients (170 males). At 30 minutes, and 1, 2, 3, and 4 hours after administration, patients rated the

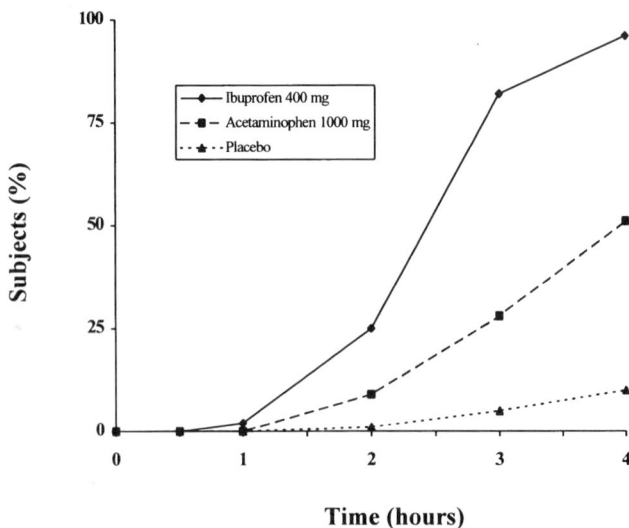

Time (hours)

FIGURE 3.—Number of participants reporting no pain on the 100-mm Headache Pain Intensity Scale at each time point after administration. Participants receiving ibuprofen at 400 mg reported experiencing no pain in a significantly shorter period than those receiving acetaminophen at 1,000 mg ($P < 0.001$). (Courtesy of Schachtel BP, Furey SA, Thoden WR: Nonprescription ibuprofen and acetaminophen in the treatment of tension-type headache. *J Clin Pharm* 36:1120–1125, 1996. Copyright © American Society of Clinical Pharmacology.)

intensity of their headaches on the 100-mm Headache Pain Intensity Scale and the pain on the 5-point Headache Pain Severity Scale.

Results.—The mean headache score for participants was 3.4 with an intensity of 71 mm. Patients experienced significantly more pain and intensity relief with ibuprofen and acetaminophen than with placebo (63% vs. 34% vs. 7%). Patients treated with ibuprofen experienced significantly more complete relief and achieved it faster than with acetaminophen (Fig 3). One placebo-treated patient had nausea.

Conclusion.—Whereas both acetaminophen and ibuprofen are effective at treating the pain and intensity of tension-type headache, ibuprofen provided significantly more complete relief significantly faster than acetaminophen.

▶ Headache is really a difficult clinical model in which to study analgesics. First of all, there is generally a high placebo effect because, as we all know, headaches get better. Then, there is a difficulty in getting a pure tension-type headache and separating it from sinus headache or migraine headache of a milder type, so you have to be really certain as to what kind of headache you're dealing with. As shown in the graph that accompanies this abstract, ibuprofen, in this study, was superior both to placebo and to acetaminophen. The graph shows the number of participants reporting no pain, a very important and too rarely noted outcome.

M. Weintraub, M.D.

Pharmacokinetic and Pharmacodynamic Profiles of Sumatriptan in Migraine Patients With Headache Recurrence or No Response
Visser WH, Burggraaf J, Muller LM, et al (Leiden Univ, The Netherlands; Ctr for Human Drug Research, Leiden, The Netherlands; Glaxo Group Research Ltd, Ware, England)
Clin Pharmacol Ther 60:452–460, 1996   16–21

Background.—For most patients, sumatriptan is effective in the acute treatment of migraine. However, as many as 15% of patients do not obtain relief from sumatriptan, and 40% may have recurrent headache within 24 hours. The available evidence suggests that this phenomenon may be related to patient characteristics, rather than to some characteristic that is present during attacks only. Pharmacokinetic or pharmacodynamic differences involved in nonresponse to sumatriptan were studied.

Methods.—Three groups of patients were studied: 14 patients who had lasting relief of migraine after taking a 6 mg subcutaneous dose of sumatriptan, 12 patients who consistently had recurrent headache after taking sumatriptan, and 6 patients with no relief after taking sumatriptan. For practical reasons, the patients were studied when not having migraine attacks. The pharmacokinetic profiles of these groups were compared. Changes in the diameter and blood velocity of the common, internal, and external carotid arteries were assessed as well.

Results.—There were no significant differences in the pharmacokinetic and pharmacodynamic profiles of the 3 groups, even though the study had sufficient power to detect substantial differences. Neither were there any differences in the adverse event rate.

Conclusion.—No differences were found in the pharmacokinetic or pharmacodynamic profiles of migraine patients with differing patterns of response to sumatriptan. There were no differences in the effects of sumatriptan on blood flow velocity or blood vessel diameter. The results suggest that the newer sumatriptan-like drugs will be no more effective than sumatriptan in terms of initial response or prevention of recurrent headache.

▶ Only about half of patients with migraine who use sumatriptan respond optimally to this drug, and the response is said to be "patient-dependent," i.e., the response varies among patients but not among each individual (patients do not respond differently at different times, for example).

These authors attempted to explain the different therapeutic responses either by different pharmacokinetics or by different cerebral blood flow dynamics. They failed, but the research idea was admirable.

L. Lasagna, M.D.

Chronic Pain in Cystic Fibrosis
Ravilly S, Robinson W, Suresh S, et al (Children's Hosp, Boston; Harvard Med School, Boston; Children's Mem Hosp, Chicago)
Pediatrics 98:741–747, 1996   16–22

Introduction.—In the last few decades, survival has improved substantially for patients with cystic fibrosis (CF). This has led to the emergence of various chronic nonpulmonary manifestations of CF, including arthritis, headache, and chest pain. Little information about the management of chronic pain in CF is available, however. The incidence and treatment of chronic pain among patients with CF were examined in a retrospective study.

Methods.—Two groups of patients with CF were studied: 55 patients older than 5 years of age who died during follow-up between 1984 and 1993 and 23 patients who were evaluated by the authors' pain treatment service. The records of these patients were reviewed to gain insight into the management of serious pain in a relatively older and sicker population of patients with CF.

Findings.—The posthumous survey found a sharp increase in the incidence of chronic pain in the 6 months before death in patients with CF. Sixty-five percent of patients had chest pain and 55% had headache. Back pain was present in 19% of patients, abdominal pain in 19%, and limb pain in 16%. The major causes of headache were hypercarbia or hypoxia, migraine, and sinusitis. Most of the chest pain was musculoskeletal in origin, although pleuritis, pneumothorax, and rib fracture also occurred.

Most patients had at least 1 attempt at nonpharmacologic therapy, such as acupuncture, transcutaneous electrical nerve stimulation, relaxation, and biofeedback. These were generally tried before opioid therapy. Opioid treatment was eventually required in 53% of patients and continued for more than 3 months in 13% of patients. Regional analgesia was effective in 8 patients with very severe pain.

Conclusions.—Many patients with CF, particularly older patients, have chronic pain problems. Nonpharmacologic approaches are of value in this population. Opioid treatment is effective and safe, if used with caution. Regional anesthesia can be very effective in treating severe pain while preserving pulmonary toilet.

▶ Cystic fibrosis, although still a dread disease, is no longer fatal at a median age of 14 years (as it was in 1969). Median survival has at least doubled in the 1990s, as a result of better nutritional management and aggressive antibiotic treatment. Chronic pain seems to be a considerable problem in patients with CF, especially in the last 6 months of life. Chest pain and headaches are the most common manifestations of this tendency, but pain in the back, abdomen, and limbs also occurs. The authors achieved good results with regional analgesia and opioids.

L. Lasagna, M.D.

Case Report: Pain Relief With Oral Cannabinoids in Familial Mediterranean Fever
Holdcroft A, Smith M, Jacklin A, et al (Hammersmith Hosp, London; Maudsley Hosp, London; Univ of London)
Anaesthesia 52:483–488, 1997   16–23

Introduction.—Cannabinoids may have analgesic and anti-inflammatory effects, but their medicinal use has been limited by licensing regulations and a lack of standardized preparations. Clinical trials of licensed pharmaceutical extracts of cannabis may help overcome these problems. A double-blind, placebo-controlled trial of a standardized pharmaceutical preparation of cannabinoids in capsular form was conducted in a patient with familial Mediterranean fever.

> *Case Report.*—Man, 29, had experienced severe abdominal pain for more than 10 years. In 1992, sigmoidoscopy, endoscopy, and ultrasonography were normal. Conservative treatment and analgesia were somewhat effective in relieving his symptoms. Familial Mediterranean fever was diagnosed. The patient's pain was less severe and frequent in response to colchicine. In 1993, he was prescribed a modified-release morphine sulfate because of increased pain, and he had reasonable pain relief with 30 mg twice per day. When he was referred to the pain clinic, the patient had continuous pain of 4 cm or 5 cm, with sporadic increases to 10 cm,

on a 10-cm Visual Analogue Scale. He took temazepam at night in order to sleep. A suitable analgesic dosage of orally given cannabinoids was determined. The patient was administered tetrahydrocannabinol 50 mg per day in 5 divided doses. The patient's regular medication was maintained. Tetrahydrocannabinol did not reduce inflammation but significantly reduced the need for additional analgesic.

Discussion.—This is the first report in the United Kingdom of a standardized pharmaceutical preparation of naturally occurring cannabis. Its use in treating chronic inflammatory pain of gastrointestinal origin has not been previously documented. There are potential problems and legal restrictions in conducting clinical trials of naturally occurring substances with therapeutic potential but with known psychomotor effects in high dosage. The conditions under which manufacturers would prepare such preparations for legitimate clinical use have not been determined.

▶ It seems at times impossible to have a discussion about the medical benefits of marijuana without politics and drug abuse interests contaminating the playing field. This study nicely shows that tetrahydrocannabinol was effective in managing the pain of a patient with familial Mediterranean fever.

L. Lasagna, M.D.

17 Psychiatric Disorders

Chronological Milestones to Guide Drug Change: When Should Clinicians Switch Antidepressants?
Quitkin FM, McGrath PJ, Stewart JW, et al (Columbia Univ, New York)
Arch Gen Psychiatry 53:785–792, 1996   17–1

Introduction.—Antidepressant treatment is ineffective in 30% to 40% of patients. There are few data on the important decision of when to switch a depressed patient to a new treatment. Some authors maintain that patients who are or are not going to respond can be identified within a short time. The time at which patients who have not responded to antidepressant treatment are unlikely to benefit and should have their treatment changed was determined.

Methods.—The study used data from 8 antidepressant studies performed at a university-affiliated outpatient clinic over 10 years. Each study included an initial, single-blind placebo run-in period followed by a 6-week double-blind trial. There were 5 drug-placebo comparisons and 3 drug-drug comparisons. Drugs evaluated included monoamine oxidase inhibitors, tricyclic antidepressants, and mianserin. The patients' clinical condition was analyzed by the Clinical Global Impression Scale at the end of the run-in period. The current analysis included 593 patients who did not improve with placebo and proceeded to the double-blind comparison. The course of this 6-week treatment period was analyzed to identify the week at which patients were more likely to respond by the end of the study than patients receiving placebo.

Results.—The percentage of patients who had no improvement in response to treatment by the end of week 3 but were rated as responders by week 6 was 32% in the drug-treated groups and 10% in the placebo-treated groups. Drug and placebo treatment were equally effective in patients who were still unimproved by week 4. Until that point, the prognosis was better with active treatment for drug-treated patients who had not improved significantly but had had minimal improvement at some point.

Conclusions.—Patients who have not had at least minimal improvement after 4 weeks of treatment with an adequate dose of antidepressant should have their treatment changed. Such patients accounted for only about 10% of drug-treated patients in this placebo-controlled analysis. Treatment also should be changed for patients who have had minimal improvement previously but not after week 5. In patients with minimal improvement in week 5, treatment should continue for another week.

▶ Depressed patients who need an antidepressant drug must put up with delays in improvement because several weeks usually go by before any significant change occurs. Even when improvement starts (as gauged by observers or the physician), the patient may deny any change for the better. Failure to respond is often a result of inadequate dosage, but the failures described in this paper presumably were not plagued by this factor. The described results provide good advice to the physician faced with the question posed in the article's title.

L. Lasagna, M.D.

Pharmacological Choices After One Antidepressant Fails: A Survey of UK Psychiatrists
Shergill SS, Katona CLE (Maudsley Hosp, London; UCL Med School, London)
J Affect Disord 43:19–25, 1997   17–2

Introduction.—Approximately one third of patients with depression fail to respond to first-line antidepressants, and up to 21% have not recovered after 2 years of adequate dosage and compliance. A popular option in such cases is lithium augmentation, but it is not known whether most psychiatrists are aware of treatment choices for refractory depression. This question was examined in a survey of practicing psychiatrists in the United Kingdom.

Methods.—The survey, sent to 300 randomly selected physicians on the membership roll of the Royal College of Psychiatrists, presented a detailed vignette of a "typical" case of depression with initial treatment failure. The patient was a white woman, aged 40 years, who had been depressed for about 4 months. She sought treatment after intrusive suicidal thoughts led her to consider crashing her car. Her history included sexual abuse by her stepfather, migraine headaches, and a sister who had been treated for an episode of major depression. Treatment consisted of amitriptyline, 150 mg daily, and intensive individual, group, marital, and occupational therapy. No improvement was seen after 6 weeks.

Results.—Surveys were returned by 175 psychiatrists (63%). Respondents were predominantly men (61%) working as consultants (51%) in general psychiatric practice (62%). They had spent a mean of 13 years in the field and saw a mean of 9 patients per year with refractory depression. The most popular treatment choices in such cases were increasing dosages of tricyclic medication and change of medication to selective serotonin reuptake inhibitors; augmentation with tri-iodothyronine or with tryptophan or monoamine oxidase inhibitors was rarely chosen. Psychiatrists with elderly patients were more likely to choose lithium augmentation; electroconvulsive therapy was the preferred choice of those seeing more patients with resistant depression.

Conclusion.—The best established treatments for resistant depression were underused by psychiatrists in the United Kingdom, many of whom (39%) expressed a lack of confidence in treating this problem. Resistant depression should be included as a topic in continuing professional development courses.

▶ Just to show you that every expert can easily locate 3 other experts with different opinions, I happen to think that the United Kingdom psychiatrists who were changing to a specific serotonin reuptake inhibitor rather than augmenting with triiodothyronine, tryptophan, monoamine oxidase inhibitors, or even with lithium were absolutely correct. I think they were giving the patients an oral drug and one that was simple to give and highly effective.

M. Weintraub, M.D.

Dose Escalation vs. Continued Doses of Paroxetine and Maprotiline: A Prospective Study in Depressed Out-patients With Inadequate Treatment Response
Benkert BO, Szegedi A, Wetzel H, et al (Univ of Mainz, Germany; Smith Kline Beecham Pharma GmbH, Munich)
Acta Psychiatr Scand 95:288–296, 1997   17–3

Introduction.—The therapeutic response to some antidepressant agents increases as the dosage is increased within certain limits, whereas dose escalation offers no advantage with other antidepressants. A study of 544 outpatients with various degrees of severity of depression compared the possible benefits of dose escalation of paroxetine and maprotiline.

Methods.—The multicenter study was conducted in a randomized, double-blind manner. Eligible patients were aged 18 to 71 years and had major or minor depression and a total score of 13 or greater on the 17–item Hamilton Depression Rating Scale (HAMD-17). Paroxetine was started at 20 mg daily, given in a single oral dose in the morning; the other subjects received maprotiline (100 mg) divided into 3 doses per day. Patients who failed to have sufficient clinical improvement after 3 weeks had the dosage increased or continued with the previous dosage for an additional 3 weeks.

Results.—Thirty-six nonresponders to paroxetine were randomized to continue the previous dosage and 50 to an increase to 40 mg daily; 48 nonresponders continued to receive 100 mg of maprotiline and 40 were given the increased dosage (150 mg). Dose escalation did not significantly increase therapeutic response with either antidepressant. Response was defined as a reduction of 50% or greater from baseline in the HAMD-17. Results were unchanged after patients were stratified according to baseline severity of depression. The incidence of adverse events was not increased by the larger doses.

Conclusion.—This prospective study using explicit criteria for dose escalation found no significant benefit when the dosages of paroxetine and maprotiline were increased for nonresponders (from 20 mg to 40 mg and from 100 mg to 150 mg daily, respectively). For most patients with acute depression, a dose of 20 mg of paroxetine is optimal.

▶ Several psychiatric medications exhibit a "window" of dosage and an inverse high end of the dose response curve. This means that as the dose increases beyond the optimal or window, adverse effects or a decrease in effect become more apparent. Of course, another possibility is that the patients at the higher doses are refractory to treatment. This, unfortunately, can happen as patients are titrated up to high doses.

One way to show this very clearly is to do a study like the one reported here. Roughly a third of the patients had not responded by the third week of the study and met the criteria for a possible dose escalation in the next 3 weeks of the study. It is difficult to show that a dose of 10 mg of paroxetine is different from placebo. Twenty milligrams, however, is not only different from placebo and the higher doses, such as 30 and 40 mg, but it appears to act with well-tolerated side effects. This study did not show a difference with an increase of 20 mg of paroxetine and 50 mg of maprotiline. Now these patients, perhaps, should have had lithium added, or triiodothyronine as recommended in Abstract 17–2. However, randomizing subjects to more of the same drug dose or to an increased dose remains a valid method for studying nonresponders as well as responders.

M. Weintraub, M.D.

General Practitioners' Perceptions of the Tolerability of Antidepressant Drugs: A Comparison of Selective Serotonin Reuptake Inhibitors and Tricyclic Antidepressants
Martin RM, Hilton SR, Kerry SM, et al (St George's Hosp, London)
BMJ 314:646–651, 1997   17–4

Background.—Although the routine use of selective serotonin reuptake inhibitors (SRIs)as first-line agents is controversial, they are being increasingly prescribed in general practice. General practitioners' perceptions of the tolerability of these agents, compared with that of tricyclic antidepressants, were examined.

Methods.—Data were obtained from an ongoing cross-sectional postal survey. Every 3 months, a representative sample of 250 physicians were asked to record their prescribing activity for 4 weeks.

Findings.—A total of 13,619 inceptions and 3,934 discontinuations of selective SRIs and tricyclic antidepressants were recorded during 4,000 general practitioner weeks per year. Newly prescribed courses of antidepressants rose by 116%, mostly because of an increase in SRI prescriptions. The ratio of total discontinuations to inceptions was 22% for SRIs and 33% for tricyclic antidepressants, a significant difference. These differences persisted after adjustments for patient age, sex, and depression severity. However, there was more switching away from SRIs when they failed than from tricyclic antidepressants, those rates being 72% and 58%, respectively.

Conclusions.—Selective serotonin reuptake inhibitors appear to be better tolerated than tricyclic antidepressants. These findings may have important implications for cost-effectiveness.

▶ Selective serotonin reuptake inhibitors are very popular and have certain advantages over tricyclic antidepressants, but they are a lot more expensive. As this study shows, discontinuation of treatment is not uncommon with either class of antidepressants, but it is a bit more likely with the older tricyclics.

L. Lasagna, M.D.

Resistance to Antidepressant Medications and Short-term Clinical Response to ECT
Prudic J, Haskett RF, Mulsant B, et al (New York State Psychiatric Inst, New York; Western Psychiatric Inst and Clinic, Pittsburgh, Pa; Carrier Found, Belle Mead, NJ)
Am J Psychiatry 153:985–992, 1996   17–5

Objective.—The clinical response to electroconvulsive therapy was investigated in patients who are resistant to antidepressant medication and in patients who have not failed prior medication trials.

Background.—Electroconvulsive therapy was used to treat major depression well before antidepressant medications were introduced, and early studies reported a response rate of 80% to 90%. Currently, a lack of response to pharmacologic treatment is the most common indication for electroconvulsive therapy. It is important to know whether resistance to antidepressant medication will affect a patient's response to electroconvulsive therapy. Uncontrolled studies have reported that resistance to antidepressant medication is not predictive of the outcome of electroconvulsive therapy, but these studies did not compare patients resistant to medication and patients who had not failed adequate medication trials.

Methods.—One hundred patients with primary, unipolar, nonpsychotic major depression were treated with electroconvulsive therapy at 3 sites. The patients scored at least 20 on the Hamilton Depression Rating Scale. Medication resistance was evaluated with the Antidepressant Treatment History Form. Patients were assessed immediately after and 1 week after electroconvulsive therapy.

Results.—Analysis showed that 91.4% of the patients with inadequate pharmacotherapy before electroconvulsive therapy had a response immediately after the cessation of electroconvulsive therapy, whereas 63.1% of the patients who were resistant to medication had a response immediately after the cessation of electroconvulsive therapy. This was observed at all 3 sites. Patients who were medication-resistant scored higher on the Hamilton Depression Rating Scale immediately after electroconvulsive therapy.

Immediately after the cessation of electroconvulsive therapy, scores on the Hamilton Depression Rating Scale decreased less than 40% in 10 patients who were medication resistant. From baseline to immediately after cessation of electroconvulsive therapy, there was a significant inverse relation between scores from the most potent medication trial and the percent change in scores on the Hamilton Depression Rating Scale.

Discussion.—The predictive value for outcome of electroconvulsive therapy after various antidepressant medications may vary. A lower response rate to electroconvulsive therapy was predicted by resistance to heterocyclic or bupropion medications. Resistance to an adequate selective serotonin reuptake inhibitor (SSRI) or monoamine oxidase inhibitor trial had no predictive value. Medication resistance was most common for SSRIs. Heterocyclic antidepressants, SSRIs, and monoamine oxidase inhibitors are all effective for major depression, but they may act through different mechanisms. These findings suggest that the mechanisms of action of heterocyclic antidepressants and electroconvulsive therapy may be more similar than the mechanisms of action of SSRIs or monoamine oxidase inhibitors and electroconvulsive therapy. Selective serotonin reuptake inhibitors are being used more frequently for major depression, and it is important to distinguish between SSRI resistance and resistance to other classes of antidepressants.

▶ Electroconvulsive therapy (ECT) is indicated in severe depression that has not responded to adequate trials of antidepressants, but it doesn't always work, and some patients who respond to ECT may relapse. Continuing antidepressant treatment after response to ECT seems to be of questionable value.

L. Lasagna, M.D.

Fluoxetine Versus Phenelzine in Atypical Depression
Pande AC, Birkett M, Fechner-Bates S, et al (Univ of Michigan, Ann Arbor; Lilly Research Centre, Surrey, England)
Biol Psychiatry 40:1017–1020, 1996   17–6

Background.—Although monoamine oxidase inhibitors are effective antidepressants, certain medications and foods must be restricted to prevent hypertensive crises, which limits monoamine oxidase inhibitor use. Fluoxetine, an effective and well-tolerated antidepressant with serotonergically mediated effects on mood and appetite, may be an alternative for atypical depression. Previous research has shown that the presence of atypical features in a depressive illness predicts a better response to fluoxetine. The efficacy and safety of fluoxetine were compared with those of phenelzine in patients with atypical depression.

Methods and Findings.—Forty-two patients were enrolled in the randomized, double-blind trial. All met the criteria for major depressive disorder, dysthymic disorder, or depressive disorder not otherwise specified in the *Diagnostic and Statistical Manual of Mental Disorders*, ed 3, revised; met the Columbia criteria for atypical depression; and scored 10 or more on the 17-item Hamilton Depression Rating Scale. After a single-blind placebo lead-in, patients were given fluoxetine 20–60 mg/day or phenelzine 45–90 mg/day for 6 weeks. Thirty-eight patients completed the 6-week study. Response rates between treatment groups did not differ. Phenelzine produced more frequent adverse effects than did fluoxetine, with a few exceptions (such as tremor).

Conclusions.—In this group of patients with atypical depression as defined by the Columbia criteria, fluoxetine and phenelzine both effectively reduced depressive symptoms. Response and remission rates did not differ between groups. The frequency of adverse effects was greater with phenelzine, but both treatments were fairly well accepted.

▶ "Atypical" depression is a term applied to depressed patients with hyperphagia or weight gain, hypersomnia, extreme fatigue, and rejection sensitivity. Phenelzine, a monoamine oxidase inhibitor, works better than imipramine in such patients. Fluoxetine seems like a good addition to the therapeutic armamentarium and may be better tolerated.

L. Lasagna, M.D.

A Comparison of Fluvoxamine and Fluoxetine in the Treatment of Major Depression
Rapaport M, Coccaro E, Sheline Y, et al (Univ of California, San Diego; Med College of Pennsylvania, Philadelphia; Washington Univ, St Louis; et al)
J Clin Psychopharmacol 16:373–378, 1996   17–7

Background.—Selective serotine reuptake inhibitors are generally as effective as tricyclic antidepressants but have a better safety profile, perhaps especially in medically unstable or elderly patients with depression. Whether the incidence and severity of adverse events differ with the different selective serotine reuptake inhibitors has not been established. The efficacy and tolerability of fluvoxamine and fluoxetine were compared.

Methods.—By random assignment, 51 patients received fluvoxamine and 49, fluoxetine, for 7 weeks. Eighty-four percent of each group completed treatment.

Findings.—Both treatment groups had a 60% improvement in Hamilton Rating Scale for Depression scores after the trial. The 2 groups did not differ significantly on any efficacy parameter. Only 2 patients in each group quit the study because of adverse effects. The side-effect profiles associated with the 2 treatments did not differ. Less nausea occurred with fluvoxamine than with fluoxetine.

Conclusions.—Fluvoxamine and fluoxetine were equally effective in decreasing depressive symptoms in these patients. The side-effect profiles of the 2 drugs differed slightly.

▶ These drugs were identical in their efficacy; however, there may have been some differences in the side-effect profile. For example, although there was less insomnia in the fluoxetine group, there appeared to be more nausea, diarrhea, and "agitation." Both of these specific serotonin reuptake inhibitors were generally excellent medications. The real question is have they bypassed the tricyclic antidepressants? I think the answer is generally yes, because of their side effects, which seem to be less than with the tricyclics.

M. Weintraub, M.D.

Combining Serotonin Reuptake Inhibitors and Bupropion in Partial Responders to Antidepressant Monotherapy
Bodkin JA, Lasser RA, Wines JD Jr, et al (Harvard Med School, Boston; Massachusetts Gen Hosp, Belmont)
J Clin Psychiatry 58:137–145, 1997   17–8

Objective.—A significant number of patients with affective disorders fail to achieve full remission of symptoms or improvement in all symptoms in controlled trials. Possibly these patients may benefit from combinations of antidepressants. A review of 27 patients treated with combinations of serotonin reuptake inhibitors (SRIs) and bupropion is presented. Five cases are discussed.

Methods.—Between February 1991 and April 1996, 27 incompletely recovered patients (16 women), aged 20 to 83 years, were treated with a combination of an SRI and bupropion for an average of 11 months. Mood, energy level, anxiety or panic, obsessive-compulsive symptoms, sleep disturbance, motivation, cognitive function, and sexual dysfunction were analyzed clinically. Responders and nonresponders to combination therapy were compared.

Results.—Patients were diagnosed with unipolar major depression ($n = 9$), dysthymic disorder ($n = 6$), bipolar disorder type II ($n = 5$) or type I ($n = 3$), attention deficit/hyperactivity disorder ($n = 3$), and generalized anxiety disorder with obsessive-compulsive disorder ($n = 1$). Twenty patients had at least 1 additional comorbid psychiatric disorder. Nineteen (70.4%) patients were considered responders to a mean daily dose of 243 mg of bupropion and a mean daily fluoxetine-equivalent dose of 31 mg. At least 10% of patients had adverse events including sexual dysfunction (40.7%), insomnia (22.2%), reduced energy level (14.8%), and tremor (11.1%). Adverse events were similar to those encountered with monotherapy. Treatment of 4 patients was discontinued because of adverse events.

Conclusion.—Combinations of SRIs and bupropion can be beneficial in incompletely recovered patients with affective disorders. Drug selection and dosing must be done carefully and closely monitored.

▶ Although I am a fan of combining medications, it must be done very carefully, taking into account the lack of interaction studies between the medications. Usually, neither drug sponsor wants to do interactions, either clinical or pharmacologic, in patients with a competitor's medication. This is particularly true when the medications aren't being used for monotherapy but as part of a regimen for treating failures. The authors of this open series of patients really do recommend a number of ways of making sure that the drugs don't interact to the patient's detriment. They recommend conservative dosing and close clinical and laboratory monitoring. I think, in addition, the search for measures of drug interactions is important. Perhaps they should also be checking on the blood levels of serotonin or dopamine. As an unlabeled use of the 2 medications, the safety of the combination would not have been established.

M. Weintraub, M.D.

Gradual Discontinuation of Lithium Augmentation in Elderly Patients With Unipolar Depression
Hardy BG, Shulman KI, Zucchero C (Univ of Toronto)
J Clin Psychopharmacol 17:22–26, 1997   17–9

Objective.—As many as 25% of patients with unipolar depression receive long-term lithium treatment. In the elderly, however, there is a high incidence of side effects including CNS, renal, and thyroid toxicities. A prospective, double-blind, placebo-controlled, parallel-design study was conducted to evaluate the effect of gradual discontinuation of adjunct lithium therapy in elderly patients with unipolar depression and to investigate the usefulness of patient demographics in predicting recurrent risk.

Methods.—Twelve patients (2 men), aged 69–85 years, with unipolar depression, who failed to show improvement after at least 6 months of maximal doses of antidepressant therapy but who were without depressive symptoms for at least 1 year while on lithium therapy, were randomly assigned to the active or placebo group. Patients' attitudes toward lithium withdrawal were assessed prior to beginning the study. Lithium was withdrawn at a maximum of 150 mg/day/week in the withdrawal group. Patients were seen 14 times over a 2-year period. Demographic information was obtained at the first visit. A depression self-assessment, side-effect profile, and renal and thyroid toxicities were recorded at each visit. Recurrences of depressive episodes were recorded. Serum lithium levels were determined throughout the study.

Results.—One patient died and 2 were withdrawn for noncompliance. Two placebo patients had a recurrence of depression at 7 and 92 weeks. Two withdrawal patients, who had a recurrence of depression at 61 and 96 weeks, did not respond to reinstituted lithium therapy for 3 months and 9 months. No patient characteristics predictive of outcome were discovered. Patients withdrawn from lithium had improved renal function but unchanged thyroid function. The placebo group had a significantly lower mean composite side-effect symptom score than did the withdrawal group.

Conclusion.—Withdrawal of lithium therapy from elderly patients can result in serious consequences. Reinstitution of lithium therapy in withdrawal patients who experienced a recurrence was a lengthy process involving several months before the patients were stabilized.

▶ One of my colleagues includes the "randomized withdrawal" study as a way of enriching the patient population so that you can do a clinical trial and get an answer quickly without putting too many people at risk. In this particular case, there were only 12 patients to be given either the placebo or continued lithium. With such a small population, unless some beneficial or adverse effect happens very quickly, you really wouldn't be able to tell much. I think this study was valuable for telling when the side effects would stop after discontinuation of lithium. That's not a small thing. It happened quickly, but fortunately, the investigators kept the patients under observation for a long time, looking for a bad outcome—a recurrence of depression. As in all studies of geriatric patients, however, life events caught up with the investigators. Patient losses dampened their ability to see clear-cut results.

M. Weintraub, M.D.

How Safe Are Serotonin Reuptake Inhibitors for Depression in Patients With Coronary Heart Disease?

Sheline YI, Freedland KE, Carney RM (Washington Univ, St Louis, Mo)
Am J Med 102:54–59, 1997   17–10

Purpose.—Patients with coronary heart disease (CHD) are at risk of depression, which carries significant risk of additional cardiac morbidity and mortality. However, for unclear reasons, patients with CHD are rarely treated for depression. Although the cardiac effects of the tricyclic antidepressants are well documented, little is known about the potential cardiac effects of the selective serotonin reuptake inhibitors (SSRIs). Available data on the cardiac effects of the SSRIs were reviewed, including recommendations for their use in patients with CHD.

Findings.—All articles on the cardiac effects of SSRIs from 1986 to 1996 were analyzed. Case reports have suggested some cardiac effects of SSRIs in patients without known cardiac disease. These include arrhythmias such as atrial fibrillation and flutter, bradycardia, supraventricular tachycardia, and heart block. However, the rate of arrhythmias and other cardiovascular effects of SSRIs seems to be very low (less than 5,000 reported out of an estimated 15 million treatment cases). In overdose, these drugs have a remarkable safety record. Through their effects on metabolism, however, they have the potential to affect plasma levels of other drugs. Interactions with tricyclic antidepressants and type IC antiarrhythmic agents are possible.

In deciding to administer SSRIs to patients with CHD and depression, the risks associated with drug interactions must be assessed against the benefits of treating depression. However, there are few data on the effectiveness of SSRIs in elderly patients or in patients with cardiac disease. The lack of data would suggest the need for caution in using SSRIs for cardiac patients, especially elderly patients receiving certain types of antiarrhythmic drugs. On the other hand, as long as due consideration is given, the risks of not treating depression in patients with CHD probably exceed the risks of SSRI treatment. More study is needed to compare the antidepressant effects of tricyclic antidepressants and SSRIs in patients with cardiovascular disease.

Summary.—Depression is a common and serious problem in patients with CHD. The SSRIs appear to have very few adverse cardiovascular effects, although they do have the potential for interaction with other drugs, including certain antiarrhythmic drugs. There are insufficient data on the effects of SSRIs in elderly patients and in patients with CHD.

▶ Selective serotonin reuptake inhibitors are very popular for treating depression, a not uncommon problem in cardiac patients. These compounds are remarkably safe in overdose and produce adverse cardiac events only rarely. They can, however, affect the metabolism and, hence, the plasma levels of other drugs by way of SSRI effects on the cytochrome P450 system. Certain antiarrhythmic drugs fall into this category. A word to the wise may or may not be sufficient, but this article provides good advice.

L. Lasagna, M.D.

Serotonin Reuptake Inhibitor Withdrawal
Coupland NJ, Bell CJ, Potokar JP (Univ of Alberta, Edmonton, Canada; Univ of Bristol, England)
J Clin Psychopharmacol 16:356–362, 1996   17–11

Objective.—It is generally recommended that antidepressant treatment with serotonin reuptake inhibitors continue for months or years. Such long-term treatment may bring out previously unrecognized adverse effects. Symptoms related to the discontinuation of therapy with selective serotonin reuptake inhibitors (SSRIs) have been reported, particularly dizziness and paresthesia, but also asthenia, nausea, visual disturbances, and headache. The incidence of withdrawal symptoms and associated factors was assessed in patients discontinuing treatment with serotonin reuptake inhibitors.

Methods.—The retrospective study included 352 of 380 patients discontinuing treatment with clomipramine or an SSRI—fluoxetine, fluvoxamine, paroxetine, or sertraline. One hundred seventy-one of these patients were monitored closely during the drug discontinuation period.

Data collected included the effects of restarting medication and whether the patient was considered to have clinical relapse. Cases were identified according to a published definition of withdrawal syndrome, i.e., those with 1 or more new symptoms qualitatively and quantitatively different from their index illness.

Findings.—Many patients experienced adverse effects of drug withdrawal, the most frequent symptoms being dizziness, paresthesia, lethargy, and nausea. Some patients with dizziness also had slight eye or head movements associated with jerking or blurred vision. The symptoms started within 5 days of the end of treatment and sometimes during the dose-tapering period. Patients who stopped taking fluvoxamine, paroxetine, or clomipramine were more likely to experience symptoms than those who had taken sertraline or fluoxetine. No patient treated for less than 7 weeks had withdrawal symptoms. The risk of symptoms was not increased by treatment periods of longer than 6 months, however. Most patients did not have relapses.

Conclusions.—Withdrawal symptoms are common after cessation of serotonin reuptake inhibitor treatment. Withdrawal is more likely for patients taking clomipramine or one of the shorter–half-life SSRIs. The symptoms occur despite dose tapering and resolve when the medication is restarted; relapses are unusual, however. The occurrence of withdrawal symptoms may be related to serotonin's role in the coordination of sensory, autonomic, and motor activity.

▶ Nobody questions the utility of antidepressants for a variety of psychiatric disorders. Nor are they devoid of adverse effects. What has been relatively neglected are the withdrawal phenomena that can occur after stopping serotonin reuptake inhibitor therapy. These include dizziness, paresthesias, asthenia, lethargy, nausea, visual disturbances, and headache and seem to occur mostly after 1 or more months of uninterrupted treatment. The exact mechanisms remain to be elucidated.

L. Lasagna, M.D.

Decreased Efficacy of Combined Benzodiazepines and Unilateral ECT in Treatment of Depression
Jha A, Stein G (Mayday Univ, Croydon, England; Farnborough Hosp, Kent, England)
Acta Psychiatr Scand 94:101–104, 1996   17–12

Purpose.—Previous studies have suggested that benzodiazepine treatment may reduce the efficacy of unilateral or bilateral electroconvulsive therapy (ECT). Other studies find no such effect. The effects of concomitant benzodiazepine therapy on the efficacy of ECT were assessed.

Methods.—The retrospective study included 124 patients receiving concomitant benzodiazepines and ECT over a 10-year period. Most patients received a 3- to 4-second treatment with an electricity dose of 112 to 234

Mc. Patients who received unilateral and bilateral ECT were included. A second shock at a higher level sometimes was administered if the patient did not respond to the first treatment. The efficacy of ECT was assessed from the case notes; the results were compared to those of a matched group of patients who received ECT but not benzodiazepines. *Diagnostic and Statistical Manual of Mental Disorders*-IV criteria were applied where possible.

Findings.—The rate of improvement on ECT was 84% in the patients who received benzodiazepines and 89% in those who did not receive benzodiazepines. However, among patients who received unilateral ECT, the response was much poorer with benzodiazepines. The hospital stay also was longer. The response to unilateral ECT was worse with both long- and short-acting benzodiazepines.

Conclusions.—The response to unilateral ECT is not as good in patients taking benzodiazepines. This effect may arise from a benzodiazepine-induced increase in seizure threshold, in addition to inadequate energy dosing and insufficient seizure duration. Prospective randomized studies of concomitant benzodiazepines and ECT are needed.

▶ This was *not* a prospective, randomized, controlled trial, but it does support the concern voiced in earlier studies that benzodiazepines may somehow interfere with the therapeutic benefits of ECT (at least for the unilateral type). Why this interference occurs remains a mystery.

L. Lasagna, M.D.

Renal Side-effects of Long-term Lithium Treatment
Coşkunol H, Vahip S, Mees ED, et al (Ege Univ, Bornova, Izmir, Turkey)
J Affect Disord 43:5–10, 1997   17–13

Objective.—Polyuria is a common side effect of lithium treatment, and renal insufficiency is a concern for patients treated with lithium. Results of a study of the relation between excretion of 2 indicators of renal damage, β_2-microglobulin (β_2-Mg) and glycosaminoglycan (GAG), with various parameters of treatment and with degrees of concentration defect, polyuria, and creatinine clearance to detect their value as indicators of lithium-induced renal damage are presented.

Methods.—During 3 days of hospitalization, urine output and fluid consumption were measured for 2 days in 107 patients, average age 39, diagnosed with bipolar disorder, prophylactic lithium use, in remission, no history of renal or rheumatic disease, and no history of hypertension or diabetes mellitus lithium intoxication, and in 29 control patients diagnosed with other psychiatric, somatic, or psychogenic disorders. Fluid intake was restricted for 17 hours beginning in the evening of day 2. Urinary osmolality was determined at 9, 10, and 11 AM the next day, and β_2-Mg, GAG, blood, and creatinine levels were measured. Serum and urinary lithium concentrations were established.

Results.—Compared with the control group, the lithium group had significantly higher 24-hour urine volume, urinary GAG, and β_2-Mg, and significantly lower maximal urinary osmolality. Patients with a concentration defect also had significantly increased β_2-Mg. Serum creatinine concentrations and creatinine clearances were similar between groups. Creatinine clearance was not related to duration of illness, duration of lithium treatment, or lithium dosage.

Conclusion.—Urinary GAG and β_2-Mg were significantly elevated in patients on lithium therapy. Patients with a severe concentration defect also had significantly increased β_2-Mg.

▶ Actually, there are many levels of dealing with drug adverse effects. The first level is describing what happened; the second is searching for a mechanism; and the third is searching for some marker or tell-tale sign that physicians can use to pick up the developing toxicity before it becomes clinically manifest, or at least significant. Sometimes these laboratory tests are searching for long-term measurements of an adverse effect that has fully developed, but may be stable. That's what the investigators from Turkey found in their search for markers in patients with different degrees of manifestation of the renal side effects of lithium.

M. Weintraub, M.D.

Factors Associated With Pharmacologic Noncompliance in Patients With Mania

Keck PE Jr, McElroy SL, Strakowski SM, et al (Univ of Cincinnati, Ohio)
J Clin Psychiatry 57:292–297, 1996   17–14

Background.—Medication noncompliance can be a life-threatening problem in patients with bipolar disorder and can also be responsible for relapse or poor response to treatment. One study of relapse rates after the discontinuation of drug therapy reported that more than 50% of patients with bipolar I disorder had a recurrent manic or depressive episode within 6 months of discontinuing lithium, and that virtually all patients had a relapse within 2 years. Some patients who respond well to lithium may fail to respond to such therapy when treated again for a recurrent episode after a period of discontinuing treatment. Most studies of medication noncompliance in patients with bipolar disorder have examined outpatients treated with lithium. There is little information about rates of recurrence and hospitalization associated with medication noncompliance, reasons why patients do not comply with their medication regimen, and the effect of illness, co-morbid disorders, and psychotropic agents other than lithium on noncompliance.

Methods.—The Structured Clinical Interview for *Diagnostic and Statistical Manual of Mental Disorders*, ed 3, revised, was used to diagnose bipolar disorder and schizoaffective disorder, and to establish co-morbidity in 101 patients admitted for acute mania. Severity of manic and depressive symptoms was determined by the Young Mania Rating Scale and Hamilton Rating Scale for Depression. Medication noncompliance was determined by answers to an administered questionnaire and by plasma concentrations of mood-stabilizing agents.

Results.—In the month before their admission, 65 patients were noncompliant with their medication regimen as defined by criteria for full compliance and partial or total noncompliance. There was a significant association between more severe mania at the time of admission and treatment with combinations of mood stabilizers.

Discussion.—Almost two thirds of these patients with bipolar or schizoaffective disorder hospitalized for acute mania were partially or totally noncompliant with their medication regimen. There are many drugs available for treating bipolar disorder, but poor compliance significantly affects the effectiveness of drug therapy; poor outcome is significantly affected by medication noncompliance. Interventions to minimize or prevent noncompliance in these patients are needed.

▶ Noncompliance in medication taking would be expected to be an even bigger problem than usual in manic patients, who often don't realize that they have a serious disease problem.

L. Lasagna, M.D.

Prospective Study of Patients' Refusal of Antipsychotic Medication Under a Physician Discretion Review Procedure
Kasper JA, Hoge SK, Feucht-Haviar T, et al (Univ of Virginia, Charlottesville)
Am J Psychiatry 154:483–489, 1997   17–15

Background.—There is debate about the appropriate conditions under which a committed psychiatric patient can refuse antipsychotic medication and the process of determining when refusal can be overridden. Under a "rights-driven" approach to treatment refusal, patients who are competent have an absolute right to refuse treatment. Under a "treatment-driven" approach, patients have a right to refuse inappropriate treatment. Some studies have reported that there is no practical difference between these two approaches because almost all patients are ultimately given treatment. However, these studies may be limited by patient selection bias. There has been no study of all patients who refused treatment in a jurisdiction that uses a treatment-driven approach.

Methods.—A questionnaire on attitude toward admission and the Brief Psychiatric Rating Scale were administered to 348 psychiatric patients in a state mental health facility where psychiatrists have the right to administer treatment over a patient's objections. Data were collected on patients who refused antipsychotic medication, the length of refusal, and if the refusal ended voluntarily or involuntarily. Patients who complied with treatment made up a control group.

Results.—The rate of treatment refusal was 12.9%. Patients who refused antipsychotic medication had significantly higher scores on the Brief Psychiatric Rating Scale than patients who complied with treatment. Patients who refused treatment also had more negative attitudes toward admission and toward past, present, and future treatment. The average length of refusal was 2.8 days. All patients who refused treatment were treated later. Patients who refused treatment were more likely to be assaultive, require seclusion and restraint, and had longer hospitalization periods.

Discussion.—Although all patients who initially refused treatment were treated, they had more morbidity than compliant patients. Rapid treatment cannot eliminate the negative results of refusal of treatment with antipsychotic medication. These findings may help to inform policymakers of the rate and outcome of treatment refusal in a state facility.

▶ In this state-operated facility for mentally ill patients, the medical staff have the discretion to administer treatment over patients' objections, representing a triumph of paternalism over autonomy. The arguments over "rights-driven" vs. "treatment-driven" policy will never cease, but it's never been clear to me why a patient's refusal to take helpful medication for a serious disease is more ethically palatable than the mandated prescription of a drug by competent medical staff that have the patient's welfare in mind. This paper is worth reading in its original published version.

L. Lasagna, M.D.

Positive and Negative Symptoms: Is Their Change Related?
Czobor P, Volavka J (Nathan S Kline Inst for Psychiatric Research, Orangeburg, NY; New York Univ)
Schizophr Bull 22:577–590, 1996   17–16

Background.—There are conflicting opinions about the relation of positive and negative symptoms in schizophrenia. Crow believed that positive and negative symptoms are 2 separate entities with very different pathogenetic, prognostic, and therapeutic correlates. Andreasen believed that positive and negative symptoms represent the opposite ends of a continuum. Recent factor-analytic data suggest that positive and negative symptoms may be best described using multidimensional models; positive and negative symptoms may constitute higher-order constructs. Although it is unclear what constitutes an elementary dimension within these constructs, the basic positive-negative distinction has been shown to be clinically valid and significant.

Methods.—There were 178 patients with acutely exacerbating chronic schizophrenia taking part in a study of haloperidol. Positive and negative symptoms were measured by the positive and negative symptom clusters of the Brief Psychiatric Rating Scale and the Scales for the Assessment of Positive and Negative Symptoms. Symptom-change trajectories of positive and negative symptoms over time, and the relation between these trajectories, were evaluated by hierarchical linear model analysis.

Results.—A close association was seen in the positive and negative symptom-change trajectories over time. This finding was not dependent on extrapyramidal side effects, depression, or baseline values of positive and negative symptoms.

Discussion.—Changes in positive and negative symptoms over time in patients with acutely exacerbating chronic schizophrenia seem to be related during initial pharmacologic treatment. This relation may not apply to other treatment protocols, after initial treatment, or to other populations.

▶ Schizophrenia is seen with manifestations that usually are categorized as either "positive" or "negative" symptomatology. Antipsychotic drugs have been said by some to affect these 2 sets of symptoms differentially, perhaps because the positive symptoms are related to hyperdopaminergia, whereas the negative ones result from some structural brain deficit and therefore are not amenable to pharmacotherapy (at least of the traditional type). These authors suggest that in fact haloperidol responsiveness occurs with both sets of symptoms.

L. Lasagna, M.D.

Disrupted Pattern of D_2 Dopamine Receptors in the Temporal Lobe in Schizophrenia: A Postmortem Study
Goldsmith SK, Shapiro RM, Joyce JN (Univ of Pennsylvania, Philadelphia)
Arch Gen Psychiatry 54:649–658, 1997   17–17

Background.—The anatomical substrates for the clinical efficacy of D_2 dopamine receptor antagonism in relieving positive symptoms in schizophrenia (such as auditory hallucinations) are not clearly defined. Receptor autoradiography was used to determine whether there is a disrupted laminar pattern of D_2 receptors in the temporal cortex, including that in the D_2 bands, in postmortem tissue from schizophrenic patients.

Methods.—Tissue was obtained from 12 elderly schizophrenic patients after their death and 13 control subjects matched for age and postmortem interval. Quantitative receptor autoradiography for D_2 receptor binding with $[^{125}I]$epidepride was used to examine the tissue. All regions of the temporal lobe in all cases were assessed.

Findings.—Tissue from schizophrenic patients showed significantly disrupted patterns of D_2 receptors in the perirhinal, superior, and inferior temporal cortices. This included disrupted patterns in the modular D_2 receptor bands. Tissue from schizophrenic individuals showed decreased concentrations of D_2 receptors in the supragranular layers and increased concentrations of D_2 receptors in the granular layer in isocortical regions of the temporal lobe. Such disruption did not seem to be the result of long-term treatment with antipsychotic agents and was regionally specific, as there were no between-group differences for concentrations or patterns of expression in the hippocampal complex.

Conclusions.—A likely mechanism for the clinical efficacy of D_2 antagonists in decreasing hallucinations is blockade of the disrupted distribution of D_2 receptors in auditory and auditory-visual association cortices. The regionally specific, aberrant pattern of D_2 receptors may be an effect of abnormal cortical development in these areas.

▶ There has long been a controversy regarding whether schizophrenia is a condition that occurs because of certain factors in one's development or a disease related to anatomical disturbances. It's the old nature vs. nurture argument. I don't think this particular study settles the issue. All the patients had been on high-dose dopamine2 binding drugs. We need better methodologies for tracing the receptor activity in different parts of the brain before medications are begun. Of course, that will still not answer the question fully because, one could say that the psychic situation was such that it affected the receptor density, number, or location.

M. Weintraub, M.D.

Placebo Washout in Trials of Antipsychotic Drugs
Volavka J, Cooper TB, Laska EM, et al (New York Univ; Columbia Univ, NY)
Schizophr Bull 22:567–576, 1996   17–18

Objective.—Phase 3 clinical trials of antipsychotic drugs are usually preceded by a 1-week to 1-month washout period. Because denial of treatment to these patients raises ethical considerations, the use of placebo was compared with a prerandomization treatment period (PRTP) that replaces the patients' therapy with a standard antipsychotic at a clinically appropriate dosage.

Minimizing the Carryover Effects of Previous (Nonstudy) Drugs.—Washout periods do not completely eliminate antipsychotics from the blood. Tremor or rigidity may result and persist for months. With a PRTP, the residual drug would be the same in all patients.

Screen Out Spontaneous Remitters and Placebo Responders.—Threshold criteria excluding spurious responders are defined in advance and depend on the scale selected. The PRTP approach would preclude acceptance of spontaneous remitters, placebo responders and low-dose responders. The PRTP may also produce fewer dropouts because of acute exacerbations of patients withdrawn from their medication.

Establish a True Baseline and Enhance Diagnostic Precision.—Because antipsychotic medications mask patients' symptoms, washout periods serve to establish a baseline but can also lead to a serious deterioration in some patients. Totally unmasking a patient's symptoms is not clinically necessary. The PRTP's unmasking would be less pronounced, but it would obscure the baseline. Although fewer symptoms would be unmasked for treatment-withdrawn patients with PRTP than with placebo, the PRTP schedule would be unlikely to compromise the study. If a lead-in period is desired, then a placebo washout period is preferable.

Discussion.—For ethical reasons, and because information gleaned during a PRTP period does not compromise most studies, it is recommended that investigators carefully evaluate the need for a washout period before beginning phase 3 clinical trials of antipsychotic drugs.

▶ Throughout much of my career in clinical pharmacology, I've been impressed that psychiatrists were very innovative in trying new study designs. For example, many psychiatric drugs have been studied by establishing a dose-response relationship. Unfortunately, the investigators often push all the patients to the highest possible dose just to see what would happen. But, really they do a very careful job of checking for dose-response relationships.

One point that is a little more controversial is using a placebo washout period before studying new antipsychotic agents. This abstracted paper is not a report of a specific clinical trial or an epidemiologic study of patients. It really is a review paper discussing various ways in which one could both have and not have a placebo washout. The investigators will have to figure out which gives the better power for determining an effect between treatments. It may also allow them to check on the effect before they start, compared with the effect after they have instituted the new treatment. In many ways, as good as the abstraction of this study is, the paper might well be read in its entirety.

M. Weintraub, M.D.

Medication Noncompliance and Substance Abuse Among Patients With Schizophrenia
Owen RR, Fischer EP, Booth BM, et al (VA Med Ctr, North Little Rock, Ark; Univ of Arkansas, Little Rock; Santa Clara Univ, Calif; et al)
Psychiatric Serv 47:853–858, 1996   17–19

Background.—Medication compliance is an important factor in determining the effectiveness of treatment for schizophrenia. Among outpatients with schizophrenia, the rate of medication noncompliance may be as high as 50%. Many patients with schizophrenia are unaware of their illness and have symptoms such as suspiciousness, delusions of persecution, grandiosity, anxiety or depression; these factors may all increase medication noncompliance. Comorbid substance abuse is also common in patients with schizophrenia. Such individuals have a high reported rate of prescribed medication noncompliance.

Methods.—Individuals with schizophrenia admitted as short-term inpatients to psychiatric units were studied. At baseline and follow-up at 6 months, data from the Brief Psychiatric Rating Scale, and information on medication noncompliance, substance abuse, severity of symptoms, and side effects from medication were obtained. After discharge, patients received standard continued care. Relationships between dependent and independent variables were analyzed using logistic and linear regression models.

Results.—There were 161 subjects enrolled; complete scores from the Brief Psychiatric Rating Scale and complete information on compliance were available for 135 subjects. There was a significant association between medication noncompliance and substance abuse. Significantly greater severity of symptoms was seen in individuals who abused substances, had no outpatient contact, and did not comply with their prescribed medication regimen.

Discussion.—Individuals with schizophrenia who are substance abusers have a significantly higher risk for medication noncompliance and poor outcome. Lack of outpatient contact worsens this situation. It is important for clinicians to identify patients with schizophrenia and co-morbid substance abuse. Effective interventions for these individuals need to be identified.

▶ The rate of medication noncompliance among outpatient schizophrenic patients has been reported to be as high as 50%. Side effects are an important reason for such noncompliance, as are some of the typical symptoms of schizophrenia, such as paranoia and grandiosity. Use of alcohol or illicit drugs seems to make things worse, as does lack of outpatient contact.

L. Lasagna, M.D.

Developments in the Drug Treatment of Panic Disorder: What Is the Place of the Selective Serotonin Reuptake Inhibitors?
Westenberg HGM (Univ Hosp Utrecht, The Netherlands)
J Affect Disord 40:85–93, 1996   17–20

Introduction.—The reported incidence of panic disorder has increased as awareness of its clinical manifestations has grown. Recent studies have reported a lifetime prevalence of 3.8% to 4.2% for panic disorder and 5.6% to 15.0% for panic attacks. The consensus panel of the United States National Institutes of Health and the National Institutes of Mental Health issued a statement in 1991 that panic disorder is a distinct condition that can be treated by pharmacologic and cognitive-behavioral methods. There is evidence that dysregulation of noradrenaline and serotonin systems is involved in the production of anxiety, and that antidepressant medication that affects these systems is effective in treating panic disorder. Selective serotonin reuptake inhibitors may have an important role in panic disorder.

Co-morbidity.—Co-morbidity strongly affects the choice of drug treatment. The most common co-morbid condition in patients with panic disorder is depression. Panic disorder and unipolar depression seem to coexist more often than chance would predict. There is an association between panic disorder and major depression, seasonal depression, and bipolar disorders. Agoraphobia, other anxiety disorders, and drug and alcohol abuse may also exist.

Selective Serotonin Reuptake Inhibitors.—There is evidence that serotonergic pathways have a role in the pathogenesis of anxiety disorders. The main pharmacologic difference between the effective tricyclic antidepressants and the ineffective tetracyclic maprotiline is that tricyclics have serotonin uptake-blocking properties. The first drug with serotonin reuptake inhibitory properties that was approved for use in Europe was clomipramine. Because it is a tricyclic, it has the same disadvantages of other tricyclics. Studies have shown that zimelidine, fluoxetine, and fluvoxamine are very effective in patients with panic disorder and panic disorder with agoraphobia. Side effects include a transient initial increase in anxiety or a general increase in agitation with fluvoxamine or fluoxetine. A meta-analysis comparing selective serotonin reuptake inhibitors and imipramine and alprazolam concluded that they were all more effective than placebo, and that the selective serotonin reuptake inhibitors were more effective than imipramine and alprazolam. Paroxetine is a more selective serotonin reuptake inhibitor and may cause fewer side effects than the tricyclics. It has been used to treat depression and has been approved to treat panic disorder. There has been no evidence of initial increased anxiety after paroxetine.

Discussion.—There is much epidemiologic and pharmacologic interest in panic disorder, and a great need for safe and effective treatments. The evidence to date suggests that selective serotonin reuptake inhibitors may be effective in treating panic disorder. They are faster acting and better tolerated than tricyclic antidepressants and are not associated with dependence and the discontinuation syndromes of benzodiazepines.

▶ A lot of patients with panic disorder do not receive a correct diagnosis and as a result have not benefited from treatment with such well-studied drugs as benzodiazepines and tricyclic antidepressants. The newer selective serotonin reuptake inhibitors may be more effective or better tolerated. Time (and study) will tell.

L. Lasagna, M.D.

Predictors of Weight Loss in Children With Attention Deficit Hyperactivity Disorder Treated With Stimulant Medication
Schertz M, Adesman AR, Alfieri NE, et al (Albert Einstein College of Medicine, New Hyde Park, NY)
Pediatrics 98:763–769, 1996   17–21

Background.—Psychostimulant medications commonly used in the treatment of attention deficit hyperactivity disorder (ADHD) often result in reduced appetite and weight loss, which are of great concern to parents and physicians. The clinical predictors of weight loss in children taking stimulants for ADHD have not been established definitively.

Methods.—A retrospective chart review was performed to identify children with ADHD treated by stimulants for at least 5 months. Twenty-nine boys and 3 girls treated with methylphenidate hydrochloride (MPH) and 25 boys and 3 girls treated with dextroamphetamine sulfate (DEX) were studied. Pretreatment weight, pretreatment body mass index (BMI), treatment duration, total daily dose, and weight-adjusted dose were considered.

Findings.—In a linear regression analysis, pretreatment weight was significantly correlated with change in weight for children in both the MPH and DEX groups. Pretreatment age, weight-adjusted dose, and duration of follow-up did not contribute significantly to the variance in change of weight in either group. When the 2 treatment groups were combined, a greater proportion of heavier children had a reduction relative to their predicted BMI than did thinner children. Heavier children had an absolute reduction of -0.139 BMI, in contrast to the thinner group, which had a gain of $+0.014$.

Conclusions.—Pretreatment weight adjusted for age, gender, and height significantly predicts weight loss in MPH- or DEX-treated children with ADHD. Pretreatment age, duration of treatment, and weight-adjusted dose were not significant predictors.

▶ Attention deficit disorder afflicts perhaps 3% to 5% of school-age children and responds reasonably well to either methylphenidate, pemoline, or dextroamphetamine, but such treatment often decreases appetite and leads to weight loss.

If weight loss in fact occurs mostly in overweight children, this effect becomes a plus rather than a minus.

L. Lasagna, M.D.

Six-week, Double-blind, Placebo-controlled Study of Desipramine for Adult Attention Deficit Hyperactivity Disorder
Wilens TE, Biederman J, Prince J, et al (Massachusetts Gen Hosp, Boston; Harvard Med School, Boston)
Am J Psychiatry 153:1147–1153, 1996   17–22

Introduction.—Up to 9% of school-aged children are affected by attention deficit hyperactivity disorder, a neuropsychiatric syndrome. The disorder persists in up to 60% of adults in whom this disorder was diagnosed in childhood. Although several studies have been conducted on the treatment of this disorder in children, few have been conducted in adults. The best established alternative agents for this disorder in children and adolescents are the tricyclic antidepressants, particularly desipramine. Desipramine also may be effective for adults with attention deficit disorder. A controlled trial of desipramine was conducted in adults with attention deficit disorder.

Methods.—Forty-one patients with attention deficit hyperactivity disorder participated in a randomized, 6-week, placebo-controlled, parallel-design study of desipramine at a target daily dose of 200 mg. Standardized structured psychiatric instruments were used to establish the diagnoses. To determine outcome, separate assessments of adult attention deficit hyperactivity disorder, and depressive and anxiety symptoms at baseline and at each biweekly visit were used. Symptoms tested included difficulty remaining seated, fidgeting, difficulty working quietly, excessive talking, blurting out answers, acting before thinking, difficulty waiting turn, interrupting or intruding, difficulty sustaining attention, shifting activity, difficulty following instructions, easy distraction misplacement of objects, and difficulty listening.

Results.—Between adults receiving placebo and those receiving desipramine, there were highly significant differences in the reduction of attention deficit hyperactivity disorder symptoms. Twelve of the 14 symptoms were reduced within the desipramine-treated group, and there were decreases in the broad categories of inattentiveness, impulsiveness, and hyperactivity. No differences between baseline and end point for any of the attention deficit hyperactivity disorder symptoms were found in the placebo-treated group. Positive responders were found in 68% of the desipramine-treated group versus none in the placebo-treated group. Dose, level of impairment, gender, and lifetime psychiatric co-morbidity with anxiety or depressive disorders were factors independent of the response to desipramine.

Conclusion.—Desipramine is effective in the treatment of attention deficit hyperactivity disorder in adults, similar to the findings in children and adolescents with this disorder.

▶ Although attention deficit hyperactivity disorder (ADHD) seems to disappear in many children as they become adults, some clearly continue to exhibit related symptoms (10% to 60%, depending on which report you read). Unfortunately, only a handful of studies have been carried out in adults with ADHD, most on the efficacy of stimulants. Because tricyclic antidepressants seem to help children and adolescents with ADHD, one might well expect this class of drugs to be helpful in adult patients. The present study supports this concept. Unanswered are 2 important questions: How does desipramine compare with methylphenidate? Are there specific individuals who do much better with 1 of these drugs than with the other? If so, can we identify them in advance, or must we resort to trial and error?

L. Lasagna, M.D.

A Double-blind, Placebo-controlled Study of Fluvoxamine in Adults With Autistic Disorder
McDougle CJ, Naylor ST, Cohen DJ, et al (Yale Univ, New Haven, Conn)
Arch Gen Psychiatry 53:1001–1008, 1996   17–23

Background.—Patients with autistic disorder are impaired in social functioning and communication and have a markedly restricted repertoire of activities and interests. Some patients have abnormalities in their serotonin neurotransmitter system. Currently there are no consistently effective, safe drugs for treating the symptoms of autism. Fluvoxamine was tested in a double-blind, placebo-controlled trial.

Methods.—Thirty adults with autistic disorder completed the 12-week trial. Behavioral ratings were obtained before treatment and after 4, 8, and 12 weeks of therapy.

Findings.—Fifty-three percent of the 15 patients receiving fluvoxamine responded, compared to none receiving placebo. Fluvoxamine was better than placebo in decreasing repetitive thoughts and behavior, maladaptive behavior, and aggression. Active treatment was also superior in improving some aspects of social relatedness, especially language usage. Treatment response was unassociated with age, level of autistic behavior, or full-scale intelligence quotient. Fluvoxamine was well tolerated; a few patients experienced mild sedation and nausea.

Conclusions.—In adults with autistic disorder, fluvoxamine is more effective than placebo in the short-term treatment of symptoms. Further studies of this agent and other potent selective serotonin uptake inhibitors appear to be warranted in autistic children and adolescents.

▶ Autistic disorder is troubling and at present incurable. Fluvoxamine seems to offer the possibility of some amelioration.

L. Lasagna, M.D.

Maximizing Function in Alzheimer's Disease: What Role for Tacrine?
Smucker WD (Northeastern Ohio Univs, Rootstown)
Am Fam Physician 54:645–652, 1996   17–24

Objective.—Tacrine has been shown to provide modest therapeutic benefit in the treatment of Alzheimer's disease. The decision to use tacrine must be predicated on a comprehensive elevation of the patient and a thorough understanding of the effects of the drug.

Confirming the Diagnosis.—A dementia evaluation should be made. Confounding factors such as alcoholsim, medication interaction, and depression must be ruled out. Diagnostic criteria for Alzheimer's disease include memory deficits and cognitive disturbances of language, learned motor behaviors, and planning and organizing skills that begin gradually and progress in the absence of systemic illness.

Patient and Caregiver Functioning.—The goal of treatment is to enable patients to function as well and as independently as possible. Patient function must be monitored regularly, and caregivers must be provided with a support system that regularly assesses their mental and physical well-being.

Pathophysiology of Alzheimer's Disease and the Actions of Tacrine.—Neuronal and synaptic loss and abnormal protein deposition characterize the disease. Tacrine increases the availability of acetylcholine to neuronal receptors.

Measuring the Effectiveness of Therapy in Alzheimer's Disease.—Because tacrine slows only the degeneration of memory, memory and cognitive testing are the only ways of evaluating the effectiveness of therapy. Treating other patient problems and reducing anxiety, depression, and the caregiving time of caregivers are also necessary.

Effectiveness of Tacrine.—Tacrine is approved for use in Alzheimer's disease patients scoring between 10 and 26 on the Mini-Mental State Examination. Improvements are dose related and are seen in about 50% of patients who can take the drug.

Monitoring Tacrine Therapy.—Efficacy is measured by improvement or lack of deterioration in cognition and behavior. Adverse effects include liver toxicity and cholinergic symptoms.

Titrating the Tacrine Dose.—Tacrine is administered as a 10-mg dose 4 times a day for 6 weeks, preferably between meals. If bilirubin and liver transaminase levels remain within a safe range, the dosage is increased in 10-mg increments every 6 weeks to a maximum of 40 mg/dose. Liver transaminase levels should be monitored every 2 weeks until dosage is stable; monitoring should then be gradually extended to every 3 months, provided that liver transaminase levels remain within the safe range.

Conclusion.—Tacrine has been shown to benefit about 25% of patients with Alzheimer's disease who are able to tolerate the drug. One month of therapy with monitoring costs $300. Any treatment plan must include treatment of other symptoms of Alzheimer's disease and must provide medical, psychological, and time-off support for caregivers.

▶ Tacrine modestly helps patients with Alzheimer's disease, and only a minority of patients at that. It would appear that the drug both delays progressive deterioration of cognitive function and improves cognition over baseline, with a return to baseline when the drug is stopped.

L. Lasagna, M.D.

Relation of Prescription Nonsteroidal Antiinflammatory Drug Use to Cognitive Function Among Community-dwelling Elderly
Hanlon JT, Schmader KE, Landerman LR, et al (Duke Univ, Durham, NC; Ctr for Health Services Research in Primary Care; Veterans Affairs Med Ctr, Durham, NC; et al)
Ann Epidemiol 7:87–94, 1997   17–25

Background.—Nonsteroidal anti-inflammatory drugs (NSAIDs) are commonly prescribed in the United States, especially in the elderly. These drugs can have protective, negative, or no effects on the CNS in the elderly. Case reports have indicated that certain NSAIDs can cause psychosis or delirium or exacerbate cognitive impairment. Other reports indicate that

NSAIDs can protect against severe cognitive impairment from Alzheimer's disease.

Methods.—Data were obtained from 2,765 elderly individuals from the Duke University Established Populations for Epidemiologic Studies of the Elderly. These individuals had normal cognitive function at baseline and were alive for follow-up evaluation at 3 years. The Short Portable Mental Status Questionnaire and the individual domains of the Orientation-Memory-Concentration Test were used to evaluate cognitive function. Information was obtained on use of NSAIDs, including dose, frequency of use, and prescription status.

Results.—Continuous, regular prescription use of NSAIDs was associated with preservation of concentration only, after controlling for demographic factors, health status, and behavior. There was no consistent dose-response relation. There was no correlation between current and previous use of NSAIDs and level of cognitive functioning across all 5 measures; current users taking moderate or high doses made more errors on the memory test than current users taking low doses.

Discussion.—In this large sample of community-dwelling elderly individuals, no significant or consistent protective effect of use of prescription NSAIDs on cognitive function was found. These inconclusive results suggest an association between sustained use of NSAIDs and a slight reduction in cognitive function.

▶ The lay press has carried several reports linking chronic NSAID ingestion with a decreased incidence of Alzheimer's dementia. These stories are based on some positive case-control studies, but contradictory data also have been reported.

This study not only is not encouraging, but it also suggests that at least with higher-dose NSAID usage, memory may actually be worse.

L. Lasagna, M.D.

18 Pulmonary Disorders

Antibiotics: Neither Cost Effective nor 'Cough' Effective
Hueston WJ (Univ of Wisconsin, Madison; Eau Claire Family Practice Residency, Wis)
J Fam Pract 44:261–265, 1997
18–1

Introduction.—Physicians commonly prescribe antibiotics for acute bronchitis, despite reports that this approach is not beneficial. Viral infections are more common than bacterial infections in acute bronchitis. A small number of patients with acute bronchitis have *Mycoplasma pneumoniae* or *Chlamydia pneumoniae* bacterial infections. The cost of various treatment strategies for acute bronchitis was assessed to determine which is the most cost-effective strategy in patients with persistent cough.

Methods.—The following 3 treatment strategies were evaluated: (1) withholding antibiotics and treating only patients with persistent cough, (2) screening patients for *M. pneumoniae* or *C. pneumoniae* and treating all patients with positive results with antibiotics, and (3) treating all patients with antibiotics. The antibiotic of choice was erythromycin. Cost was determined on the basis of what charges would be assumed by the patient. Outcome was determined by cost per patient in whom acute bronchitis was diagnosed.

Results.—Using the baseline assumptions described, the most cost-effective strategy was withholding antibiotics and treating only patients with persistent cough. The average cost per patient to treat acute bronchitis was $43.01, $50.06, and $61.65, respectively, for treatment strategies 1, 2, and 3.

Conclusions.—Empirical antibiotic use for acute bronchitis is not cost-effective. Further work is needed to better determine patients most likely to respond to antibiotic treatment. For some patients, the trade-off in higher costs for the possibility that improvement may be more rapid may be worth the additional expense.

▶ This is a counterintuitive outcome of a cost-effectiveness study. Usually when the analysis is done, what works out as the cheapest strategy very often is that you should treat all the patients without screening them. Perhaps this particular strategy of not treating any patients initially can also decrease antibiotic overusage. We'd have to carry out another study, however. We have to find out how patients feel about their doctors carrying out a "no treatment" strategy. Patients may have to learn that a cough will persist in bronchitis without being too damaging, but the problem of losing sleep, missing work, and the withholding of antibiotics by the physician may increase the patients' anxiety and result in poorer overall treatment outcomes.

M. Weintraub, M.D.

Double Blind Placebo Controlled Trial of Nebulised Budesonide for Croup

Godden CW, Campbell MJ, Hussey M, et al (Poole NHS Trust Hosp, Dorset, England; Southampton Gen Hosp, England)

Arch Dis Child 76:155–158, 1997   18–2

Background.—Authorities continue to disagree about the treatment of croup. The efficacy of nebulized budesonide in improving symptoms or shortening the duration of stay of children hospitalized with a clinical diagnosis of croup was investigated.

Methods.—Eighty-seven children, ages 7 to 116 months, were enrolled in the prospective, randomized, double-blind, placebo-controlled trial. Nebulized budesonide or placebo was given every 12 hours.

Findings.—Nebulized budesonide was associated with significant improvement in symptoms at 12 and 24 hours. Patients with an initial croup score exceeding 3 had a significant improvement in symptoms at 2 hours. Active treatment was also associated with a 33% decrease in length of stay, after adjustment for age, initial croup score, and coryzal symptoms.

Conclusions.—The use of nebulized budesonide in children hospitalized with croup is of significant clinical benefit. Croup scores obtained periodically and length of hospital stay were significantly improved with active treatment.

▶ The inspiratory stridor, barking cough, and respiratory distress that constitute croup are well-known to many parents, but treatment of croup is controversial. When mild, kindly neglect is usually enough. Humidification has been used since the nineteenth century, but doesn't always work well, and nebulized adrenaline's benefits are short-lived. Oral or nebulized steroids seem better at relieving symptoms, as attested to in a number of well-conducted studies.

These authors, reasonably enough, argue in favor of oral dexamethasone over nebulized budesonide because (a) it's lots, lots cheaper and (b) kids with croup often are made very apprehensive by a mask placed over their face.

L. Lasagna, M.D.

An Evaluation of Salmeterol in the Treatment of Chronic Obstructive Pulmonary Disease (COPD)

Boyd G, Morice AH, Pounsford JC, et al (Stobhill Hosp, Glasgow, Scotland; Royal Hallamshire Hosp, Sheffield, England; Frenchay Hosp, Bristol, UK; et al)

Eur Respir J 10:815–821, 1997   18–3

Objective.—Respiratory failure, as a consequence of chronic obstructive pulmonary disease (COPD), is one of the leading causes of death worldwide. Although salmeterol is effective in the treatment of asthma, there have been few studies of its efficacy in patients with COPD. The efficacy and safety of the addition of 2 doses of salmeterol xinafoate to the existing regimen of patients with COPD were compared with placebo in a multicenter, multinational, randomized, double-blind, parallel group study.

Methods.—Either 50 or 100 µg salmeterol twice a day or placebo was administered to 674 patients with COPD, in addition to their non-β_2-agonist medication, for 16 weeks. Patients were assessed at recruitment; at 1 week before recruitment; at randomization; and at 4, 8, 16, and 18 weeks after randomization. Daily day and night symptom scores were recorded in diaries. Safety and lung function were assessed at each clinic visit. Symptom scores, bronchodilator use, and Borg scores were statistically analyzed.

Results.—There were 21 placebo patients, 23 of the lower dose salmeterol patients, and 27 of the higher dose salmeterol patients withdrawn from the study. Day and night-time symptom scores of both salmeterol treatment groups were significantly lower than the scores of the placebo group. Day and night-time bronchodilator use was significantly lower in the salmeterol treatment groups than in the placebo group. Forced expiratory volume is 1 second improved at each visit for both salmeterol treatment groups, compared with the placebo group. Although the distribution of the breathlessness scores after a 6-minute walk at 8 and 16 weeks was significantly lower in the 50-µg group than in the placebo group, there was no difference between treatment groups. There was no significant difference in adverse events among groups, except for tremor which was significantly higher in the 100-µg group than in either of the other groups.

Conclusion.—Treatment with salmeterol significantly improved day and night symptoms, day and night bronchodilator use, and distribution of breathlessness scores. The incidence of tremor was significantly higher in the high-dose salmeterol treatment group, compared with the other 2 groups.

▶ This was an international study done everywhere in the world except the United States. In any case, the medication was effective in lowering the amount of other bronchodilators used. It was, however, an "add-on" study, and this has its own detriments as well as values. The patients took salmeterol with a variety of therapies, which included theophylline and other inhaled bronchodilators. The reason why this study may not be accepted—

particularly by the pharmaceutical industry—is that one cannot tell where the adverse effects might be coming from if they occur. They could be related to the new drug, the old drug, or the combination of the 2, so the investigators are usually left swimming in a morass, trying to figure out where things, bad and good, happened.

M. Weintraub, M.D.

Quality of Life Changes in COPD Patients Treated With Salmeterol
Jones PW, Bosh TK (St George's Hosp Med School, London; Glaxo Wellcome R&D, Greenford, Middlesex, England)
Am J Respir Crit Care Med 155:1283–1289, 1997   18–4

Objective.—Changes in health-related quality of life were evaluated by patients with chronic obstructive pulmonary disease (COPD) taking either 50 or 100 µg salmeterol twice daily or placebo, using the St. George's Respiratory Questionnaire (SGRQ) and the Medical Outcomes Study Short Form 36 (SF-36).

Methods.—In a double-blind, randomized, parallel-group, placebo-controlled study, after a 2-week run-in period, 283 patients (41 women) with an average age of 63 years, received either 50 ($n = 94$) or 100 µg ($n = 94$) salmeterol or placebo ($n = 95$) twice daily via metered-dose inhalers for 16 weeks. Patients were clinically and subjectively assessed at 0, 2, 4, 8, and 16 weeks. Patients rated symptoms, activity, and psychosocial impact of the disease on SGRQ and SF-36 scales at weeks 0 and 16. Differences between baseline and final questionnaire answers for the intent-to-treat group were analyzed statistically.

Results.—Compared with placebo, there was a statistically and clinically significant improvement in SGRQ Total and Impact scores and in SF-36 scores in the 50-µg salmeterol group but not in the 100-µg salmeterol group. Physicians rated both doses of salmeterol to be equally effective and significantly more effective than placebo. The SGRQ Activity and Total scores were modestly correlated with, and SF-36 scores were significantly correlated with, baseline forced expiratory volume is 1 second (FEV_1). Changes in scores at 16 weeks were significantly correlated with FEV_1.

Conclusion.—Modest improvements in lung function after 16 weeks of treatment with salmeterol significantly improved the quality of life for patients with COPD.

▶ This study was part of an international study of salmeterol. Part of a randomized clinical trial, it meets many of the criteria that I and several others demand from quality-of-life and other kinds of studies with so-called "soft" end points. The patients were receiving placebo or other medications in double-blind fashion, and the assessment techniques (the SF-36 and the SGRQ) were pretty good.

In analyzing the data, the investigators included an analysis of variance which not only controlled for age, gender, and baseline score, but also took into account the country where the patient lived. Unfortunately, the SF-36 contains some items that really are not very important for patients with COPD. That reduced its value in this study. The SGRQ is a specific measurement instrument for respiratory diseases and the psychosocial effects of the medication, and its results were statistically significant in this study. Perhaps because of adverse effects of the 100-µg dose given twice daily, the scores tended not to be as positive on the SGRQ.

M. Weintraub, M.D.

A Comparison of Nebulized Budesonide With Oral Prednisolone in the Treatment of Exacerbations of Obstructive Pulmonary Disease
Morice AH, Morris D, Lawson-Matthew P (Royal Hallamshire Hosp, Sheffield, England)
Clin Pharmacol Ther 60:675–678, 1996   18–5

Introduction.—Many studies confirm inhaled corticosteroids to be safe and effective in the treatment of chronic asthma and steroid-responsive chronic obstructive pulmonary disease (COPD). Yet parenteral corticosteroids are recommended for the treatment of acute asthma and exacerbations of COPD, despite a potential for systemic side effects. The hypothesis that treatment of acute bronchospasm with nebulized corticosteroids would lead to improvements in the biochemical markers characteristic of corticosteroid side effects was tested.

Methods.—Nineteen consecutive adult patients, all with previously diagnosed asthma or COPD, who were responsive to corticosteroids, took part in the study. They were randomly assigned to 30 mg of oral prednisolone once daily or 2 mg of nebulized budesonide twice daily. Additionally, all received 5 mg of nebulized albuterol 4 times daily. Blood was drawn, urine was collected, and lung function studies were performed on study days 1 and 5.

Results.—All patients tolerated the treatment well and the 2 groups responded similarly to therapy. Biochemical variables did not differ between groups on day 1, but mean urinary corticosteroid metabolites were significantly higher on day 5 in the nebulized budesonide group. Urinary androgen metabolites and urinary hydroxyproline to creatinine ratios were similar in the 2 groups. Serum osteocalcin was elevated and 24-hour urinary calcium to creatinine ratios were lower in those patients receiving budesonide.

Conclusion.—Nebulized budesonide led to fewer systemic effects in patients with acute bronchospasm than did conventional treatment with oral prednisolone. The improvement in biochemical markers associated with nebulized budesonide was achieved without a reduction in clinical benefits relative to oral prednisolone.

▶ Although much of an inhaled dose of corticosteroid is swallowed, rapid first-pass hepatic metabolism results in little systemic bioavailability, so inhaled corticosteroids are relatively free from the systemic effects that plague continued treatment with oral corticosteroids. This study supports the argument of those who recommend nebulized corticosteroid for treatment of acute exacerbations of COPD.

L. Lasagna, M.D.

Treatment of Malignant Pleural Effusions With a Combination of Bleomycin and Tetracycline: A Comparison of Bleomycin of Tetracycline Alone Versus a Combination of Bleomycin and Tetracycline
Emad A, Rezaian GR (Shiraz Univ, Iran)
Cancer 78:498–501, 1996   18–6

Introduction.—Bleomycin and tetracycline are the most commonly used agents for the treatment of malignant pleural effusions. A combination of these 2 drugs was found to be more effective than either drug used alone in patients with pleurodesis.

Methods.—The randomized study included 60 patients, mean age 54 years. All had histologically or cytologically proved massive malignant pleural effusions and remained symptomatic despite treatment with chemotherapy. The 3 treatment groups received a single intrapleural instillation containing either tetracycline, bleomycin, or a combination of tetracycline and bleomycin. Patients were followed-up for 6 months for recurrence of pleural effusions.

Results.—Breast carcinoma and lung malignancies were the most common causes of malignant pleural effusions, accounting for 40 of 60 cases. Complete response (CR) was defined as the absence of an accumulation of pleural effusion, as determined by chest X-ray and clinical examination. Rates of CR were similarly high in the 3 groups at 1 month (70% to 95%) and did not differ significantly at 3 months. At 6 months, however, CR rates were reduced significantly in the tetracycline and bleomycin groups (35% and 25%, respectively) compared with the combination therapy group (70%).

Conclusion.—The short-terms benefits of bleomycin, tetracycline, and their combination were similar, but administration of both drugs brought about more lasting freedom from malignant pleural effusions in patients receiving palliative therapy.

▶ I think that using medications of different mechanisms of action will be helpful in diseases with poor response to therapy. This is an instance where the early effects of the medication are much less important than the later effects. Since 6 patients died during the course of this study, the interim results could be accurately gauged. Pretty soon, someone is going to do a study adding talc to the combination of tetracycline and bleomycin.

M. Weintraub, M.D.

19 Rheumatic and Arthritic Diseases

Response to Therapy in Rheumatoid Arthritis Is Influenced by Immediately Prior Therapy

Fries JF, Williams CA, Singh G, et al (Stanford Univ, Calif)

J Rheumatol 24:838–844, 1997   19–1

Objective.—Clinicians do not routinely use a washout period when they change therapy for their patients with rheumatoid arthritis. Therefore, observed efficacy can actually represent effectiveness of the new drug minus residual effectiveness of the old drug. Results of an evaluation of the empirical effectiveness of new drug starts in subgroups of patients receiving different therapies were presented.

Methods.—The effects after new-disease-modifying antirheumatic drug (DMARD) starts were evaluated in 2,898 patients with rheumatoid arthritis from 8 Arthritis, Rheumatism and Aging Medical Information System (ARAMIS) data bank centers. Patients were divided into subgroups based on prior therapy. The null hypothesis stated that the chance that the therapy was observed effective depended on the preceding therapy. Results of a Health Assessment Questionnaire and disability and pain scores of the intent-to-treat group was evaluated at an average of 9 months after the new drug start.

Results.—Prior therapy significantly influenced the effectiveness of the new treatment. Methotrexate significantly reduced disability, except after IM gold therapy or hydroxychloroquine. Methotrexate reduced pain after all treatments. Hydroxychloroquine reduced disability after nonsteroidal anti-inflammatory drug (NSAID) therapy, increased disability after IM gold therapy, and decreased pain after NSAID therapy. Prednisone decreased pain only. Treatment with DMARDs was most effective when started after NSAID therapy. Disability increased when gold therapy was followed by hydroxychloroquine treatment.

Conclusion.—The effectiveness of a new drug start may be dependent on the previous drug therapy. Because of the small size of the study and the approximate nature of the methodology, these observations may not be generalizable. However, the dependence of 1 therapy on the identity of the previous therapy may explain some clinical contradictions.

▶ This study from ARAMIS is of interest both to people who make their living studying the antirheumatic drugs and those who have to digest the information and make patient care decisions regarding the same drugs. The basis of the analysis is shown in the figure. Disability or pain is shown as increasing monitonically, something that we know is not true, but, more importantly, the clinical situation is quite well laid out on the figure by showing where the second drug is begun.

Often, the first drug is stopped in the clinical situation. That may account for at least some of the beneficial effect of almost every new drug just after the start, because it will contain effects of the new medication plus a residual effect of the medication the patient was taking. There are really a lot of things to be learned by looking at the way in which physicians practice medicine and the patient responses. Every year, we seem to include an ARAMIS paper because of their study of a physician's treatment of patients.

M. Weintraub, M.D.

Measurement Methods of Drug Consumption as a Secondary Judgement Criterion for Clinical Trials in Chronic Rheumatic Diseases
Constant F, Guillemin F, Herbeth B, et al (Univ Henri Poincaré, Nancy, France; Ctr for Preventive Medicine, Nancy, France)
Am J Epidemiol 145:826–833, 1997   19–2

Objective.—Determining whether it is possible to reduce drug treatment after it becomes effective requires quantifying drug consumption. Different methods of measurement are neither comparable nor uniform. Various methods of measurement were compared to determine an easy and practical method for detecting a significant drug consumption change over time.

Methods.—Anti-inflammatory and analgesic drugs were classified into their respective therapeutic subclasses. Consumption was measured in 4 ways: number of tablets taken per week in every main therapeutic class; units of defined daily dose; milligrams of active principle taken per week; and a nonsteroidal anti-inflammatory drug (NSAID) equivalence score per week. These measurement methods were studied in a controlled clinical trial to assess the overall effectiveness of spa therapy vs. routine drug therapy in 121 patients with chronic low back pain. Consumption was recorded in a diary. Effects were assessed at 3-week and 6-month intervals. Measurement methods were compared on the basis of sensitivity to change, and the standardized response mean was calculated for each therapeutic class.

Results.—At 3 weeks and 2 months, analgesic drug consumption declined significantly in the treatment group but not in the control group. According to methods 1, 2, and 4, NSAID consumption declined significantly in the treatment group at all time points. Functional disability decreased more in the treatment group than in the control group at 3 weeks and 2 months. Analgesic drug consumption measures by all 3 methods were positively correlated; NSAID consumption score changes were correlated except between methods 1 and 3 at 3 weeks, but at 2 months, score changes by methods 1, 2, and 4 were correlated. When sensitivity to change of analgesic drug consumption was examined, method 1 was significantly more sensitive than method 3 at 3 weeks and significantly more sensitive than method 2 at 2 months. For NSAIDs, method 1 was significantly more sensitive than method 3 at 3 weeks and significantly more sensitive than methods 2 and 3 at 2 months. Method 4 provided inconsistent results.

Conclusion.—Of the 4 methods evaluated, daily tablet count was the best measurement method for determining drug consumption. The method is also simple to use and makes results easy to compare.

▶ All the methods for measuring drug consumption in this study represented essentially patient reports rather than electronic monitoring. Although it may be a fault of this particular study, we cannot berate the investigators too much, as they managed to do a lot with the data they had. However, an electronic monitoring system might have provided the opportunity to tell what days the patients did or did not take the therapy in a clinical trial. One could have also calculated pharmacokinetic parameters and been more certain that the patients did not throw the medication down the toilet the night before. These latter items would more easily been obtained if the date and time of opening the medicine container were known.

M. Weintraub, M.D.

Effect of Resumption of Second Line Drugs in Patients With Rheumatoid Arthritis That Flared Up After Treatment Discontinuation
ten Wolde S, Hermans J, Breedveld FC, et al (Univ Hosp, Leiden, The Netherlands; Free Univ Hosp, Amsterdam)
Ann Rheum Dis 56:235–239, 1997   19–3

Objective.—In 1 study, in the first year after discontinuing second-line antirheumatic drugs, 38% of patients with rheumatoid arthritis experienced a flare. Nonetheless, if resumption of treatment results in improvement, discontinuing second-line treatment to reduce side effects is an alternative. The effect of treatment resumption of second-line drugs in patients whose disease flared up after ending treatment was investigated.

Methods.—Patients who experienced a flare after participating in the placebo arm of a placebo-controlled discontinuation study were given, preferably, the same second-line drug they were taking before the study started. Patients were assessed at flareup and 3 and 12 months later. Demographic and disease characteristics were recorded, as were side ef-

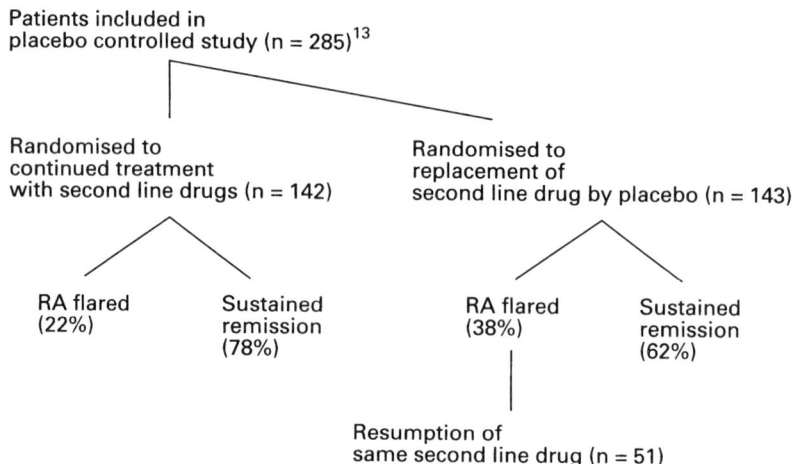

FIGURE 1.—Flow diagram illustrating patient numbers and percentages at all stages of the placebo-controlled treatment discontinuation study until the inclusion of 51 patients whose disease flared into the present second-line treatment resumption study. (Courtesy of ten Wolde S, Hermans J, Breedveld FC, et al: Effect of resumption of second line drugs in patients with rheumatoid arthritis that flared up after treatment discontinuation. *Ann Rheum Dis* 56:235–239, 1997. By permission of BMJ Publishing Group.)

fects and adverse reactions. Changes in disease activity parameters were analyzed statistically.

Results.—Of the 53 patients who experienced a flare, 24 had severe flare (Fig 1). Two did not resume treatment. Of the 51 who did resume treatment, 26 required higher doses after flare than they had needed previously, and 37 were also taking nonsteroidal anti-inflammatory drugs (NSAIDs). Whereas disease activity parameters improved significantly after 3 months, disease activity remained at a significantly higher level than when drugs were discontinued. Although 24 patients were classified as responders at 3 months, only 25% had reached the prediscontinuation erythrocyte sedimentation rate level. Ten of 22 patients with a severe flare and 14 of 29 with a mild flare responded, which indicated that there was no relationship between severity of flare and occurrence of a response. The response rate for patients taking and not taking NSAIDs was similar. The number of responses for various drugs were as follows: antimalarials, 15 of 25; sulphasalazine, 5 of 8; methotrexate, 2 of 2; azathioprine, 1 of 2; parenteral gold, 1 of 10; and penicillamine, 0 of 4. After 12 months, treatment was discontinued for lack of efficacy in 2 patients taking parenteral gold and 2 taking sulphasalazine, and the patients were treated with another drug. At 12 months, disease activity was absent in 18 patients, mild in 22, and moderate or severe in 11. No patients discontinued treatment because of side effects.

Conclusion.—Resumption of treatment of rheumatoid arthritis flares with second-line therapy is safe and effective, with approximately half the patients classified as responders 3 months after resumption.

▶ As seen in the figure, 62% of the patients who were receiving the placebo after an initial period of second-line agents sustained a remission that lasted for the course of the study. Unfortunately, we cannot tell who would be in this 62% without giving them placebo or stopping therapy first The second group of interest are the patients who were randomized to continue treatment with second-line drugs and had a rheumatoid arthritis flare. We also do not know how to pick this group of patients. We have no good ways of deciding on the basis of presence or absence of nodules, severity of disease, or other factors whether these patients would be different from those who maintained a remission. Side effects were not a major issue once the rheumatoid arthritis flared, so no one should worry about restarting the same therapy that the patient had been on before.

There are a number of "prices" to be paid by removing patients from second-line drugs that are working. Initially, a greater percentage will flare. This group will also be more or less incapacitated for a certain time while waiting for the drugs to take effect. The third price, although it is not terribly important, is the adverse effects that might occur with continued therapy. Until that day—sometime in the future when we can tell which group a patient might fall into once the initial therapy has been stopped—we will just have to decide whether, for a specific patient, it would be better to continue therapy or to stop it and see whether the patient has remitted.

M. Weintraub, M.D.

Limited Effect of Sulphasalazine Treatment in Reactive Arthritis: A Randomised Double Blind Placebo Controlled Trial
Egsmose C, Hansen TM, Andersen LS, et al (Copenhagen Municipal Hosp; Herlev Univ, Denmark; King Christian X Rheumatism Hosp, Graasten, Denmark; et al)
Ann Rheum Dis 56:32–36, 1997   19–4

Objective.—Current treatments for reactive arthritis are palliative in nature. Sulphasalazine (SSZ) has shown some benefit in treating inflammatory lesions of the ileum and colon in these patients and in the treatment of psoriatic arthritis. Results of a prospective, double blind, placebo controlled, multicenter study evaluating the effect of SSZ in patients with reactive arthritis were presented.

Methods.—One 500 mg tablet of SSZ ($n = 37$; 13 women) twice daily during week 1, followed by 2 tablets twice daily during week 2, and 3 tablets twice daily during week 3 and thereafter or placebo ($n = 42$; 8 women) was administered for 6 months. Pain, joint tenderness, erythrocyte sedimentation rate (ESR), entesopathy, extra-articular manifestations, and working ability were evaluated monthly.

Results.—Although there were significant improvements in pain, joint swelling, and ESR in both groups, there was no significant difference between groups. The incidence of adverse events was 22 in the SSZ group and 11 in the placebo group. Of the 53 patients who completed the study,

10 patients in the SSZ group and 11 in the placebo group were in complete remission. Compliance was assessed by asking patients if they had taken the medication as prescribed.

Conclusion.—Results of this study show that SSZ may confer some beneficial effect in patients with reactive arthritis. There was a 30% dropout rate, mainly because of gastrointestinal side effects.

▶ This was a failed study. This was also the first time that I had ever heard of reactive arthritis. I am not sure that the diagnosis exists in the United States as clearly as it does in Europe. It may be closer to ankylosing spondylitis and psoriatic arthritis, although it may also include lesions in the colon. Because of its mild nature, and perhaps because of its gastrointestinal effects, the patients with reactive arthritis decided that the treatment was not worth the candle.

M. Weintraub, M.D.

Calcium and Vitamin D₃ Supplementation Prevents Bone Loss in the Spine Secondary to Low-dose Corticosteroids in Patients With Rheumatoid Arthritis
Buckley LM, Leib ES, Cartularo KS, et al (Med College of Virginia, Richmond; Univ of Vermont, Burlington)
Ann Intern Med 125:961–968, 1996   19–5

Purpose.—Patients with allergic and autoimmune diseases are commonly treated with low-dose corticosteroids. Over time, this treatment can lead to reduced bone mineral density, with a corresponding increase in the risk of vertebral fracture. Supplemental calcium and vitamin D_3, which improves calcium absorption, have been suggested for use in reducing bone loss. However, there are few data to support the efficacy of this intervention. Patients receiving low-dose corticosteroids were studied to determine whether supplemental calcium and vitamin D_3 can prevent spinal bone loss.

Methods.—The randomized, controlled trial included 96 patients with rheumatoid arthritis, 65 of whom were being treated with corticosteroids. The mean corticosteroid dosage was 5.6 mg/day. The patients were randomly assigned to receive supplementation with calcium carbonate, 1,000 mg/day, and vitamin D_3, or placebo for 2 years. At 1 and 2 years, they underwent measurement of bone mineral density in the spine and femur.

Results.—The rate of bone mineral density loss in patients taking prednisone who were assigned to placebo was 2.0% per year in the lumbar spine and 0.9% per year in the trochanter. In contrast, patients taking prednisone who received supplemental calcium and vitamin D_3 had increasing bone mineral density: 0.72% per year in the lumbar spine and 0.85% per year in the trochanter. This group showed no increase in bone mineral density in the femoral neck or the Ward triangle, however. Patients who were not taking corticosteroids showed no improvement in bone mineral density with calcium and vitamin D_3 supplementation.

Conclusions.—In patients taking low-dose corticosteroids, supplementation with calcium carbonate and vitamin D_3 prevents declining bone mineral density in the spine and hip. These supplements are available over the counter and have few toxic effects. They may help to reduce the risk of vertebral fracture in patients who require long-term corticosteroid treatment.

▶ Although this was a very well done study and the results were positive, it didn't answer the crucial question, which was what was the rate of spinal fractures in this population? The bone density in the vertebral spine is a surrogate measure for fracture rates. In addition, the authors name a number of important factors for stratification of future studies. These include age and sex, presence of menstrual periods or postmenopausal state, and many others.

M. Weintraub, M.D.

Androgens as Adjuvant Treatment in Postmenopausal Female Patients With Rheumatoid Arthritis
Booij A, Biewenga-Booij CM, Huber-Bruning O, et al (Univ Hosp Utrecht, The Netherlands)
Ann Rheum Dis 55:811–815, 1996   19–6

Introduction.—Sex hormones predispose a person to and modulate rheumatoid arthritis. Androgens are natural immunosuppressants, and estrogens enhance the immune response. In vitro studies have shown that androgens inhibit the production of cytokines by activated murine lymphocytes and increase suppressor cell activity in thymocytes and lymphocytes. Previous studies have also shown improvement in patients with active rheumatoid arthritis who were given testosterone propionate. The effects of testosterone on disease activity were determined in a double-blind, placebo-controlled study of postmenopausal women with rheumatoid arthritis.

Methods.—To evaluate the effect of 50 mg of testosterone propionate administered intramuscularly every 2 weeks and 2.5 mg of progesterone given every other week for 1 year, 107 women participated in the double-blind, placebo-controlled trial. The women had at least 6 tender joints, 3 or more swollen joints, erythrocyte sedimentation rate greater than 28 mm in the first hour, a C reactive protein level of more than 30 mg/L, and morning stiffness that exceeded 30 minutes. Patients were evaluated at baseline, 6 months, and 12 months. Outcome measures were an unweighted 28 joint count, erythrocyte sedimentation rate, functional disability with a Dutch version of the Stanford health assessment questionnaire, pain, and general well-being.

Results.—Noted improvement was seen in the erythrocyte sedimentation rate, health assessment questionnaire results, and pain scores in the group that received testosterone. After 1 year, 21% of patients treated with testosterone fulfilled the American College of Rheumatology improvement criteria compared with only 4% of the placebo group. Sixty-seven percent of the treated group wanted to continue treatment compared with only 37% of the placebo group. The most common side effects of testosterone were hypertrichosis and hoarse voice.

Conclusion.—The general well-being of postmenopausal women with active rheumatoid arthritis may be improved by testosterone. Improvement of the catabolic state that is prevalent among so many elderly patients with active rheumatoid arthritis seems to be the main indication for androgen treatment because more potent disease-modifying agents are available.

▶ Treatment with testosterone dates back to the 1950s. The father of the lead author of this study apparently studied this treatment in the 1960s. Surprisingly, the current authors did find an improvement in the patients who received testosterone. However, the widespread use, even in postmenopausal women, of androgen therapy is probably not a reasonable alternative. Other, less worrisome, hormonal approaches to the treatment of rheumatoid arthritis may be available. If there are, I hope that brave and competent physicians and pharmaceutical firms can find them. We certainly do need new treatments for rheumatoid arthritis.

M. Weintraub, M.D.

Treatment of Early Rheumatoid Arthritis With Minocycline or Placebo
O'Dell JR, Haire CE, Palmer W, et al (Univ of Nebraska, Omaha; Omaha VA Hosp, Neb)
Arthritis Rheum 40:842–848, 1997   19–7

Background.—Rheumatologists currently emphasize the importance of early control of rheumatoid arthritis (RA). Evidence suggests that tetracyclines may have anti-arthritic action. The efficacy of minocycline in the treatment of seropositive RA within the first year of diagnosis was investigated.

Methods.—Forty-six patients with RA were enrolled in the 6-month study. The patients received 100 mg of minocycline twice a day or placebo.

Findings.—Eighteen patients met 50% improvement criteria at 3 months and maintained at least a 50% improvement for 6 months. No significant toxicity was documented. These responders included 65% of the patients receiving minocycline and only 13% of the patients receiving placebo.

Conclusions.—Minocycline is effective in the treatment of patients with seropositive RA in the first year of disease. Further research is needed to establish optimal treatment duration and to investigate the mechanism(s) of action.

▶ The possibility that RA might be related in some way to an infectious agent has been discussed for decades. In addition, tetracyclines are thought by some to have anti-arthritic effects that are not of an antibacterial nature.

This study is now the third controlled trial to conclude that minocycline can provide clinical improvement to such patients. The authors speculate that the benefit may result from an inhibition of matrix metalloproteinases.

L. Lasagna, M.D.

A Systematic Review of Randomized Controlled Trials of Pharmacological Therapy in Osteoarthritis of the Hip
Towheed TE, Hochberg MC (Univ of Maryland, Baltimore)
J Rheumatol 24:349–357, 1997   19–8

Objective.—Patients with osteoarthritis (OA) of the hip have severe pain and functional limitations. Whereas NSAIDs are effective for treating pain, they also have significant toxicity particularly in the elderly. Randomized clinical trials (RCTs) of NSAID therapy for OA of the hip were reviewed to determine which NSAID is the most effective and which is the most toxic.

Methods.—A Medline search of published studies from 1966 to August 1994 yielded 43 RCT that evaluated the effect of NSAIDs on OA of the hip. The quality of design and analysis aspects of each study were rated on a scale from 0 (poor quality) to 8 (highest quality). The ratio of improvement produced by 1 NSAID was compared with another NSAID to get the relative efficacy for pain relief. Reported toxicities were compared.

Results.—There were 29 studies that evaluated NSAIDs and 4 that evaluated analgesics. The average number of patients in these studies was 95, with an average of 81 completing each study. There were 20 trials that used a crossover design, 22 that employed a parallel group design, and 1 that used patients as their own controls. Most design and analysis scores ranged from 2 to 4. Indomethacin was used 13 times, naproxen 8 times, ketoprofen and phenylbutazone 6 times each, and diclofenac 5 times. Of the 20 NSAID comparison studies, indomethacin was more effective in 5 of 7 trials. Of the 29 studies that evaluated toxicity, indomethacin was more toxic in 7 of 9 studies. Six of 29 trials found significant differences in efficacy.

Conclusion.—A review of RCTs of NSAID therapy for OA of the hip was unable to establish an efficacy or toxicity ranking primarily because of a lack of standardization of outcomes.

▶ These authors carried out a type of meta-analysis looking for quality clinical trials in osteoarthritis using NSAIDs. Unfortunately, the trials very rarely demonstrated a difference between active medications, perhaps with the exception of indomethacin. This is because, in general, the experimenters wanted to show equivalence of the 2 medications, except in toxicity, when they were doing comparative studies of one or the other. A second reason may be that it's very difficult to show superiority of one NSAID over another because it's very difficult to know the exact dose and to use an appropriate dose which will demonstrate efficacy. If it's almost impossible to show the difference between doses double or triple the standard dose of an NSAID vs. other doses of that same NSAID, it will be difficult to show them across trials. Another thing that this paper demonstrated was that the measure of the quality of the studies may have been too rigorous and the investigators, perhaps, should have taken a less rigid design to choose the trials. More studies might have been brought into review for evaluation. Still, this systematic review was an important, good try and does really relate some of the adverse effects, for example, those on indomethacin with good effect. Whenever there was a placebo, however, the standard drug beat placebo in most, if not all, of the studies.

M. Weintraub, M.D.

Comparison of Sulfasalazine and Placebo in the Treatment of Psoriatic Arthritis: A Department of Veterans Affairs Cooperative Study
Clegg DO, Reda DJ, Mejias E, et al (Veterans Affairs Med Ctr, Salt Lake City, Utah; Hines CSP Coordinating Ctr, Ill; Veterans Affairs Med Ctr, San Juan, Puerto Rico; et al)
Arthritis Rheum 39:2013–2020, 1996   19–9

Objective.—Although nonsteroidal anti-inflammatory drugs (NSAIDs) are the therapy of choice for treating active psoriatic arthritis (PsA), some patients continue to have active disease. Some small studies have suggested that sulfasalazine (SSZ) might be helpful in treating these patients. The safety and efficacy of SSZ for the treatment of PsA were evaluated.

Methods.—In a 36-week, multicenter, double-blind, randomized, placebo-controlled parallel trial, patients with PsA received either 1 tablet daily (500 mg) of enteric-coated SSZ ($n=109$) or placebo ($n=112$) for week 1, 2 tablets for week 2, 3 tablets for week 3, and 4 tablets for week 4 and beyond. Patient and physician global assessments, joint pain/tenderness and swelling, and erythrocyte sedimentation rate (ESR) were recorded and radiographs were taken at every visit. Cutaneous psoriasis was evaluated. Adverse drug reactions and compliance were monitored.

Results.—Response rates were 57.8% in the SSZ group and 44.6% in the placebo group. The physician global assessment demonstrated that 41.3% of the SSZ group and 38.4% of the placebo group improved, whereas 6.4% of the SSZ group and 10.7% of the placebo group worsened. The patient global assessment showed that 45.9% of the SSZ group and 41.1% of the placebo group improved, whereas 7.3% of the SSZ group and 9.8% of the placebo group worsened (Fig 3). In the SSZ group, there were significant decreases in total neutrophils, platelet count, and

ESR, compared with the placebo group. There were 35 withdrawals in the SSZ group and 25 in the placebo group, including, respectively, 14 and 6 for adverse reactions, and 5 and 7 for no improvement or worsening of their condition. Side effects were mainly gastrointestinal.

Conclusion.—Sulfasalazine had a beneficial effect in patients with PsA as determined by joint pain/tenderness and swelling scores and by patient and physician global assessments.

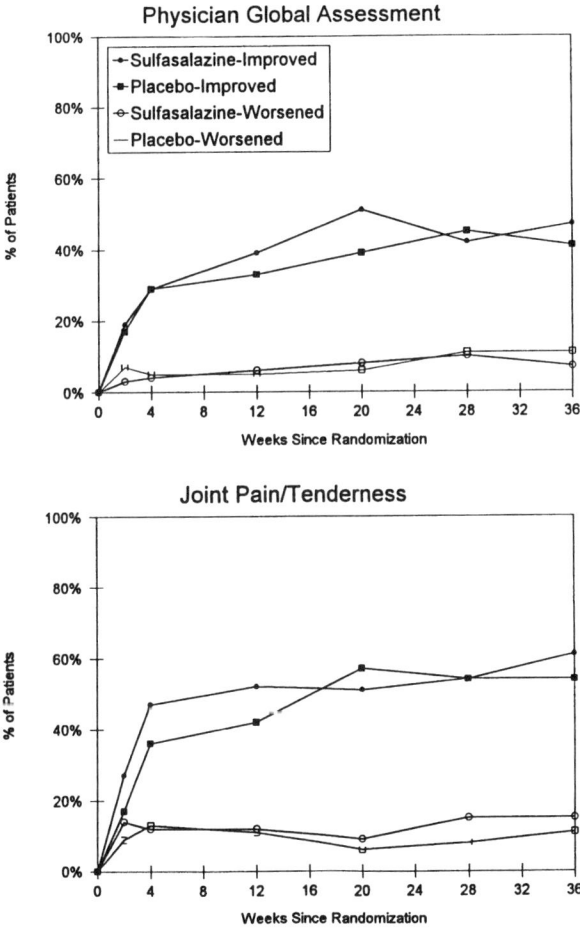

FIGURE 3.—Changes in physician global assessment, patient global assessment, morning stiffness, and back pain among patients with psoriatic arthritis treated with sulfasalazine or placebo, by response group. (Courtesy of Clegg DO, Reda DJ, Mejias E, et al: Comparison of sulfasalazine and placebo in the treatment of psoriatic arthritis. *Arthritis Rheum* 39:2013–2020, 1996. Copyright American College of Rheumatology.)

(*Continued*)

FIGURE 3 (cont.)

Patient Global Assessment

Joint Swelling

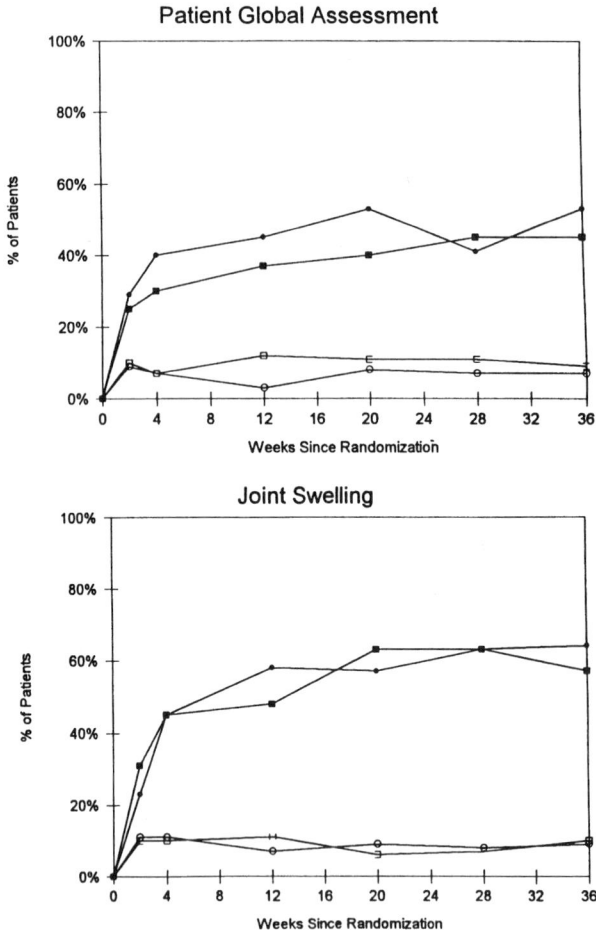

▶ This analysis used a 2–point scale, "response" or "no response," in the analysis of whether the patients improved. I think this is an excellent technique as long as the patients can get up over the benchmark and get into the response group. Unfortunately, the overall effect of SSZ was not statistically significant. However, one can worry about whether SSZ would work more quickly, as it does in 3 of the graphs. A second possibility, not revealed by these graphs, is that the SSZ was becoming more effective over time and that the lines continued to diverge. This is shown in the pattern of treatment response for the whole group in terms of the "response/no response" paradigm. The interpretation would be different, in this case, and we would ask for a longer study to show the beneficial effects.

Nonetheless, although there was only a trend, the drug is already on the market for inflammatory bowel disease and for other forms of arthritis, so if you would select the treatment, you would have to understand a little about the side effects. Fortunately, the side effects are fewer than one would expect and were gastrointestinal in nature. I do not think we will see another study of SSZ in PsA. However, if I had a patient with persistent, active PsA, I would really think long and hard about trying SSZ.

M. Weintraub, M.D.

Treatment of Plantar Fasciitis by Iontophoresis of 0.4% Dexamethasone: A Randomized Double-blind, Placebo-controlled Study
Gudeman SD, Eisele SA, Heidt RS, et al (Specialty Ctrs for Orthopaedic & Rehabilitative Excellence, Indianapolis, Ind; Univ of Cincinnati, Ohio)
Am J Sports Med 25:312–316, 1997   19–10

Background.—Plantar fasciitis is a common cause of heel pain in athletes, especially runners; in persons who stand for long periods; and in overweight persons. Pain is often worse after periods of inactivity, but lessens as activity progresses. Conservative treatment includes orthoses, nonsteroidal anti-inflammatory drugs, stretching and strengthening, ultrasound, friction massage, and night splints. Several methods are often combined. Treatment must also include correction of the foot abnormalities, including forefoot abnormalities and hindfoot instability. When conservative treatment fails, steroid injection and surgical release can be considered. Iontophoresis of corticosteroids is a process in which ions in solution are transferred through intact skin via electrical potential with bipolar electrodes. Ionizable material in solution, such as dexamethasone sodium phosphate, migrates toward the poles of opposite charge. There have been no reports of iontophoresis in the treatment of plantar fasciitis.

Methods.—Patients were randomly assigned to one of two groups. In group 1, feet received traditional treatment and sham iontophoresis. In group 2, feet received traditional treatment plus iontophoresis of 0.4% dexamethasone sodium phosphate USP. After dropouts, there were 20 patients and 40 feet treated in each group. Patients were treated 6 times in 2 weeks.

Results.—Outcome was evaluated with the Maryland Foot Score. At the end of the treatment period, patients in group 2 had improved significantly more than patients in group 1. At 1-month follow-up, improvement in both groups was similar.

Discussion.—In these patients with plantar fasciitis, iontophoresis provided greater immediate relief of symptoms than traditional treatment alone. Iontophoresis of corticosteroids is noninvasive, painless, and results in local tissue concentrations that are lower than with injection but higher than with oral administration. Iontophoresis may also be less expensive.

Clinical Significance.—Because functional outcome is the same if iontophoresis is used or not, it is recommended for patients who need immediate relief of symptoms, such as performance athletes or other active patients. Treatment must also address the underlying cause of the disorder.

▶ With the increasing weight in the American population and increase in athletic undertakings, the incidence of plantar fasciitis will increase. If people don't warm up properly, they may have a higher incidence of plantar fasciitis. Iontophoresis in a double-blind, randomized, prospective study, was added to standard therapy. Thus everybody received a physical intervention (ice), a health professional intervention (physical therapy), and a home exercise program (REST [*resume exercises below the soreness threshold*]). It may be harder to test both the effectiveness of therapy and its adverse effects in add-on studies. However, it is much more important to use what the world is using as the best current therapy. The study also attempted to assess the total cost of the various interventions and their adverse effects. The additional cost may be only $50 per session for approximately 6 sessions. The authors point out that iontophoresis could be most effective for performance athletes. However, I see this as having a wider effect, making certain that the patients receive the other interventions as well as the iontophoresis.

M. Weintraub, M.D.

A Randomized Controlled Trial of Piroxicam in the Management of Acute Ankle Sprain in Australian Regular Army Recruits: The Kapooka Ankle Sprain Study
Slatyer MA, Hensley MJ, Lopert R (1st Recruit Training Battalion, Kapooka, Australia; Univ of Newcastle, New South Wales, Australia)
Am J Sports Med 25:544–553, 1997   19–11

Background.—Ankle sprains represent a substantial burden of injury in active populations. The efficacy of the nonsteroidal anti-inflammatory drug (NSAID) piroxicam in the management of acute ankle sprain was investigated in Australian Regular Army recruits.

Methods and Findings.—Three hundred sixty-four recruits with acute ankle sprains sustained during training were assigned randomly to receive piroxicam or placebo. Compared with placebo recipients, piroxicam recipients had less pain, were able to resume training more rapidly, were treated at lower cost, and had increased exercise endurance on resumption of activity. Nausea was the only adverse effect reported significantly more often in the treatment than in the placebo group, with incidences of 6.8% and 0.3%, respectively. Patients given piroxicam showed some evidence of local abnormalities, such as instability and decreased range of motion.

Conclusions.—Piroxicam use resulted in better recovery at a lower cost in these army recruits with acute ankle sprain. Piroxicam treatment reduced pain, shortened time lost from training, and increased exercise endurance. Although piroxicam recipients also had more instability, less range of motion, and increased swelling, overall the use of NSAIDs was beneficial.

▶ This randomized controlled clinical trial tested a very common clinical occurrence, ankle sprain. By day 14 almost everything was in favor of piroxicam, such as the lower use of acetaminophen, the ability to walk without pain, and the ability to march (after all, these were soldiers). Patients treated with piroxicam also had less pain at rest and less pain on walking by day 3. In addition, the economic costs were more than double in the placebo-treated patients. Fortunately, the stomachs of these young men were relatively immune to the toxicity of piroxicam. This study demonstrates how it's always nice to support something that many physicians do without much data (treat sprains with piroxicam) but is based on good thinking and extrapolation of what is known about medication. In addition, the treatment is cost-effective.

M. Weintraub, M.D.

Randomised Controlled Trial of Hydroquinine in Muscle Cramps
Jansen PHP, Veenhuizen KCW, Wesseling AIM, et al (Ziekenhuis Gelderse Vallei, Ede, The Netherlands; Catholic Univ of Nijmegen, The Netherlands; ASTA Medica BV, Diemen, The Netherlands)
Lancet 349:528–532, 1997   19–12

Background.—Quinine and hydroquinine are often prescribed for muscle cramps. However, the results of studies of these agents' efficacy have been mixed.

Methods.—One hundred twelve patients with 3 or more muscle cramps per week were enrolled in a randomized, double-blind, placebo-controlled, parallel-group trial. Patients received 300 mg of hydroquinine hydrobromide dihydrate or placebo daily for 2 weeks.

Findings.—In both groups, the total number of muscle cramps and of cramp days declined during the treatment period compared with the preceding 2-week period. However, the active treatment group had a median of 8 fewer cramps and 3 fewer cramp days, compared with only 3 and 1, respectively, in the placebo group. Sixty-five percent of the participants in the hydroquinine group had a 50% or greater decrease in the number of muscle cramps. Hydroquinine did not decrease the severity or duration of cramps after cramp onset. A sustained effect was noted after therapy was stopped. The adverse effects associated with hydroquinine were mild.

Conclusion.—This dose of hydroquinine is safe and effective in the short term for preventing frequent ordinary muscle cramps. The therapeutic effect of this agent continued beyond the treatment period.

▶ Although the literature is a bit controversial regarding quinine and muscle cramps, I have long been persuaded that quinine derivatives help prevent such cramps, presumably because of a curare-like action on skeletal muscle and the neuromuscular junction. Side effects are not common. This article suggests an interesting (and beneficial) carryover effect.

L. Lasagna, M.D.

Muscle Cramps and Magnesium Deficiency: Case Reports

Bilbey DLJ, Prabhakaran VM (Trinity Med Clinic, Trinity Bay, Newfoundland, Canada; Mem Univ of Newfoundland, Trinity Bay, Canada)
Can Fam Physician 42:1348–1351, 1996   19–13

Introduction.—The functions of magnesium in the body are either structural (in the bone) or biochemical (primarily neuromuscular transmission and muscle contraction). An experience with 2 patients with magnesium deficiency who initially were seen for muscle cramps was reported.

Case Report 1.—Boy, 17, was seen for aching in his muscles and thighs and generalized skeletal muscle tenderness after intense military training. His first symptom was weakness in the legs, followed by muscle spasms so intense he could "hardly move." He was unable to walk because the gastrocnemius-soleus muscles were in spasm. Tendon reflexes were brisk. His serum magnesium concentration was 0.54 mmol/L. He was hospitalized and placed on bed rest. He received orphenadrine and acetaminophen for muscle relaxation and analgesia. An IV infusion with 3 g of magnesium sulfate was administered, followed the next day by an infusion with 5 g of magnesium sulfate. Within 48 hours, the tetany was resolved and the muscle pains were diminished. He was pain free within 4 days, and was able to resume military training within 2 weeks.

Case Report 2.—Woman, 81, was admitted with severe abdominal pain and some pain in the lower legs. She had a 2-year history of congestive heart disease. Analgesics (including meperidine), tranquilizers, and muscle relaxers were administered with no relief for the intermittent bouts of severe abdominal pain. There was no indication of need for surgery. Morphine and muscle relaxers provided temporary relief. The only remarkable laboratory findings were serum magnesium levels of 0.49 and 0.51 mmol/L. Oral magnesium caused fluid diarrhea. She received an IV infusion with 5 g of magnesium sulfate over a 24-hour period. Her symptoms resolved completely by the third day. A week later, she was discharged "never feeling better for years."

Conclusions.—Magnesium deficiency rarely is suspected in clinical situations. It should be considered in patients with persistent or severe muscle pain.

▶ Because serum magnesium levels have not been easy to measure over the years, and because the element often gets short shrift in the medical curriculum, magnesium deficiency as the cause of clinical problems rarely is suggested. As these 2 interesting cases show, muscle cramps can be a consequence of magnesium deficiency, whether as the result of an inadequate intake of green vegetables, induced magnesium loss from the body by diuretics, or both.

L. Lasagna, M.D.

Bisphosphonate Therapy of Reflex Sympathetic Dystrophy Syndrome
Adami S, Fossaluzza V, Gatti D, et al (Univ of Verona, Valeggio, Italy)
Ann Rheum Dis 56:201–204, 1997   19–14

Objective.—Reflex sympathetic dystrophy syndrome (RSDS), a painful limb disorder, is associated with patchy osteoporosis. Because bisphosphonates are powerful inhibitors of bone resorption, intravenous alendronate was administered to RSDS patients for several years in a double-blind study.

Methods.—Twenty RSDS patients (8 females), aged 39 to 80, received 7.5 mg of IV alendronate in 250 mL saline or placebo saline infusions daily for 3 days. After 2 weeks, all patients were given alendronate at the same dosage. Patients were assessed twice before treatment and weekly thereafter. Pain was assessed on a visual analog scale from 1 for no pain to 10 for worst pain.

Results.—Patients treated with alendronate in the first arm of the study had significant improvement in pain, tenderness, and swelling compared with baseline scores, the placebo group, and from week 2 to week 4. Placebo-treated patients were unchanged, but improved when treated with alendronate. Bone scans showed increased activity and uptake in affected limbs of alendronate-treated patients compared with baseline scans. Bone mineral content (BMC) of affected arms of alendronate-treated patients averaged 426 mg/cm at baseline compared with 688 mg/cm for the contralateral arm. At 6 weeks after treatment, BMC in the affected arm had increased significantly by an average of 77 mg/cm, but was unchanged in the contralateral arm. Patients tolerated the treatment well.

Conclusion.—Intravenous bisphosphonates are an effective treatment for RSDS, relieving symptom and increasing BMC of the affected arm.

▶ RSDS is a very painful problem that has as its hallmarks autonomic dysfunction, osteoporosis, swelling, and, after months or years, formation of contractures. Therapy has been singularly unsuccessful. These investigators tried alendronate, which is an inhibitor of bone resorption. Their study was positive after 3 days of IV administration vs. placebo given for the same period in 20 patients. Obviously, this study has to be replicated by other investigators using different administration schedules, etc. But the finding is quite exciting, particularly given the lack of response to most therapeutic attempts.

M. Weintraub, M.D.

Tranexamic Acid Radically Decreases Blood Loss and Transfusions Associated With Total Knee Arthroplasty

Hiippala ST, Strid LJ, Wennerstrand MI, et al (South Carelian Central Hosp, Lappeenranta, Finland)
Anesth Analg 84:839–844, 1997   19–15

Objective.—Use of a pneumatic tourniquet during orthopedic procedures even for a short period enhances fibrinolytic activity. Tranexamic acid (TA) has been shown in preliminary studies to reduce blood loss in total knee arthroplasties (TKA). Results of a larger study using a larger dose of TA to evaluate the risk of possible thromboembolic complications are presented.

Methods.—Between September 1994 and April 1996, 77 patients (12 men) with 80 TKAs were randomly allocated to receive, in a blinded fashion, either an injection of normal saline (NS) ($n = 39$) or of TA (15 mg/kg) ($n = 38$) just before the pneumatic thigh tourniquet was deflated, and 2–10 mg/kg injections, 3 to 4 and 6 to 7 hours later. Blood loss was measured, and the frequency of thromboembolic events was recorded. Outcomes for the 2 groups were compared statistically.

Results.—Two patients were withdrawn from the study for taking aspirin 2 days before surgery. On average, the NS group lost significantly more blood than did the TA group (1,509 vs. 689 mL) and required significantly more transfusion units (3.1 vs. 1). Significantly more TA patients than NS patients were treated without transfusions (22 vs. 4). Two patients in each group had a thromboembolic event. One patient in the NS group died of a pulmonary embolus.

Conclusion.—The use of TA during TKA performed with a tourniquet significantly reduces blood loss and is not associated with excess complications.

▶ This was a remarkably clean study with a clear outcome. In fact, if you set up a threshold and say OK, the patients who do well can get over it and the people who don't do well can't. The score is 22 patients receiving TA and 4 patients in the normal saline group didn't require any transfusion. It's interesting that TA was so helpful because there was a time, some years ago, when it was thought that the value of fibrinolytic therapy with TA was not going to be helpful because of liver toxicity. However, it didn't seem to "pan" out that way and the golden nuggets are there today, years later.

M. Weintraub, M.D.

Antibiotic Prophylaxis in Total Hip Arthroplasty: Review of 10,905 Primary Cemented Total Hip Replacements Reported to The Norwegian Arthroplasty Register, 1987 to 1995
Espehaug B, Engesaeter LB, Vollset SE, et al (Univ of Bergen, Norway; Haukeland Univ, Norway; Buskerud Central Hosp, Norway)
J Bone Joint Surg Br 79-B:590–595, 1997   19–16

Objective.—One study suggested that the combination of systemic antibiotics and antibiotic-containing bone cement increased the survival of total hip implants. The effect on implant survival of the different regimes of antibiotic prophylaxis for hip arthroplasty in Norway was compared.

Methods.—Time to revision was compared for 10,905 patients with primary total hip replacements (THRs) performed in Norway between 1987 and 1995. There were 5,804 patients who received the combined regime, 4,586 received systemic antibiotics, 239 who were treated with antibiotics in the bone cement only, and 276 who did not receive antibiotics. The most commonly used systemic antibiotics were cephalothin, cefuroxime, dicloxacillin, and cloxacillin. Antibiotics used in bone cements were gentamicin and erythromycin/colistin. Cox analysis was used to calculate failure rate ratios (FRR). Risk factors for failure were determined.

Results.—The revision rate was lowest in patients who received the combined regimes. Compared with the combined regime with 39 revisions for infection, the revision rate was 4.3 times higher with systemic antibiotics (p=0.001), 6.3 times higher with cement-containing antibiotics (p=0.003), and 11.5 times higher when no antibiotics were used (p=0.002). There were 109 patients who had aseptic loosening. Compared with the combined regimes, there was a FRR of 1.8 (p=0.01) with systemic antibiotics and an FRR of 2.6 with antibiotic-containing cement. Adjusting for the total amount of antibiotics administered systemically did not alter the results.

Conclusion.—A combination of systemic and antibiotic-containing cement was more effective than either method alone in reducing the number of THR revisions resulting from infection or aseptic loosening.

▶ This study is one of a gigantic case series followed in Norway and the results are—hand me the envelope please—that antibiotic prophylaxis is unquestionably effective in preventing the need for revisions of the surgery. When the antibiotic is in the bone cement as well as administered systemically, the results are even better. Also, the antibiotic used is not terribly important; both cloxacillin and dicloxacillin and various cephalosporins, including cephalothin and cefuroxime, were all used to good effect. The antibiotic was only rarely administered for more than 3 days. It looks as if we've finally learned how to do antibiotic prophylaxis in hip surgery. We've learned how to do prophylaxis for deep-vein thrombosis. We've also got the surgical technique down pretty well, and the anesthesia is also quite good. Next we have to learn how to avoid the need for hip surgery for osteoarthritis and to be able to treat it with safe, effective medications.

M. Weintraub, M.D.

20 Skin Diseases

Deaths Associated With Ivermectin Treatment of Scabies
Barkwell R, Sheilds S (McMaster Univ, Hamilton; Ont, Canada; Univ of Toronto)
Lancet 349:1144–1145, 1997   20–1

Background.—Ivermectin was used for control of a scabies outbreak in the 47-bed closed ward of a long-term care institution. During the ensuing 6 months, a pattern of excess deaths was suspected among the treated residents.

Methods.—The apparent excess deaths were retrospectively investigated through case-control analysis, matching by age and sex. The control cohort was designed to maximize deaths. Symptoms and mortality rates were compared.

Results.—Between November 10, 1995 and May 10, 1996, 15 of the 47 ivermectin-treated residents died, vs. 5 control residents. Deaths in the ivermectin group were preceded by changes in behavior, including lethargy, anorexia, and listlessness. Difference in mortality was significant ($P = 0.001$), and relative risk was 3.00.

Discussion.—Ivermectin treatment for scabies is not recommended in elderly populations in light of the strong association between ivermectin and excess deaths in this cohort. The causality of this association, and any potential interactions of medications, should be investigated.

▶ "Deaths associated with ivermectin treatment of scabies"—worrisome, but not yet proved, even in this epidemiologic survey with a maximization of deaths in the control cohort. Still, there are several drugs for the treatment of scabies. They should probably be tried first in an elderly population.

M. Weintraub, M.D.

Topical Calcipotriene in Combination With UVB Phototherapy for Psoriasis
Hecker D, Lebwohl M (Mount Sinai School of Medicine, New York)
Int J Dermatol 36:302–303, 1997   20–2

Introduction.—A controlled, investigator-blinded study was designed to evaluate the benefits of topical calcipotriene in combination with ultraviolet B (UVB) in patients with psoriasis.

317

Methods.—Twenty patients with symmetric plaque-type psoriasis were recruited for the trial. All had a negative antinuclear antibody and all had shown improvement during previous exposure to sunlight or ultraviolet light. None had received other therapies, except for emollients, during the previous 2 months. Each patient was treated twice daily, with mineral oil on 1 side and with calcipotriene 0.005% ointment on the opposite side. Target areas were sites of equal severity. Both sides were treated with broad-band UVB 3 times weekly.

Results.—The examiner rated each of 4 features of psoriasis on a 4-point scale of severity: erythema, scaling, plaque elevation, and pruritus. After 12 weeks of therapy, 11 patients (55%) showed a greater decrease in the severity of psoriasis on the UVB-plus-calcipotriene–treated side than on the UVB–plus–mineral-oil side. The difference in severity scores was statistically significant at as early as 1 week and peaked between weeks 3 and 6. Three patients experienced mild photosensitivity on both sides, but there were no instances of local cutaneous irritation.

Conclusion.—Some patients with psoriasis may benefit from the combination of calcipotriene ointment and UVB. The vitamin D analogue was previously shown to be effective as a monotherapy in the treatment of psoriasis, and this small trial suggests that an additive improvement occurs when given with UVB phototherapy.

▶ The design of this study (investigator-blinded, right-left study) is a reasonable approach to mixtures of a physical treatment, UVB, and a medication (calcipotriene or mineral oil). Although the *P* values were always in favor of UVB plus calcipotriene, the authors note that not all patients benefited, and the degree of benefit really did vary between patients. It would have been nice to have carried the study out for a longer time to see whether the benefit persisted beyond medication or UVB administration.

M. Weintraub, M.D.

Oral Terbinafine in Toenail Dermatophytosis: A Double-blind Placebo-controlled Multicenter Study With 12 Months' Follow-up
Svejgaard EL, Brandrup F, Kragballe K, et al (Natl Hosp, Copenhagen; Odense Univ Hosp, Denmark; Univ Hosp of Aarhus, Denmark; et al)
Acta Derm Venereol 77:66–69, 1997   20–3

Objective.—Onychomycosis, infection of the toenails, is particularly difficult to cure. Terbinafine has been shown to be effective in curing 42% to 100% of infections after 3 to 6 months. The efficacy of 250 mg terbinafine taken daily for 3 months was compared with placebo in the treatment of dermatophytosis and in an additional treatment, results of terbinafine were evaluated in nonresponders.

Methods.—A double-blind, controlled, multicenter study evaluated the effectiveness of terbinafine (n=75) vs. placebo (n=73) in the treatment of toenail dermatophytosis. Patients were evaluated at baseline, 6 weeks, and at 3, 6, 9, and 12 months.

Results.—Of the 127 patients who completed the study, 63 received terbinafine and 64 received placebo. At 3 months, the terbinafine group had significantly greater clinical improvement than the placebo group with respect to nail length, subungual keratosis, and percent of nail affected (49 vs. 16). Sixteen placebo-treated patients improved. After 3 months significantly more patients in the terbinafine group than the placebo group had a negative culture and a growth of 2 mm or more of unaffected nail (31 vs. 4). After 12 months, the clinical cure rates for patients treated for 3 and 6 months with terbinafine were 63% and 81%. Nonresponders treated for 3 months with terbinafine had a clinical cure rate of 67%. The placebo group had a clinical cure rate of 44%. The mycological cure rate at 12 months was 33% in the placebo group, 49% for nonresponders, 40% for patients treated with terbinafine for 3 months, and 47% for patients treated with terbinafine for 6 months. Combined clinical and mycological cure rates were 25% for the placebo group, 40% for the nonresponders, 38% for patients treated with terbinafine for 3 months, and 42% for patients treated with terbinafine for 6 months. Side effects were reported by 5.4% of placebo-treated patients and 13.5% of terbinafine-treated patients after 3 months.

Conclusion.—At 12 months of follow-up, terbinafine (250 mg for 3 months) is significantly more effective than placebo for treatment of ony-chomycosis of the toenail. Side effects, reported by 13.5% of terbinafine-treated patients and 5.4% of placebo-treated patients, were not serious.

▶ The treatment of fungus of the toenails, particularly, is really very difficult. In this study, the authors followed the patients for 12 months to make sure that patients cured after 6 months would have achieved and maintained the cure. There are several ways of viewing a cure. One can look at the clinical picture and make sure that the patient feels well and has no evidence of disease. One can look at it on a microscopic level and decide whether there are organisms still present. There can also be a culture cure, which is, of course, the highest hurdle to overcome by not having any mycological growth on the culture plates. The mycelia seen by microscopy may not be infectious because of treatment. One interesting aspect of this study is that 4 people on placebo maintained a clinical as well as a mycological cure after 12 months. One of the patients had had disease in his toenails for 10 years. Isn't placebo wonderful!

M. Weintraub, M.D.

Penciclovir Cream for the Treatment of Herpes Simplex Labialis

Spruance SL, for the Topical Penciclovir Collaborative Study Group (Univ of Utah, Salt Lake City; Westover Heights Clinic, Portland, Oregon; Wenatchee Valley Clinic, Wash)

JAMA 277:1374–1379, 1997   20–4

Background.—No antiviral drug has been found to be consistently effective in large, well-controlled clinical trials involving otherwise healthy patients with herpes labialis. Topical 1% penciclovir cream was compared with vehicle control cream in a randomized, double-blind, patient-initiated, 2-arm parallel clinical study of immunocompetent patients with recurrent herpes simplex labialis.

Methods.—Thirty-one ambulatory U.S. clinics enrolled a total of 2,209 patients, 1,573 of whom initiated treatment for a recurrence. Treatment consisted of topical 1% penciclovir cream or placebo applied every 2 hours during waking hours for 4 consecutive days.

Findings.—In the patients receiving active treatment, classical lesions (such as vesicles, ulcers, and/or crusts) healed 0.7 day faster than those in the placebo recipients. In addition, pain and lesion virus shedding resolved more rapidly in the penciclovir recipients. Penciclovir cream was effective whether treatment was initiated early or late. The incidences of adverse events were comparable in the 2 groups.

Conclusions.—Penciclovir cream is the first treatment to have a clear impact on the course of recurrent herpes labialis in immunocompetent patients. All clinical and laboratory measures of the disease were improved with this treatment. Faster healing and pain resolution were evident in patients applying the cream in the prodrome and erythema stages as well as in those starting treatment in the papule and vesicle lesion stages.

▶ One person in 5 is alleged to suffer at some time from cold sores. Frequency of attacks varies enormously, as does the duration of the episodes. The search for a consistently effective anti-herpes simplex drug has largely been disappointing.

The present study has positive conclusions, but the clinical benefit is modest indeed on average.

L. Lasagna, M.D.

Treatment of Chronic Urticaria With Ketotifen

Egan CA, Rallis TM (Univ of Utah, Salt Lake City)

Arch Dermatol 133:147–149, 1997   20–5

Background.—Chronic urticaria is a difficult problem to treat. The lesions are caused by local increase in capillary permeability, induced by histamine and other local mediators from mast cells or basophils. Most patients have no specific allergic trigger. Most of the available treatments for urticaria target the symptoms and block the receptors. The potent antiasthma and antiallergic drug ketotifen was used to treat a resistant case of chronic, severe urticaria.

> *Case.*—Woman, 43, had a 5-month history of urticaria and pruritus after an influenza vaccination and an episode of pneumonia. She had seen many dermatologists and received many treatments. She had episodes of breathing difficulty that led to several emergency department visits, and had become depressed and suicidal. An extensive workup identified no source of her urticaria. Her condition improved on IV ranitidine hydrochloride and hydroxyzine hydrochloride, along with an elemental diet, in the hospital. However, the urticaria recurred after her discharge. After another severe exacerbation, the patient showed moderate improvement in response to high-dose pulse methylprednisolone acetate, but there was no response to a second course. She also had moderate improvement to plasmapheresis and supplemental oral cyclophosphamide but was unable to tolerate the cyclophosphamide.
>
> The patient was then treated with ketotifen fumarate, which she had bought in Mexico. The dosage was 2 mg orally twice daily. All other drug treatments were withdrawn except for fluoxetine and levothyroxine. This treatment rendered the patient free of urticaria for the first time in 9 months. Her pruritus resolved with time, and she was able to return to a normal diet. She has required no further hospitalizations since starting ketotifen. Similarly good results with ketotifen treatment have been obtained in 3 other patients with chronic urticaria.

Discussion.—Ketotifen appears to be a safe and effective treatment for chronic urticaria that does not respond to other treatments. Unlike other drugs that merely treat the symptoms, ketotifen acts to stabilize the mast cells and prevent the release of mediators. Ketotifen is currently unavailable for use in the United States. Double-blind research studies assessing ketotifen treatment for chronic idiopathic urticaria are warranted.

▶ These doctors really tried everything, and I mean everything, in an attempt to control the patient's urticaria. They even tried oral cyclophosphamide with plasmapheresis. The patient then bought ketotifen at a pharmacy in Mexico, which seemed to have had an effect. However, it is likely that even in a foreign country the purchase of a medication not available in the United States really didn't have anything to do with a response, or nearly as much as the medication itself had to do with her therapeutic outcome. Occasionally, patients may be able to do the right thing when they seek therapy in another country or from drugs outside the United States. It's a fine line, however, and, unlike in this case, it can be crossed to the patient's and doctor's detriment.

M. Weintraub, M.D.

Double-blind Crossover Study of High-dose Cetirizine in Cholinergic Urticaria

Zuberbier T, Münzberger Ch, Haustein U, et al (Humboldt Univ, Berlin; Univ of Leipzig, Germany; UCB Pharma, Braine-L'Alleud, Belgium)
Dermatology 193:324–327, 1996   20–6

Introduction.—Patients with cholinergic urticaria exhibit highly pruritic wheals of pinpoint size when body temperature rises during physical exercise. Systemic reactions such as dizziness and nausea affect about 10% of patients. Because the condition is difficult to treat with ordinary antihistamines, a trial of cetirizine, a new antihistamine, was conducted.

Methods.—The double-blind, crossover, placebo-controlled trial enrolled 13 patients, mean age 26.5 years, mean duration of disease 89 months. They were randomized to start with either placebo or cetirizine (20 mg/day) for 3 weeks. Rescue medication, consisting of 20 cetirizine tablets, were supplied at the start of each treatment period. Patients were asked to record attacks in a diary and to grade erythema, wheals, and pruritus on a scale of 0 (none) to 3 (severe).

Results.—Most patients had moderate or severe disease which could be provoked by vigorous exercise or a hot shower. Two patients were excluded for lack of compliance. Among the remaining 11 patients, cetirizine brought about reductions in each symptom and in the total symptoms score that were statistically significant compared with placebo. There were no adverse events in either cetirizine or placebo treatment periods.

Conclusion.—Cetirizine, at twice the normally recommended dose, was highly effective in relieving the symptoms of cholinergic urticaria. The drug's benefits in such cases may be related to its antiallergic and antieosinophilic properties.

▶ Cholinergic urticaria is a rare condition where wheals are brought on by an increase in body temperature, such as with physical exercise. Some patients also have dizziness and nausea. One valid reason for doing crossover studies is if all the patients in a specific area are available for your study, and there are not likely to be any other populations you can easily get your hands on.

M. Weintraub, M.D.

Systemic Scleroderma: Multicenter Trial of 1 Year of Treatment With Recombinant Interferon Gamma

Hunzelmann N, Anders S, Fierlbeck G, et al (Univ of Cologne, Germany; Univ of Tübingen, Germany; Univ of Regensburg, Germany; et al)
Arch Dermatol 133:609–613, 1997   20–7

Background.—The pathogenesis of systemic scleroderma is unknown. Several studies have reported increased expression of collagen type I by in situ hybridization or in fibroblasts of affected skin. Transforming growth factor-β may be instrumental in the pathogenesis of systemic scleroderma.

Interferon-γ has a strong inhibitory effect on collagen synthesis by normal dermal and scleroderma fibroblasts in vitro. This inhibitory effect is not overcome by transforming growth factor-β.

Methods.—There were 32 patients with diffuse or limited systemic sclerosis. The mean duration of the disease was 5.3 years. Recombinant interferon-γ 50 μg, was administered subcutaneously 3 times a week for 1 year. Follow-up evaluation at 12, 24, 36, and 48 months was completed for 20 patients.

Results.—In the 20 patients who completed the study, unchanged median skin scores after 1 year of treatment were noted. Similar collagen type I messenger RNA levels were seen in biopsy specimens of affected skin before and after treatment. Adverse reactions included headache, fatigue, weight gain, nausea, arthralgia, fever, renal crisis, skin ulcers, and myositis. It is unclear if these reactions resulted from treatment. Headache was the most common reaction.

Discussion.—In these patients, treatment with 50 μg of interferon-γ 3 times a week for 1 year was associated with stabilization of skin scores and visceral involvement. Skin scores probably did not improve because interferon-γ inhibits matrix deposition but does not enhance matrix degradation, which could decrease fibrosis.

▶ Systemic scleroderma is a bad disease. Effective therapy is badly needed. Recombinant interferon-γ seems to provide some benefit.

L. Lasagna, M.D.

Healing of an Ulcer Caused by Ischemia Under Treatment With *Ginkgo biloba* EGb 761
Steins A, Zuder D, Hahn M, et al (Univ Hosp, Liebermeisterstrasse, Tübingen, Germany)
Eur J Dermatol 7:109–111, 1997   20–8

Background.—Alhough there is no consensus in the medical literature about the efficacy of *Ginkgo biloba* extract EGb 761 in the treatment of peripheral arterial occlusive disease (PAOD), there have been several reports of the positive effects of this agent on PAOD. A patient in whom an ulcer caused by ischemia healed after *Ginkgo biloba* EGb 761 treatment is described.

> *Case Report.*—Man, 75, had Fontaine stage IV PAOD in the right leg. This pretibial ulcer had been triggered by a minor trauma. In the 3 years after the trauma, the ulcer showed no signs of healing, despite intensive conservative and operative treatment. The patient's cardiac condition precluded implantation with a Y-or femoral-popliteal bypass. Thus *Ginkgo biloba* EGb 761 therapy was begun. The size of the ulcer decreased significantly after 2 weeks. After 4 months, the ulcer was completely healed.

Conclusions.—In this patient, *Ginkgo biloba* EGb 761 was effective in resolving an ulcer caused by ischemia. Good granulation and a rapid reduction in ulcer size were noted.

▶ One of traditional medicine's fears is that the herbal extracts that so many patients now use may be adulterated either with other herbal medications or with chemicals that were not in the initial product. The very high adulteration rate of almost one fourth of the substances tested in Chinese hospitals in Taiwan[1] is worrisome. For example, the finding that prednisolone was present in 91 of 618 samples collected from 8 hospitals could be very detrimental to the patients who take the supposedly nontoxic medications. We really do need to know what is in the herbal preparation and how high the dose may be because certain products have a dose-response effect and are very seriously toxic at higher doses. Of course, we have to remember that some pretty potent drugs are found in plants and that they can, as every other thing can, hurt you.

Closer to home, in Canada, it has turned out to be very difficult to tell whether an herbal product has caused an adverse reaction.[2] The Canadians have an interesting system. They permit generally accepted uses for traditional herbal medicines as the basis of effectiveness claims. We'll have to wait to see how the system works out.

▶ On the other hand, a patient avoided a femoral-popliteal bypass by using *Ginkgo biloba* therapy to help heal a leg ulcer. Obviously, 1 patient very rarely, except perhaps for rabies, makes a powerful argument for a therapy. Still and all, this case report needs to be followed up.

M. Weintraub, M.D.

References

1. Huang WF, Wen KC, Hsiao ML: Adulteration by synthetic therapeutic substances of traditional Chinese medicines in Taiwan. *J Clin Pharmacol* 37:344–350, 1997.
2. Kozyrskyj A: Herbal products in Canada. How safe are they? *Can Fam Physician* 43:697–702, 1997.

21 Surgery

Academic Surgeons' Knowledge of Food and Drug Administration Regulations for Clinical Trials
Rutan RL, Deitch EA, Waymack JP (Univ of Medicine and Dentistry of New Jersey)
Arch Surg 132:94–98,1997
21–1

Objective.—The Food and Drug Administration (FDA) must approve new products before they are marketed. The agency also regulates the conduct of clinical trials. Few medical schools provide instruction to physicians about the regulations applicable to clinical trials and the role of Institutional Review Boards (IRBs). A study assessed the level of knowledge of academic surgeons about FDA and IRB regulations.

Methods.—A 20-item questionnaire was sent to 12 faculty members at each of 20 university-affiliated departments of surgery to assess awareness of FDA regulations of clinical studies and composition and purpose of IRBs.

Results.—There were 65 (27%) of 240 questionnaires returned from 14 institutions. Three responders were department chairs; 18, professors; 21, associate professors; 20, assistant professors; and 3, clinical instructors. Seventeen had served on an IRB, 14 had participated in clinical trials, 18 were primary investigators, and 17 had been consultants to pharmaceutical companies. The average number of correct answers was 6.7 of 20, with no significant difference between academic group responses Primary investigators scored somewhat higher, with an average of 7.9 correct answers of 20. All respondents were unaware in at least 1 clinical scenario that FDA approval was required before a study could be conducted. Approximately 25% of responders were willing to conduct clinical studies without obtaining IRB approval, patient consent, or both.

Conclusion.—Surgeons appear to be unfamiliar with FDA requirements for clinical studies and the need for IRB approval and patient consent before beginning studies.

▶ Surgeons in general rarely come to an IRB with research protocols, and one suspects that a lot of what might well be termed "research" is considered acceptable surgical flexibility instead. I am not surprised that surgeons are not very knowledgeable about FDA regulations for clinical trials.

L. Lasagna, M.D.

Quantitative Measurement of the Effects of Caffeine and Propranolol on Surgeon Hand Tremor

Humayun MU, Rader RS, Pieramici DJ, et al (Johns Hopkins Hosp, Baltimore, Md)

Arch Ophthalmol 115:371–374, 1997   21–2

Background.—Instrument stability is critical to the success of microsurgery. Instrument stability is significantly affected by surgeon hand tremor. Various hand and wrist rests have been developed to reduce the effects of tremor and to improve stability. Many surgeons do not ingest caffeine before surgery because of the belief that it increases hand tremor. Stress, anxiety, and physical exertion can also affect tremor. Propranolol has been shown to reduce essential tremor.

Methods.—Hand tremor was tested in 17 ophthalmic surgeons on 3 separate days in a double-blind, placebo-controlled study. Hand tremor was measured immediately before and 1 hour after each surgeon ingested 200 mg caffeine, 10 mg propranolol hydrochloride, or placebo. The Microsurgery Advanced Design Laboratory Stability, Activation, and Maneuverability tester was used to measure tremor.

Results.—The average percent magnitude change from baseline measurements of hand tremor was +31% for caffeine, −22% for propranolol, and +15% for placebo. Analysis of variance techniques accounting for effects of individuals, drugs, and day order showed that only drug effects on the percent magnitude change in hand tremor were significant. In a comparison of the groups that ingested caffeine or propranolol with the group that ingested placebo, only the mean decrease in tremor from propranolol was statistically significant, after adjusting for individual and order effects. The larger mean increase in percent magnitude change in tremor seen with caffeine than with placebo was not statistically significant. There were statistically significant drug effects on percent change in systolic and diastolic blood pressure and pulse rate. There were no significant individual or day order effects. No side effects occurred.

Discussion.—Ingestion of caffeine increased hand tremor. A low dose of propranolol reduced hand tremor by 22% from baseline in these subjects. Propranolol is a noncardioselective drug.

▶ A shaky microsurgeon would not be my choice for these delicate procedures. Lots of things can cause tremor, and β-blockers can improve tremor-affected performance in actors, musicians, and athletes. Surgeons who want to avoid hand tremor would be wise to avoid caffeine and take a modest dose of propranolol before operating.

L. Lasagna, M.D.

Premedication in the United States: A Status Report

Kain ZN, Mayes LC, Bell C, et al (Yale Univ, New Haven, Conn)
Anesth Analg 84:427–432, 1997   21–3

Background.—Preoperative anxiety has been associated with various adverse outcomes. Both pharmacologic intervention with premedication and psychological interventions have been used to treat this anxiety. The current survey was done to determine premedicant usage patterns in the United States.

Methods.—A total of 5,396 members of the American Society of Anesthesiologists were randomly selected and mailed a questionnaire. After 2 mailings, 46% returned questionnaires.

Findings.—The use of sedative premedication varied widely according to patient age and geographic location. Premedicant sedative agents were used least often in children younger then 3 years and most often in adults younger than 65 years. Midazolam was the agent most commonly given, used in more than three fourths of both children and adults. Premedicant use in adults was least common in the Northeast and most common in the Southeast. In a multivariate analysis, HMO penetration was found to be an independent predictor of premedicant use in adults and children.

Conclusions.—The substantial variation in premedicant use among geographic regions emphasizes the lack of consensus among anesthesiologists on the need for premedication. Premedicant usage patterns were associated with HMO penetration.

▶ There is obviously a lot of variation among anesthesiologists with regard to use of premedication, and U.S. physicians differ from their British colleagues. What is not clear is what difference these variations make in quality of care.

L. Lasagna, M.D.

Inhalation Induction With Sevoflurane: A Double-blind Comparison With Propofol

Thwaites A, Edmends S, Smith I (North Staffordshire Hosps, Stoke-on-Trent, UK)
Br J Anaesth 78:356–361, 1997   21–4

Objective.—Inhalation induction of anesthesia avoids many of the problems associated with IV induction. Earlier studies with inhalation induction of anesthesia with sevoflurane were not blinded and used 5% rather than the 8% output currently used. A randomized, double-blind induction of anesthesia in unpremedicated patients compared 8% sevoflurane and IV propofol, the most commonly used induction agent.

Methods.—A 20-gauge IV cannula was inserted into the nondominant hand of each of 102 patients, aged 18 to 85, who were breathing oxygen at 5 L/min, and 2 mL of 1% lignocaine were administered. A blinded observer administered either 20-mL propofol (n=51) or 10% intralipid as placebo. Anesthesia was induced in the treatment group (n=51) with 8% sevoflurane but maintained in all patients with 2% sevoflurane delivered by face mask and adjusted up or down as needed. Occurrence of apnea, movements, and coughing were recorded. After the procedure, patients were asked about their recollections of the face mask, smells, tastes, pain of injection, and asked to guess if their anesthesia had been induced by gas or injection. Patients were asked to rate their experiences.

Results.—Induction of anesthesia with propofol was significantly faster than with sevoflurane (57 vs. 84 seconds). Apnea occurred significantly more frequently in the propofol group than in the sevoflurane group (65% vs. 16%). Time from start of induction to spontaneous breathing was significantly shorter with sevoflurane than with propofol (94 vs. 126 seconds). Coughing after induction occurred in 24% of the propofol group and in 8% of sevoflurane group. There was less hypotension in the sevoflurane group during the transition to maintenance. Sevoflurane patients emerged from anesthesia significantly sooner than propofol patients (5.2 vs. 7.0 minutes). Induction costs associated with propofol were significantly higher than for sevoflurane (£3.88 vs. £1.95). Significantly more sevoflurane than propofol patients found the face mask (10% vs. 2%) and smell (29% vs. 8%) unpleasant and would prefer a different induction technique in the future (24% vs. 6%).

Conclusion.—Whereas induction of anesthesia provides several objective advantages over propofol, a significant minority of patients found the procedure objectionable.

▶ The exigencies of modern, day-case surgery, where the patient goes home on the same day as the surgery, requires new types of anesthetic agents. In this case, sevoflurane was given by inhalation and the propofol was given intravenously. More patients preferred the IV administration. Several found the smell and wearing the mask unpleasant. While the mask was put on both groups of patients, the propofol group mentioned a smell, in any case, which may have persisted in the mask or machinery used for administering sevoflurane. I don't know about these anesthesiologists, but when I was a kid I had my tonsils out, and I still remember the smell of the anesthetic. Later, when I was an adolescent and had my appendix removed, I had IV induction and remember it as being much more acceptable. I say let the patients choose.

M. Weintraub, M.D.

Dose-response to Anaesthetic Induction With Sufentanil: Haemodynamic and Electroencephalographic Effects

Sareen J, Hudson RJ, Rosenbloom M, et al (Univ of Manitoba, Winnipeg, Canada)

Can J Anaesth 44:19–25, 1997

21–5

Background.—Hemodynamic stability is important in patients with coronary artery disease undergoing general anesthesia. Sufentanil and other synthetic opioids are frequently used in patients having coronary artery bypass grafting because they are usually accompanied by hemodynamic stability. Bradyarrhythmias and hypotension have been reported after the administration of sufentanil in humans, although the relationship between opioid dose, opioid serum concentration, and hemodynamic response has not been examined.

Methods.—There were 34 patients scheduled for coronary artery bypass grafting. Thirty patients were men; the mean patient age was 64 years. Patients in group L were given sufentanil, 3 µg/kg, and patients in group H were given sufentanil, 15 µg/kg. Patients were premedicated with lorazepam by mouth, 60 µg/kg. Anesthesia and neuromuscular blockade were induced by IV sufentanil and 0.15 mg/kg vecuronium. Hemodynamic data and electroencephalographic (EEG) response were compared at baseline, induction, and intubation.

Results.—Hemodynamic data and EEG response at end induction were not affected by the dose of sufentanil. No patient had bradyarrhythmia. In both groups, the rate of hypotension was 12%. In group H, electromyographic artifacts and a transient greater increase in heart rate occurred. At induction, the serum sufentanil concentration was 6.1 ng/mL in group L and 25.4 ng/mL in group H. There was no correlation between these concentrations and hemodynamic changes.

Discussion.—A variation in dose of sufentanil from 3 to 15 µg/kg did not affect the hemodynamic response to anesthesia in these patients. In patients having coronary artery bypass grafting, sufentanil, 3 µg/kg, plus lorazepam premedication and vecuronium produces rapid near-maximal opioid effects and is adequate for induction of anesthesia and tracheal intubation.

▶ In this particular study, there was no improved dose response with a fivefold change in the sufentanil dose. There were some adverse effects, however, although they probably were not terribly important. The point is that it is incredibly important to be able to assess a dose response to anesthetic agents, because less is no doubt better than more in this case. We would like to have patients be more responsive and wake up from their anesthetic more quickly. A higher dose, in addition to not being more efficacious, certainly would not accomplish that.

M. Weintraub, M.D.

Prophylactic Intravenous Administration of Caffeine and Recovery After Ambulatory Surgical Procedures

Weber JG, Klindworth JT, Arnold JJ, et al (Mayo Clinic Rochester, Minn)
Mayo Clin Proc 72:621–626, 1997   21–6

Objective.—Patients who consume caffeinated beverages may have symptoms of withdrawal when having to fast before surgery. Consumption of caffeinated beverages before or after a procedure lessens the risk of a postoperative headache. The potential beneficial effect on frequency of headaches and recovery time after ambulatory surgery of prophylactic postoperative intravenous administration of caffeine was investigated in a prospective, randomized, double-blind study.

Methods.—Saline or 200 mg caffeine in isotonic saline was administered preoperatively to 300 ambulatory surgery patients, aged 18 to 80. Daily intake of caffeine, nicotine, history of headaches, postoperative symptoms, postoperative well-being, severity of postoperative headache, and postoperative pain were determined by survey. Incidence of headaches between groups was compared using the χ^2 test.

Results.—There were 234 completed questionnaires (56% female), and 44% said they had headaches at least weekly. Risk factors for postoperative headache were a history of frequent headaches, age younger than 50, and lack of caffeine before surgery. High intake of caffeine was not a risk factor. Patients receiving placebo and no caffeinated beverages had a headache rate of 23%. Patients receiving IV caffeine only had a significantly lower (10%) headache rate. Patients receiving caffeinated beverages after surgery and placebo had a lower headache rate (11%) that approached significance. Patients receiving caffeinated beverages after surgery plus IV caffeine had a headache rate (20%) similar to the placebo/no caffeine beverage group. Recovery times, postoperative symptoms, postoperative well-being, and postoperative pain were similar among all groups.

Conclusion.—Prophylactic intravenous administration of caffeine to ambulatory surgery patients lessens the risk of postoperative headache in patients at risk of caffeine withdrawal.

▶ One problem that many of us have is that we don't take the patient's life into account. We only look at our procedure or our intervention as the most important aspect and forget all about the patient's life and lifestyle. This particular paper documents the helpfulness of caffeine, although the dose seemed a little high to me. Perhaps ambulatory surgical patients can be urged to drink caffeine-containing beverages when they awaken from their anesthetic and prevent caffeine withdrawal on that basis. We have to think about the implications of the patient's habits, for example, on their postoperative status.

M. Weintraub, M.D.

Efficacy of Prophylactic Antibiotics in Arthroscopic Surgery

Wieck JA, Jackson JK, O'Brien TJ, et al (Naval Hosp, Pensacola, Fla)

Orthopedics 20:133–134, 1997

21–7

Introduction.—There have been several retrospective studies of the use of prophylactic antibiotics in patients undergoing arthroscopic surgery. However, there have been no prospective studies of this issue. A prospective, double-blind study of the efficacy of prophylactic antibiotics for arthroscopic surgery is reported.

Methods.—The study included 437 patients undergoing arthroscopic diagnostic and operative procedures. Exclusion criteria included known allergy to cefazolin or penicillin and use of a metallic implant. The patients were randomized to receive either 1 g of cefazolin in 50 mL of D5W or D5W only. The patients were evaluated postoperatively at 10 to 14 days and again at 6 weeks.

Results.—No patient in either group had a deep infection. One patient assigned to the placebo group had a superficial wound infection after ankle arthroscopy. One patient in the antibiotic group had a mild allergic reaction, which resolved with Benadryl treatment.

Conclusions.—Giving cefazolin does not appear to reduce the risk of infections in patients undergoing arthroscopy. Given the high cost and slight risk of antibiotic use, cefazolin prophylaxis should not be routinely given to patients undergoing arthroscopic surgery.

▶ Here's another counterintuitive paper. These investigators said, "You don't need to give antibiotics in patients undergoing arthroscopic surgery." Of course, you can't prove a negative, but this was a relatively large, randomized, prospective, double-blind study which contained almost 450 people. It's really very convincing. However, I'm not sure it will be accepted by our colleagues who do arthroscopic surgery. After all, the *money (around* $50 for the antibiotics) was relatively unimportant and, although there were no infections, you never can tell.

M. Weintraub, M.D.

Audit of Thromboembolic Prophylaxis in Hip and Knee Surgery

Williams HR, Macdonald DA (St James's Univ Hosp, Leeds, England)

Ann R Coll Surg Engl 79:55–57, 1997

21–8

Introduction.—Thromboembolic prophylaxis is an important part of the management of patients undergoing hip and knee surgery. Although the orthopedic department at the study institution has an established policy for such cases, an audit determined that compliance with thromboembolic prophylaxis was poor.

Methods.—The audit was carried out unannounced during the course of an afternoon. Data collected on inpatients under the care of the department included reason for admission, use of TED stockings, subcutaneous heparin (HEP) for those without fractured neck of the femur, and inclusion of patients in a multicenter pulmonary embolism prevention trial in which the department was collaborating. A similar audit was performed 3 weeks later.

Results.—At the first audit, 35 inpatients had undergone a hip or knee arthroplasty or sustained a fractured neck of the femur. There were 39 such patients at the second audit. Overall compliance with the protocol was improved at the second audit, although there was a decline (from 70% to 25%) in the use of TED stockings in patients who had a hemiarthroplasty. Subcutaneous HEP was given to only 43% of patients having primary hip replacement and 14% undergoing revision replacement, in spite of unit policy. All patients having total knee replacement were given HEP, but 75% of these patients received an incorrect dose. Enrollment of patients in the pulmonary embolism prevention trial was increased at the second audit.

Discussion.—Established protocols are of little value unless an audit is performed, results are given to the department, and a follow-up audit is undertaken to confirm protocol compliance.

▶ Elsewhere in this edition of the YEAR BOOK OF DRUG THERAPY we present the results of a large epidemiologic study on the use of prophylactic antibiotics in hip surgery. I state that we have solved many of the problems in dealing with orthopedic surgery of the hip and knee. However, this article points out that if you've got a protocol, it really is of very slight value if you don't have an audit mechanism in place to ensure that the doctors are using it.

M. Weintraub, M.D.

Are Prophylactic Antibiotics Required for Elective Laparoscopic Cholecystectomy?
Illig KA, Schmidt E, Cavanaugh J, et al (Univ of Rochester, NY)
J Am Coll Surg 184:353–356, 1997   21–9

Background.—Some studies support the practice of routinely giving prophylactic antibiotics before laparoscopic cholecystectomy. The necessity of prophylactic antibiotic administration in low-risk patients undergoing routine laparoscopic cholecystectomy was investigated.

Methods.—Two hundred fifty patients with no evidence of acute inflammation, common duct stones, or other indications for antibiotics were assigned randomly to receive 3 perioperative doses of cefazolin or no prophylaxis. The patients were then followed up for up to 30 days.

Findings.—Only 1 major complication occurred among the 122 patients receiving no prophylaxis: an abscess occurred in the presence of a bile leak despite the administration of antibiotics when the leak was discovered several days before infectious problems began. Minor complications included 2 lower urinary tract infections and 1 superficial wound infection in a patient receiving no prophylaxis and 1 urinary tract infection in a patient receiving prophylaxis (a statistically nonsignificant difference). These minor complications were managed easily. Prophylactic antibiotics did not sterilize the bile. Infectious complications were unassociated with weight, inflammation found at the time of surgery, reported stone or bile spillage, or conversion to an open procedure.

Conclusions.—Prophylactic antibiotics are not necessary in healthy, low-risk patients undergoing elective laparoscopic cholecystectomy. Only 1 of the 250 patients in the current series (0.4%) had a major infectious problem.

▶ Before laparoscopic surgery, elective open cholecystectomy in low-risk patients was seldom associated with infection. Bile spillage is more frequent during laparoscopic cholecystectomy, but the wounds are smaller. These authors suggest that the infection rate is so low, and infections so easy to identify and treat, that routine prophylactic antibiotics are unnecessary and wasteful of millions of dollars nationwide.

L. Lasagna, M.D.

Tramadol in the Treatment of Postanesthetic Shivering

De Witte J, Deloof T, De Veylder J, et al (OLV-Clinic, Aalst, Belgium)
Acta Anaesthesiol Scand 41:506–510, 1997   21–10

Objective.—There are only 2 reports of the use of tramadol, an epinephrine and serotonin reuptake inhibitor in the spinal cord, in the treatment of postanesthetic shivering. The efficacy of tramadol and its dose-dependence was investigated in a placebo-controlled, randomized, double-blind study of postanesthetic shivering.

Methods.—Either tramadol (0.5 mg/kg, 1 mg/kg, or 2 mg/kg) or placebo was administered intravenously to 40 of 72 adult patients (17 women), ASA physical status I or II, who had anesthesia induced with droperidol, midazolam, fentanyl, thiopental, and vecuronium, maintained with 66% nitrous oxide in oxygen, enflurane or isoflurane. This group included patients who began shivering within 10 minutes of admission to recovery. A second group of 64 patients (44 females), who received arbitrary general anesthesia and shivered within 10 minutes of admission to recovery, was similarly treated. Shivering was graded 6 times, after injection and at 1-minute intervals. Nonresponders at 5 minutes were given IV pethidine (25 mg). Nausea and vomiting were recorded. Data were analyzed by ANOVA.

Results.—All patients receiving 1 or 2 mg tramadol stopped shivering within 5 minutes. All but 1 patient stopped shivering after receiving 0.5 mg tramadol. Compared with placebo, tramadol significantly reduced shivering at all time points. All 3 doses were equally effective at reducing the intensity and prevalence of shivering. Similar results were obtained with

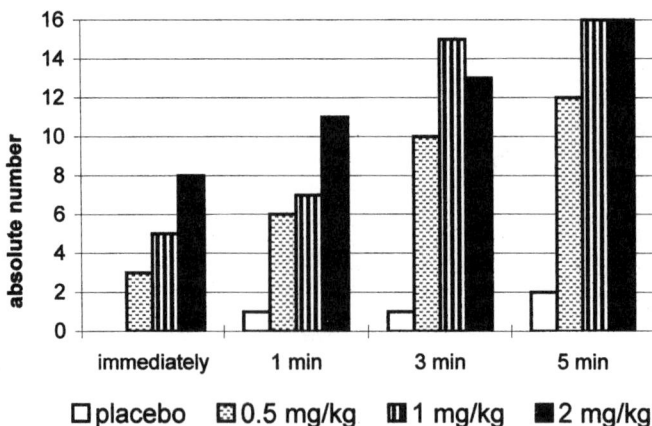

FIGURE 2.—Treatment of shivering after an arbitrary general anesthesia. Number of patients without shivering after three different doses of tramadol compared with placebo. (Courtesy of De Witte J, Deloof T, De Veylder J, et al: Tramadol in the treatment of postanesthetic shivering. *Acta Anaesthesiol Scand* 41:506–510, 1997.)

the arbitrary anesthesia group (Fig 2). One patient in the arbitrary anesthesia group experienced nausea and vomiting.

Conclusion.—Tramadol is safe and effective for postanesthetic shivering.

▶ As shown in the figure, shivering was abolished in the vast majority of patients within minutes. The 0.5 mg of tramadol was slower and incomplete compared to the 1 and 2 mg doses. However, the placebo group was very little affected. The use of the 3 active treatments and placebo was an excellent one to demonstrate pretty well that 1 mg is an effective dose. This is one of those situations where there are lots of drugs that have been tried; many drugs affect some of the aspects of postanesthetic shivering, but none of them does it perfectly. Tramadol, at least in the United States, is associated with a certain incidence of seizures, rarely, however, on the first dose. But sometimes the seizures do occur right after starting the medication. Use of specific serotonin re-uptake inhibitors and drugs such as tricyclics, including cyclobenzaprine HCl (Flexoril), are also potentiators of tramadol-induced seizures. However, it looks like tramadol is an excellent therapy for postanesthetic shivering. Investigators are to be congratulated for doing what so often is needed, and that is a dose-response study against placebo.

M. Weintraub, M.D.

Aspirin-induced Post-Gingivectomy Haemorrhage: A Timely Reminder
Thomason JM, Seymour RA, Murphy P, et al (Royal Victoria Infirmary and Associated Hospitals NHS Trust, New Castle upon Tyne, United Kingdom)
J Clin Periodontol 24:136–138, 1997   21–11

Introduction.—Aspirin can impair platelet aggregation and increase bleeding time. Because platelets do not synthesize new enzymes, the effects of aspirin on cyclooxygenase last for the 7 to 10 day life of the platelet. Aspirin-induced impairment of hemostasis can be prolonged because platelet function returns only after platelet replacement. There have been various case reports of severe aspirin-induced impairment of hemostasis, but few have involved periodontal procedures, and none have involved low-dose aspirin. The case of severe postoperative hemorrhage resulting from low-dose aspirin after gingivectomy in a patient who had undergone organ transplantation is described.

Case Report.—Man, 30, had undergone renal transplantation in 1992 and was scheduled for gingivectomy. The gingival surgery was to be done in stages, using local anesthetic. Initial gingivectomy around the lower anterior teeth was performed without incident. About 40 minutes after gingivectomy around the upper anterior teeth was completed, the patient complained of persistent bleeding. A continuous ooze was seen coming from the surgical site under the dressing. Further pressure and local injection of adrenaline and anesthetic did not control the bleeding. At this point, it was believed that an aspirin-induced impairment of platelet function was involved. The patient was transferred to a hemophilia center, and within 40 minutes of platelet transfusion, the bleeding was controlled, and the patient was discharged after 24 hours. The patient was advised to stop aspirin therapy before invasive procedures.

Discussion.—Aspirin-induced bleeding after gingival surgery is rare. This patient was prescribed low-dose aspirin to prevent primary and secondary arterial thromboembolic disorder. Even low-dose aspirin can cause significant impairment of platelet function.

▶ It's useful to be reminded that aspirin's potential for producing serious adverse effects, although rare, is all too real.

L. Lasagna, M.D.

Should Heparin Be Reversed After Carotid Endarterectomy? A Randomised Prospective Trial

Fearn SJ, Parry AD, Picton AJ, et al (Univ Hosp of South Manchester, England)

Eur J Vasc Endovasc Surg 13:394–397, 1997   21–12

Introduction.—Patients undergoing carotid endarterectomy for prevention of stroke are treated with aspirin and heparin, a combination that may contribute to the risk of postoperative hemorrhage or wound hematoma. A randomized prospective trial examined the benefits of heparin reversal after carotid endarterectomy.

Methods.—Sixty-three patients were enrolled in the trial, and 1 had a bilateral procedure. Protamine was randomized for heparin reversal in 31 cases; 33 control cases did not receive protamine. Carotid endarterectomy was performed under care of the same surgeon and the same anesthetist in all cases. Serial activated clotting times were obtained at baseline, 3 minutes after the heparin bolus, after endarterectomy, and 3 minutes after protamine administration. Perioperative aspirin was given to all patients; none received postoperative heparin or protamine.

Results.—The use of protamine reversal significantly reduced wound drainage compared with no protamine (35 mL vs. 68.5 mL), but neck swelling was similar in the 2 groups (73 mm vs. 72 mm). Neck hematomas requiring evacuation developed in 2 control patients, but 2 patients given protamine died after internal carotid artery thrombosis developed within 12 hours of surgery. During a median follow-up of 4 months, 1 patient had occluded his carotid Dacron graft and another had a 70% restenosis; neither patient had received protamine.

Conclusion.—Postoperative wound drainage after carotid surgery was reduced by heparin reversal with protamine, but this strategy may increase the risk of internal carotid artery thrombosis and stroke.

▶ There are not always many randomized prospective trials of commonly utilized procedures. This study really shows the trade-offs that need to be made between the reversal of anticoagulation and not having enough heparin effect present. Without protamine, 2 patients needed to have neck hematomas evacuated. The same number of patients developed strokes. Of course, the blood loss was much higher in patients who received the control rather than protamine to reverse the heparin. These authors claim that heparin reversal should not be undertaken due to the predisposition to thrombosis and stroke. Other groups of physicians should look at their carotid endarterectomy data and make a judgement based on the risk/benefit relationship. It may be different depending on the patient population, or the drugs may be different, such as aspirin, warfarin, or subcutaneous heparin.

M. Weintraub, M.D.

A Randomized, Prospective Trial of Deep Venous Thrombosis Prophylaxis in Aortic Surgery

Killewich LA, Aswad MA, Sandager GP, et al (Univ of Maryland, Baltimore)
Arch Surg 132:499–504, 1997   21–13

Objective.—Because of the significant morbidity and mortality resulting from deep vein thrombosis (DVT), identifying patients at high risk for thromboembolic complications before surgery is important. Studies have documented the effectiveness of DVT prophylaxis, but results are inconsistent. The incidence of major proximal DVT after elective aortic surgery and the effect of aggressive DVT prophylaxis on that incidence were investigated in a randomized prospective trial.

Methods.—One group of 50 patients undergoing elective surgery received 5,000 U of unfractionated heparin sodium subcutaneously every 12 hours and calf-length IMC devices from the time of surgery for 7 days or until the patient was ambulatory. Another group of 50 patients received no DVT prophylaxis. Intravenous heparin sodium was administered to all patients before aortic cross clamping. Venous duplex ultrasound scanning was performed on both legs preoperatively and on postoperative days 1, 3, and 7 to detect formation of DVT. Costs associated with DVT prophylaxis were tallied.

Results.—Two patients in the control group died postoperatively. Deep vein thrombosis developed postoperatively in 1 control patient and 1 DVT prophylaxis patient. Both recovered uneventfully. One control patient had a nonfatal pulmonary embolus. Heparin prophylaxis cost $392 per patient and the pneumatic compression device cost $144 per patient.

Conclusion.—The incidence of DVT in this study was 2%. Aggressive DVT prophylaxis made no difference in the occurrence of DVT or pulmonary embolus. Whereas these patients were not at high risk for DVT, prophylaxis would be beneficial for patients who are at high risk.

▶ This study, although done properly, is relatively small for an attempt at distinguishing between heparin and no prophylaxis. The overall incidence, in any case, was only 1 patient in each treatment group. I am not sure that the authors would have found a true difference had one existed. They defended themselves by saying that they knew the study was "underpowered" (did not contain enough patients to statistically show a true difference). Another point made was that the patients received systemic anticoagulation as part of the surgery and that this protects them against development of DVT. Perhaps the fact that patients routinely have, on average, only a 4% rate of DVT means that we could not see a difference until several hundred or a thousand patients had participated in the study. More importantly, it would not make much difference because the patients are already systemically anticoagulated.

M. Weintraub, M.D.

Aprotinin in Primary Valve Replacement and Reconstruction: A Multicenter, Double-blind, Placebo-controlled Trial

D'Ambra MN, Akins CW, Blackstone EH, et al (Massachusetts Gen Hosp, Boston; Univ of Alabama, Birmingham; Miles Inc, West Haven, Conn; et al)
J Thorac Cardiovasc Surg 112:1081–1089, 1996   21–14

Background.—Aprotinin can decrease the need for blood transfusions during coronary artery bypass graft operations. The efficacy and safety of aprotinin in reducing the use of allogeneic blood and postoperative mediastinal chest tube drainage were evaluated.

Methods.—Two hundred twelve patients undergoing primary sternotomy for valve replacement or repair were enrolled in the multicenter, randomized, prospective, double-blind, placebo-controlled trial. Seventy-one patients received high-dose aprotinin; 70, low-dose aprotinin; and 71, placebo. Aprotinin was administered as a loading dose followed by a continuous infusion and pump prime dose.

Findings.—Compared with placebo, aprotinin did not reduce the proportion of patients receiving transfusions, which were needed in 63% of patients receiving high-dose aprotinin, 52% receiving low-dose aprotinin, and 48% receiving placebo. A reduced volume of mediastinal shed blood was associated with aprotinin administration. Adverse events were comparable among the groups, except for postoperative renal dysfunction, which occurred in 11% of the patients in the high-dose group, 7% in the low-dose group, and none in the placebo group. A disproportionate number of patients receiving high-dose aprotinin who had postoperative renal dysfunction also had diabetes mellitus.

Conclusion.—In these patients, aprotinin administration did not decrease allogeneic blood use. However, there were significant reductions in the volume of mediastinal shed blood. The incidence of renal dysfunction after surgery was significantly higher in the aprotinin recipients than in the placebo recipients.

▶ This article is one of an increasing number of negative studies which, contrary to past experiences, are now published. Aprotinin did not decrease the use of blood transfusions. Doctors could say, "Look, why study this drug in a placebo-controlled experiment, why not just do the dose response study present in this design with no placebo group? In fact, why do an experiment at all? Shouldn't we just depend on so-called 'priors,' which really are pretty strong in other cardiac operations?" Unfortunately, this is one of those cases in which extrapolation probably would not be okay because of the great difference between bypass graft operations and valve replacement surgery.

M. Weintraub, M.D.

Possible Prevention of Postangioplasty Restenosis by Ascorbic Acid

Tomoda H, Yoshitake M, Morimoto K, et al (Tokai Univ, Japan)
Am J Cardiol 78:1284–1286, 1996
21–15

Objective.—A study of patients who underwent percutaneous transluminal coronary angioplasty (PTCA) examined the possibility that ascorbic acid could prevent post-PTCA restenosis. No agent has been found that reduces coronary restenosis, a significant problem after PTCA.

Methods.—The study enrolled 119 patients who had stable or unstable angina and in whom PTCA achieved a residual diameter of less than 50%. Coronary angiograms were obtained before and immediately after angioplasty and at follow-up. Fifty-nine patients were randomized to oral ascorbic acid (500 mg/day, divided 3 times) to be started immediately after successful PTCA. The 60 controls did not receive this treatment. All patients were given aspirin, calcium antagonists, and nitrates. Restenosis was defined as a greater than 50% diameter narrowing of the target vessel at follow-up angiography.

Results.—Treatment and placebo groups were similar in patient characteristics and morphologic features of the dilated coronary arteries. The 2 groups did not differ significantly in reference coronary diameters immediately before or after PTCA or at follow-up. Minimal luminal diameter was significantly larger in the ascorbic acid group than that in the placebo group at follow-up, and late loss and loss index were significantly less after ascorbic acid treatment. The incidence of restenosis was greater in the control group (43%) than in the treatment group (24%). Repeat interventions were also reduced with ascorbic acid.

Conclusion.—A number of studies have reported antioxidants to have a beneficial effect on plasma lipid levels and atherogenesis. Ascorbic acid, the most potent water-soluble antioxidant, is inexpensive and without significant side effects. The positive results in this series of patients suggest that ascorbic acid may be effective in reducing post-PTCA restenosis.

▶ Provocative! Ascorbic acid is an antioxidant and, as such, might have a favorable effect on low-density lipoprotein oxidation and, hence, atherogenesis. At these doses, ascorbic acid is cheap and safe. I hope additional studies occur, but, meanwhile, why *not* take vitamin C after angioplasty?

L. Lasagna, M.D.

Effect of Preoperative Supplementation With α-Tocopherol and Ascorbic Acid on Myocardial Injury in Patients Undergoing Cardiac Operations

Westhuyzen J, Cochrane AD, Tesar PJ, et al (Royal Brisbane Hosp, Australia; Prince Charles Hosp, Brisbane, Australia)
J Thorac Cardiovasc Surg 113:942–948, 1997
21–16

Background.—Augmentation of antioxidant defenses may help protect tissues against the ischemia-reperfusion injury that can result in surgery involving cardiopulmonary bypass. The effect of pretreating patients with α-tocopherol and ascorbic acid or placebo on myocardial injury was studied.

Methods.—Seventy-six patients undergoing elective coronary artery bypass grafting were enrolled in a double-blind, placebo-controlled, randomized study. The patients received placebo or both α-tocopherol, 750 IU/day for 7 to 10 days, and ascorbic acid, 1 g, 12 hours before surgery.

Findings.—Plasma levels of α-tocopherol, increased 4-fold by supplementation, declined by 70% after surgery in the supplemented group and to negligible levels in the placebo group. The groups did not differ significantly in release of creatine kinase–MB isoenzyme during 72 hours or in reduction of the myocardial perfusion defect determined by thallium 201 uptake. No evidence of benefit from antioxidant supplementation was observed electrocardiographically.

Conclusions.—Supplementation with α-tocopherol and ascorbic acid prevented the depletion of the primary lipid soluble antioxidant in plasma. However, it did not measurably reduce myocardial injury after surgery.

▶ Antioxidants are considered by many to prevent a variety of troubles, but this study provides little evidence of reduced myocardial injury from their use after coronary artery bypass.

L. Lasagna, M.D.

Change of Conventional Cyclosporine to Neoral Cyclosporine Formulation in Long-term Liver Transplant Recipients

Diliz HS, Olivera MA, Kershenobich D, et al (Instituto Nacional de la Nutrición "Salvador Zubirán," Mexico City)
Transplant Proc 28:3348–3350, 1996   21–17

Introduction.—The use of cyclosporine (CyA) as an immunosuppressive agent has improved the prognosis and survival of transplant patients. Absorption of CyA after oral administration is unpredictable, however, for bioavailability can range from 5% to 80% and clearance rates can vary 16-fold. A new oral formulation, neoral CyA (NOF), was evaluated in a study of long-term liver transplant recipients.

Methods.—Eligible patients had had their first liver transplant 2 months or more previously, had been receiving CyA oral solution twice daily for at least 2 weeks, and had had stable graft function with normal liver function test (LFT) results for at least 2 months. In the first part of the protocol, patients had blood samples taken for a CyA pharmacokinetic study and analysis of cytology, chemistry, and LFT. Patients were then switched to an equivalent dose of NOF and examined in an identical protocol 14 days later. Timed serum CyA determinations of CyA and NOF were compared for each patient and for each group.

Results and Conclusion.—The 3 patients studied—2 men and 1 woman—had a mean age of 42.6 years and a mean posttransplant survival time of 62.3 months. All 3 had hematologic and biochemical profiles within normal ranges before and after the switch to NOF. Pharmacokinetic profiles showed better bioavailability for the NOF formulation, as evidenced by higher and sooner peak serum levels, as well as greater area under the time-concentration curve values. Thus, the NOF formulation, which allows microemulsification in the gastrointestinal tract, improves absorption of CyA and may maintain therapeutic levels with lower doses. No adverse effects were associated with the new oral formulation.

▶ Cyclosporine has been the main agent for effective immunosuppression in organ transplant patients, but absorption after oral administration is very variable, the bioavailability ranging from 5% to 80%, with clearance rates varying as much as 16-fold. This new formulation, which contains surfactants as well as lipophilic and hydrophilic solvents, looks promising.

L. Lasagna, M.D.

Steroid Withdrawal in Tacrolimus (FK506)-Treated Pediatric Liver Transplant Recipients
McKee M, Mattei P, Schwarz K, et al (Johns Hopkins Univ, Baltimore, Md)
J Pediatr Surg 32:973–975, 1997   21–18

Background.—Steroid use in children receiving transplants results in significant adverse effects. The feasibility of steroid withdrawal in patients undergoing immunosuppression with the aid of FK506 (FK) was investigated.

Methods.—All children undergoing liver transplantation and receiving FK for more than 6 months were assessed for steroid withdrawal. Two divided doses of FK, 0.3 mg/kg/day, were administered. Steroid tapering was done as tolerated, the goal being 0.2–0.3 mg/kg/day at 6 weeks, 0.2–0.3 mg/kg every other day at 3 months, and complete withdrawal after 6 months. Steroid bolus and taper were done for enzyme increases or rejection during biopsy.

Findings.—Twenty-nine children were evaluated for steroid withdrawal. Five could not be placed on FK monotherapy, but the remaining 24 underwent withdrawal. Half of this group had no complications and continue on FK monotherapy a mean of 22 months after steroid tapering. The other 12 children need intermittent steroid therapy for presumed or biopsy-proved rejection, graft dysfunction, lymphoproliferative disease requiring a decrease in FK, or exacerbations of asthma. Five of these 12 children are currently on FK monotherapy a mean of 6 months after steroid tapering. Thus overall, 71% of the children are currently not taking steroids.

Conclusions.—In children undergoing liver transplantation, FK is an effective immunosuppressant. In most patients, steroids can be withdrawn successfully with the use of FK monotherapy.

▶ Enabling patients to be off steroids or on lower steroid dosages is a desirable effect of many other therapies. In this uncontrolled study, a very high percentage of the patients had their steroid removed or the dose intermittently lowered. One other interesting point was raised in the discussion that followed this paper. It was that, in these children with liver transplantation, the question of letting them outgrow their immunosuppressant dose by not increasing it as the children get larger, appears to be an effective way of cutting down tacrolimus. Now, that's something to think about.

M. Weintraub, M.D.

The Nordic Multicenter Double-blind Randomized Controlled Trial of Prophylactic Ursodeoxycholic Acid in Liver Transplant Patients
Keiding S, Höckerstedt K, Bjøro K, et al (Aarhus Univ Hosp, Denmark; Helsinki Univ; Rikshopitalet, Oslo, Norway; et al)
Transplantation 63:1591–1594, 1997   21–19

Introduction.—The incidence of acute rejection after liver transplantation has been reported to be dramatically reduced with prophylactic treatment using ursodeoxycholic acid (UDCA). A later trial did not confirm these findings. The incidence of acute rejection was evaluated prospectively in patients who underwent liver transplantation to determine patient outcomes after prophylactic UDCA treatment in a randomized, placebo-controlled multicenter trial.

Methods.—Of 102 patients, 54 were allocated to a UDCA treatment group receiving 15 mg/kg/day and 48 were allocated to a placebo group. The UDCA treatment was begun on the first postoperative day and was administered for 3 months. The treatment was stratified for adults with acute liver failure (n =10), adults with chronic liver failure (n = 77), and children (n = 15).

Results.—Patients were followed up for 1 year. Acute rejection occurred in 65% of patients in the UDCA treatment group and 68% of patients in the placebo group. There was no between-group difference in the incidence of steroid-resistant rejection. The probability of acute rejection did not differ between groups. Patient survival and graft survival probabilities did not differ between groups. The time course of biochemical testing indicated significantly lower values of γ-glutamyltransferase at 2 and 3 months in the treatment group, compared with the placebo group.

Conclusions.—The findings in this controlled trial do not support the initial optimistic report of beneficial effects of prophylactic UDCA treatment on acute rejection after liver transplantation.

▶ This is a negative outcome study, but it is very important in any case. The original uncontrolled studies indicating that UDCA treatment actually helped to prevent acute rejection after liver transplantation were comparisons with historical controls. This, of course, shows the weakness of historically controlled studies. Although helpful in some clinical situations, historical controls have to be viewed with suspicion. The investigators in this study tried to correct many of the faults that had been committed in other negative trials. For example, dosing at the initially successful level (15 mg/kg/day) was started very early as recommended in the first treatment attempts. Interestingly, the UDCA treatment affected cholestatic biochemistry positively, but this was a less important outcome than acute rejection.

M. Weintraub, M.D.

Effects of Pentoxifylline on Renal Function and Blood Pressure in Cardiac Transplant Recipients

Frantz RP, Edwards BS, Olson LJ, et al (Mayo Clinic and Mayo Found, Rochester, Minn)
Transplantation 63:1607–1610, 1997   21–20

Introduction.—It has been suggested that the nephrotoxic effects of cyclosporine may be ameliorated by pretreatment with pentoxifylline, a xanthine derivative. The course of renal function in the first year after cardiac transplantation using current immunosuppression was assessed, as was the ability of pentoxifylline to attenuate cyclosporine-induced renal dysfunction and hypertension in recipients.

Methods.—Twenty-nine patients undergoing cardiac transplantation were randomly assigned to receive pentoxifylline 400 mg orally 3 times a day or placebo for 1 year. Renal function was evaluated before transplantation and at 1, 6, and 12 months postoperatively. Glomerular filtration rate (GFR) and renal plasma flow, respectively, were calculated using iothalamate and para-aminohippurate. At 12 months after surgery, antihypertensives were withdrawn and ambulatory blood pressure was monitored for 3 days.

Results.—Twenty-seven of 29 patients were able to complete the trial. Mean changes in GFR, creatinine, renal plasma flow, and filtration fraction did not differ between groups; they were unchanged at 1 month postoperatively, improved at 6 months, then declined at 12 months. Changes in renal blood flow paralleled those of GFR. The treatment and placebo groups did not differ in 18-hour ambulatory blood pressure monitoring at 1 hour after transplantation.

Conclusions.—A slight decline in renal function was observed in the first year after cardiac transplantation. Pentoxifylline did not ameliorate cyclosporine-mediated nephrotoxicity or hypertension in recipients of cardiac transplantation.

▶ This is another negative study in which the findings did not confirm those found in previous clinic and laboratory studies that showed pentoxifylline can attenuate the negative effects of cyclosporine on the kidney. In this small patient population study, which took a long time to institute and complete, the renal parameters and blood pressure didn't fall greatly in the patients. It may be that the methodology of giving immunosuppressant therapy has improved since the initial studies of pentoxifylline were done. Perhaps patient care changed quicker than the studies could be done.

M. Weintraub, M.D.

L-Arginine Reverses the Antinatriuretic Effect of Cyclosporin in Renal Transplant Patients

Andrés A, Morales JM, Praga M, et al (Hosp 12 de Octubre, Madrid)
Nephrol Dial Transplant 12:1437–1440, 1997   21–21

Background.—Cyclosporin facilitates renal vasoconstriction and has an antinatriuretic effect. These effects may be caused by an interference of cyclosporin with the vasodilating properties of endothelium mediated by nitric oxide production. However, infusion of the nitric oxide precursor L-arginine induces renal vasodilation and facilitates natriuresis in normal volunteers. The renal effects of L-arginine infusion in renal transplant recipients receiving long-term cyclosporin treatment were investigated.

Methods.—Ten men were studied during 2 consecutive days after administration of the usual morning dose of cyclosporin. All were renal transplant recipients receiving long-term cyclosporin treatment, and all had stable renal function. On the first day, the patients were given an IV infusion of vehicle; on the second day, they were infused with graded doses of L-arginine—50, 100, and 150 mg/kg/hr—during 3 consecutive hours.

Findings.—During the first day after cyclosporin administration, there was a significant decline in natriuresis and kaliuresis, without changes in renal plasma flow and glomerular filtration rate. L-arginine administration was followed by significant increases in renal plasma flow, glomerular filtration rate, and natriuresis. The increase in cyclosporin blood levels after administration was similar on days 1 and 2.

Conclusions.—L-arginine facilitates renal vasodilation and natriuresis in renal transplant recipients. The increase in sodium excretion may indicate that L-arginine counteracts the antinatriuretic effect of cyclopsorin.

▶ We may have come across an important treatment of cyclosporin-induced hypertension in L-arginine, a precursor of nitric oxide. Obviously, this study has to be repeated and the findings replicated in several other groups of patients, but it is an exciting finding nonetheless.

M. Weintraub, M.D.

Treatment of Chronic Graft-Versus-Host Disease With Clofazimine

Lee SJ, Wegner SA, McGarigle CJ, et al (Brigham and Women's Hosp, Boston; Dana-Farber Cancer Inst, Boston; Harvard Med School, Boston)
Blood 89:2298–2302, 1997   21–22

Introduction.—Conventional therapies for chronic graft-versus-host disease (cGVHD) are of limited value because of their toxicity and failure to produce a complete response. Clofazimine, an antimycobacterial drug with anti-inflammatory activity, was evaluated for its safety and efficacy in the treatment of cGVHD.

Methods.—Over a 5-year period, 22 patients (median age 36 years) were treated with clofazimine. Most (77%) were transplanted for hematologic malignancies. Nine received the drug off protocol and 13 were treated in an open-label, phase II trial. Clofazimine was given orally, 300 mg in a single daily dose for 90 days, then lowered to 100 mg daily to continue indefinitely as tolerated. Patients were classified according to degree of response.

Results.—Treatment with clofazimine was generally well tolerated during treatment courses ranging from 7 to 835 days. Gastrointestinal problems and hyperpigmentation, the most common side effects, were reported by 36% and 55% of patients, respectively. More than 50% of patients with skin, joint, or mouth involvement achieved partial or complete responses in those organs. Twelve of the 22 patients achieved a partial response, but no patient had an overall complete response.

Discussion.—Clofazimine appears to be a safe and promising treatment for cGVHD. The drug was more effective in patients with skin, mouth, and lung involvement than in those with pulmonary symptoms. Some patients were able to reduce their cyclosporine and corticosteroid requirements when taking clofazimine, in some cases even when the drug did not improve their symptoms.

▶ Clofazimine is a drug used in the treatment of leprosy primarily for its effect on the actual disease, but also for its effect on erythema nodosum leprosum (ENL). Thalidomide is another medication with apparent activity against ENL, and one which may have activity against graft-versus-host disease. The activity is relatively slow in onset with clofazimine, and the inherent pigmentation of the skin, which does apparently resolve, may take many months. Gastrointestinal symptoms are also side effects of clofazimine. Graft-versus-host reaction is not very prevalent, but more trials are needed to find out what drugs can be used.

M. Weintraub, M.D.

Two Phase Randomised Controlled Clinical Trial of Postoperative Oral Dietary Supplements in Surgical Patients
Keele AM, Bray MJ, Emery PW, et al (Central Middlesex Hosp NHS Trust, London)
Gut 40:393–399, 1997
21–23

Introduction.—The incidence of hospital malnutrition has improved little in the past 20 years. Perioperative nutritional support and feeding jejunostomies have provided limited benefits. After gastrointestinal surgery, clinically significant benefits have been seen with nasojejunal feeding, simple oral dietary supplements have been beneficial after orthopedic surgery and gastrointestinal surgery. The benefits of giving postoperative oral dietary supplements to patients having gastrointestinal surgery were evaluated, and the long-term benefits of continuing supplements after the immediate postoperative period were assessed.

Methods.—One hundred patients having elective moderate or major gastrointestinal surgery were randomly assigned to receive an oral dietary supplement or no oral dietary supplement on an inpatient and outpatient basis.

Results.—During the inpatient phase, nutritional intake significantly improved and weight loss was lower among patients treated with oral supplements than among the control patients. Control patients had significantly reduced grip strength, whereas patients who received supplements maintained their grip strength. In control patients, subjective levels of fatigue increased significantly above preoperative levels when compared with supplemented patients. Twelve control patients developed complications compared with 4 patients in the supplement group. In the outpatient phase, nutrient intake improved in the supplement group; however, no significant differences in indices of nutritional status or well-being were seen between the 2 groups.

Conclusion.—Patients who have undergone gastrointestinal surgery have good results and clinically significant benefits with the prescription of oral dietary supplements. However, the benefits are restricted to the inpatient phase. The study results do not support the routine prescription of oral dietary supplements after discharge from hospital.

▶ This study should be repeated in the United States. With the shorter period of hospitalization after even major abdominal surgery, the chance for the dietary supplement to be helpful would be much increased under current managed care programs. In fact, even the outptient portion of this study might have yielded positive results. On the other hand, one could possibly see that eating one's own diet cooked at home would be acceptable.

M. Weintraub, M.D.

Infection and Allergy Incidence in Ambulatory Surgery Patients Using White Petrolatum vs Bacitracin Ointment: A Randomized Controlled Trial
Smack DP, Harrington AC, Dunn C, et al (Walter Reed Army Med Ctr, Washington, DC)
JAMA 276:972–977, 1996   21–24

Objective.—Many different ointments and dressings have been used to keep skin wounds moist, and thus to promote healing. Antibiotic ointments, usually in a base of white petrolatum, are routinely used. However, there is little research evidence to support the need for antibiotic ointments in postprocedure care of clean wounds. One possible drawback of using these ointments is that they may induce allergic contact dermatitis. Bacitracin and white petrolatum were compared for use in postprocedure wound care.

Methods.—The randomized, double-blind, placebo-controlled trial included 1,249 dermatologic surgical wounds in 922 patients. The patients were randomly assigned to postprocedure wound care with either bacitracin ointment or white petrolatum. The patients were followed up for 4 weeks to assess the incidence of infection and allergic contact dermatitis. Any effects of the 2 ointments on healing were noted as well.

Results.—Results in 884 patients were evaluable. The rate of postprocedure infection was 1.5% to 2.0% with white petrolatum and 0.9% with bacitracin. This difference was not statistically significant. However, the rate of *Staphylococcus aureus* infections was 1.8% in the white petrolatum group vs. 0% in the bacitracin group. Allergic contact dermatitis developed in 0.9% of patients in the bacitracin group vs. 0% in the white petrolatum group. There were no significant differences between groups in wound healing at any time during the study.

Conclusions.—White petrolatum on its own is a safe and effective ointment for use in wound care after dermatologic surgical procedures. It carries no risk of allergic sensitization and minimal potential for selection of resistant bacteria; it is also much less expensive than antibiotic ointments. Using white petrolatum instead of bacitracin ointment for wound care has no significant impact on infection risk or wound healing.

▶ Wound healing has long been thought to be helped by an occlusive dressing that keeps the skin moist. This study suggests that patients with such wounds do as well with white petrolatum as with a dressing that includes bacitracin. The advantages of using only the "vehicle" are obvious—decreases in cost, in antibiotic resistance, and in allergic reactions.

L. Lasagna, M.D.

Subject Index

A

Abdomen
  pain in cystic fibrosis, 260
  trauma, antibiotics in, 191
Abuse
  drug, 31
  substance, and medication
    noncompliance in schizophrenia,
    281
Academic
  surgeons' knowledge of FDA
    regulations for clinical trials, 325
Acetaminophen
  concentration increase, late, after
    overdose of Tylenol extended relief,
    40
  metabolites, plasma and urinary
    oxidative, decrease after
    consumption of watercress, 23
  overdose
    in children, outcome and factors
      contributing to hepatotoxicity, 44
    redefining level for anticipated
      hepatotoxicity in, 45
  prescribing habits in children's hospital,
    5
  -related acute renal failure without
    fulminant liver failure, 40
  vs. ibuprofen for tension-type headache,
    258
Acetylsalicylic acid (*see* Aspirin)
Acne
  steroids causing, anabolic, in men, 60
Acquired immunodeficiency syndrome (*see*
  AIDS)
ACTH
  doses for delayed emesis after high-dose
    cisplatin in cancer, 212
Adolescent
  acetaminophen overdose in, outcome
    and factors contributing to
    hepatotoxicity, 44
  minocycline-induced serious adverse
    reactions in, 48
  mivacurium in, potentiation by
    rocuronium, 26
  muscle cramps and magnesium
    deficiency in, 312
  pain in, self-administration of
    over-the-counter medication for,
    244
  propylthiouracil-induced fulminant
    hepatitis in, 57
  tuberculosis in, rifampin preventive
    therapy for, 188

Adrenaline
  alone or with human thrombin in
    endoscopic injection for bleeding
    peptic ulcer, 156
Adrenocorticotropic
  hormone doses for delayed emesis after
    high-dose cisplatin in cancer, 212
Adulteration
  by synthetic therapeutic substances of
    traditional Chinese medicines in
    Taiwan, 37
Adverse drug events
  dronabinol causing, in AIDS-associated
    anorexia, 65
  in hospitalized patients
    costs of, 32
    effects on length of stay, costs, and
      mortality, 34
  mefloquine *vs.* chloroquine/proguanil
    causing, 50
Adverse reactions, 31
  drug, earlier detection by patients *vs.*
    professionals, 33
  minocycline-induced, 47
  nondrug, update on, 35
  to thalidomide in HIV infection, 70
Advertising
  prescription drug, direct-to-consumer, 1
African Americans
  CYP2C19 phenotype in, determination
    with omeprazole, 151
  lovastatin in primary
    hypercholesterolemia in, 134
Afrin
  extended use of, 119
Age
  -dependent potentiation of mivacurium
    by rocuronium, 26
Aging
  collagen, vitamins and analgesics in
    prevention of, 21
AIDS, 63
  (*See also* HIV)
  -associated anorexia, dronabinol in, 65
  -associated wasting, growth hormone
    therapy for, 66
    with insulin-like growth factor 1, 67
  sulfadiazine-associated nephrotoxicity
    in, 48
Albuterol
  alone or with ipratropium in acute
    asthma, 78
  inhaled, regularly scheduled *vs.*
    as-needed use, in mild asthma, 76

Author Index